Neurology and Systemic Disease

Guest Editor

ALIREZA MINAGAR, MD, FAAN

NEUROLOGIC CLINICS

www.neurologic.theclinics.com

Consulting Editor
Randolph W. Evans, MD

February 2010 • Volume 28 • Number 1

SAUNDERS an imprint of ELSEVIER, Inc.

W.B. SAUNDERS COMPANY
A Division of Elsevier Inc.

1600 John F. Kennedy Boulevard • Suite 1800 • Philadelphia, Pennsylvania 19103-2899

http://www.theclinics.com

NEUROLOGIC CLINICS Volume 28, Number 1
February 2010 ISSN 0733-8619, ISBN-13: 978-1-4377-1918-5

Editor: Donald Mumford

Neurologic Clinics (ISSN 0733-8619) is published quarterly by Elsevier Inc., 360 Park Avenue South, New York, NY 10010–1710. Months of issue are February, May, August, and November. Periodicals postage paid at New York, NY, and additional mailing offices. Subscription prices are $247.00 per year for US individuals, $401.00 per year for US institutions, $124.00 per year for US students, $310.00 per year for Canadian individuals, $482.00 per year for Canadian institutions, $344.00 per year for international individuals, $482.00 per year for international institutions, and $175.00 for Canadian and foreign students/residents. To receive student/resident rate, orders must be accompanied by name of affiliated institution, date of term, and the *signature* of program/residency coordinator on institution letterhead. Orders will be billed at individual rate until proof of status is received. Foreign air speed delivery is included in all *Clinics* subscription prices. All prices are subject to change without notice. **POSTMASTER:** Send address changes to *Neurologic Clinics*, Elsevier Health Sciences Division, Subscription Customer Service, 3251 Riverport Lane, Maryland Heights, MO 63043. **Customer Service: Telephone: 1-800-654-2452 (U.S. and Canada); 314-447-8871 (outside U.S. and Canada). Fax: 314-447-8029. E-mail: journalscustomerservice-usa@elsevier.com (for print support); journalsonlinesupport-usa@elsevier.com (for online support).**

Reprints. For copies of 100 or more of articles in this publication, please contact the Commercial Reprints Department, Elsevier Inc., 360 Park Avenue South, New York, New York, 10010-1710; Tel.: (+1) 212-633-3812; Fax: (+1) 212-462-1935, and E-mail: reprints@elsevier.com.

Neurologic Clinics is also published in Spanish by Nueva Editorial Interamericana S.A., Mexico City, Mexico.

Neurologic Clinics is covered in *Current Contents/Clinical Medicine, MEDLINE/PubMed (Index Medicus), EMBASE/Excerpta Medica, and PsycINFO, and ISI/BIOMED.*

Printed in the United States of America.

Contributors

CONSULTING EDITOR

RANDOLPH W. EVANS, MD
Clinical Professor, Department of Neurology, Baylor College of Medicine, Houston, Texas

GUEST EDITOR

ALIREZA MINAGAR, MD, FAAN
Department of Neurology, Louisiana State University Health Sciences Center, Shreveport, Louisiana

AUTHORS

HODA ABDEL-HAMID, MD
Assistant Professor of Pediatrics, Division of Pediatric Neurology, Children's Hospital Pittsburgh, University of Pittsburgh School of Medicine, Pittsburgh, Pennsylvania

ALLEN AKSAMIT, MD
Associate Professor of Neurology, Department of Neurology, Mayo College of Medicine, Mayo Clinic, Rochester, Minnesota

ROBIN L. BREY, MD
Chair and Professor of Neurology, Department of Neurology, University of Texas Health Science Center at San Antonio, San Antonio, Texas

DAVID CLIFFORD, MD
Professor of Neurology and Medicine, Department of Neurology, Washington University in St Louis, St Louis, Missouri

DEBORAH COMMINS, MD, PhD
Associate Professor of Pathology (Neuropathology), Department of Pathology, University of Southern California Keck School of Medicine, Los Angeles, California

JOY E. DREIBELBIS, MD
Instructor of Neurology, Department of Neurology, University of Rochester School of Medicine and Dentistry, Rochester, New York

EDWARD J. DROPCHO, MD
Professor, Department of Neurology, Indiana University Medical Center, Indianapolis, Indiana; Director, Neuro-Oncology Program, Indiana University Simon Cancer Center, Indianapolis, Indiana

DEBRA ELLIOTT, MD
Department of Neurology, Louisiana State University Health Sciences Center, Shreveport, Louisiana

FRANCISCO FERNANDEZ, MD
Professor and Chair of Psychiatry, University of South Florida, Tampa, Florida

MARJORIE FOWLER, MD
Department of Pathology, Louisiana State University Health Sciences Center, Shreveport, Louisiana

HAROLD W. GOFORTH, MD
Assistant Professor of Psychiatry, Duke University Medical Center, Durham, North Carolina; Co-Director, Consultation-Liaison Psychiatry Service, Durham Veterans Affairs Medical Center, Durham, North Carolina; Palliative Medicine Attending Physician, GRECC, Durham Veterans Affairs Medical Center, Durham, North Carolina

JOHN J. HALPERIN, MD
Professor of Neurology, Mount Sinai School of Medicine, New York; Chair, Department of Neurosciences, Overlook Hospital, Summit, New Jersey

MEGHAN K. HARRIS, MD
Department of Neurology, Louisiana State University Health Sciences Center, Shreveport, Louisiana

EDOUARD HIRSCH, MD
Professor of Neurology, Service de Neurologie, Hôpitaux Universitaires de Strasbourg, Strasbourg, France; Professor, CTRS Fondation IDEE

SAMEEA HUSAIN, DO
Department of Neurology & Psychiatry, Saint Louis University School of Medicine, St Louis, Missouri

STEPHEN L. JAFFE, MD
Department of Neurology, Louisiana State University Health Sciences Center, Shreveport, Louisiana

CHARLES D. JOHNSON, MD, FACC
Professor of Medicine, Department of Medicine, Division of Cardiology, University of Puerto Rico School of Medicine, Medical Sciences Campus, San Juan, Puerto Rico

MARK D. JOHNSON, MD
Associate Professor of Neurology, Division of Cerebrovascular Diseases, University of Texas Southwestern Medical Center, Dallas, Texas

RALPH F. JÓZEFOWICZ, MD
Professor of Neurology and Medicine, Associate Chair for Education, Department of Neurology, University of Rochester School of Medicine and Dentistry, Rochester, New York

ROGER E. KELLEY, MD
Professor and Chairman, Department of Neurology, LSU Health Sciences Center-Shreveport, Shreveport, Louisiana

THIERRY KRUMMEL, MD
Service de Néphrologie, Hémodialyse et Transplantation Rénale, Hôpitaux Universitaires de Strasbourg, Strasbourg, France

NEERAJ KUMAR, MD
Associate Professor, Mayo Clinic College of Medicine; Consultant, Department
of Neurology, Mayo Clinic, Rochester, Minnesota

GLENDA LACERDA, MD
Serviço de Neurologia, Hospital Universitário Antônio Pedro, Universidade Federal
Fluminense, Rua Marquês do Paraná, Centro, Niterói; Electroencephalography Unit,
Hospital São Vicentede Paulo est rua Dr Satamini, Rio de Janeiro, Brazil

ANDREW LEVINE, PhD
Assistant Researcher in Neurology, Department of Neurology, David Geffen School
of Medicine at UCLA, Los Angeles, California

ALIREZA MINAGAR, MD, FAAN
Department of Neurology, Louisiana State University Health Sciences Center, Shreveport,
Louisiana

REED MURTAUGH, MD
Professor of Radiology, Oncologic Sciences, Neurology, Neurosurgery, and Psychiatry,
University of South Florida, Tampa, Florida

EYAL MUSCAL, MD
Assistant Professor of Pediatrics, Division of Pediatric Rheumatology, Texas Children's
Hospital/Baylor College of Medicine, Houston, Texas

RONALD F. PFEIFFER, MD
Professor and Vice Chair, Department of Neurology, University of Tennessee Health
Science Center, Memphis, Tennessee

ALEJANDRO A. RABINSTEIN, MD
Division of Critical Care Neurology, Department of Neurology, Mayo Clinic, Rochester,
Minnesota

AMY C. RAUCHWAY, DO
Assistant Professor of Neurology, Department of Neurology and Psychiatry, Saint Louis
University School of Medicine, St Louis, Missouri

THOMAS F. SCOTT, MD
Professor of Neurology, Department of Neurology, Drexel University College of Medicine,
Pittsburgh, Pennsylvania

ROBERT N. SCHWENDIMANN, MD
Department of Neurology, Louisiana State University Health Sciences Center, Shreveport

JOHN B. SELHORST, MD
Sylvia N. Sovers Professor of Neurology & Psychiatry, Department of Neurology
& Psychiatry, Saint Louis University School of Medicine, St Louis, Missouri

ELYSE J. SINGER, MD
Professor of Neurology, Department of Neurology, David Geffen School of Medicine at
UCLA, Los Angeles, California; Director, National Neurological AIDS Bank, Los Angeles,
California

BARNEY J. STERN, MD
Professor of Neurology, Department of Neurology, University of Maryland School of Medicine, Baltimore, Maryland

MIGUEL VALDES-SUEIRAS, MD
Assistant Professor of Neurology, Department of Neurology, David Geffen School of Medicine at UCLA, Los Angeles, California

ALAN H. YEE, DO
Department of Neurology, Mayo Clinic, Rochester, Minnesota

SAŠA A. ŽIVKOVIĆ, MD, PhD
Staff Physician, Neurology service, VA Pittsburgh Healthcare System; Associate Professor of Neurology, Department of Neurology, University of Pittsburgh School of Medicine, Pittsburgh, Pennsylvania

Contents

Accurate identification of nervous system dysfunction is vital in the assessment of any multisystem disorder. The neurologic manifestations of acid-base disturbances, abnormal electrolyte concentrations, and acute endocrinopathies are protean and typically determined by the acuity of the underlying derangement. Detailed history and physical examination may guide appropriate laboratory testing and lead to prompt and accurate diagnosis. Neurologic manifestations of primary and secondary systemic disorders are frequently encountered in all subspecialties of medicine. This article focuses on key neurologic presentations of respiratory and metabolic acid-base derangements and potentially life-threatening endocrinopathies.

Cardiac evaluation as part of the assessment of neurologic presentations is very much reflective of the diligence in the pursuit of the mechanism. Newer and more aggressive techniques as part of the evaluation process can enhance the diagnostic yield. The detection and management of cardioembolic disease remains an evolutionary process.

The respiratory and central nervous systems are intimately connected through strict control of ventilation by central mechanisms. The exquisite sensitivity of central chemoreceptors and cerebral blood vessels to changes in central nervous system oxygenation mandate this type of control to maintain proper brain function. When diseases of the lung and respiratory system interfere with this fine balance, neurologic symptoms, sometimes severe, may develop. This article deals with the effects of abnormal ventilation on the nervous system.

Renal diseases-related metabolic abnormalities cause diverse CNS disturbances, namely uremic encephalopathy, seizures, stroke, movement disorders, sleep alterations, and peripheral nervous system involvement comprising polyneuropathy, mononeuropathies, and myopathy. Some inherited and acquired renal diseases present with concomitant or precedent neurologic syndromes. Several mechanisms involved include toxic metabolic accumulation, hyperkalemia, hypercoagulability, immunologic disturbances, and tubular acido-basic disequilibrium. Clinical symptoms usually indicate severe renal dysfunction, but subtle abnormalities may occur. Judiciously tailored renal replacement therapy may avoid these complications, whereas others may emerge from these very therapies with overlapping clinical pictures. This makes an already complex management of renal patients even more difficult and asks for tight collaboration between nephrologists and neurologists.

Among the collagen vascular diseases neurologic manifestations have been most commonly recognized and well-studied in systemic lupus erythematosus (SLE, lupus). Neurologic manifestations are less prevalent in other systemic inflammatory and autoimmune disorders. This review focuses on the clinical presentation, pathophysiology, and treatment strategies of neuropsychiatric lupus (NPSLE) in children and adults.

In recent years, there has been increasing recognition of the presence of gastrointestinal (GI) dysfunction in the setting of neurologic diseases. Parkinson's disease is a particularly well-known example, but GI dysfunction also may occur in multiple sclerosis, stroke, and in various myopathic and peripheral neuropathic processes. There is much less awareness, however, that primary GI diseases may also display neurologic dysfunction as part of their clinical picture. This article focuses on some of those disease processes. Illnesses primarily targeting the GI tract are addressed and examples of primary esophageal, gastric, and intestinal disease processes are described.

Hepatic encephalopathy (HE) is a neuropsychiatric syndrome that develops in the context of portosystemic venous shunting, in the presence or absence of intrinsic hepatic disease. HE is clinically characterized by altered sensorium and a spectrum of neuropsychiatric abnormalities. Several hypotheses have been proposed to explain the underlying pathogenic mechanisms of altered brain function associated with advanced hepatic disease and portosystemic shunting. HE may lead to profound coma and death; however, in many cases it is reversible. This article discusses the most recent developments in understanding the pathophysiology of HE and its diagnosis and management.

Neurologic Presentations of Nutritional Deficiencies

Neeraj Kumar

Optimal functioning of the central and peripheral nervous system is dependent on a constant supply of appropriate nutrients. The first section of this review discusses neurologic manifestations related to deficiency of key nutrients such as vitamin B_{12}, folate, copper, vitamin E, thiamine, and others. The second section addresses neurologic complications related to bariatric surgery. The third sections includes neurologic presentations caused by nutrient deficiencies in the setting of alcoholism. The concluding section addresses neurologic deficiency diseases that have a geographic predilection.

Neurologic Presentations of Systemic Vasculitides

Alireza Minagar, Marjorie Fowler, Meghan K. Harris, and Stephen L. Jaffe

Vasculitis or angiitis refers to a group of inflammatory disorders of the blood vessels that cause structural damage to the affected vessel, including thickening and weakening of the vessel wall, narrowing of its lumen, and, usually, vascular necrosis. Systemic vasculitis is classified according to the vessel size and histopathologic and clinical features. Vasculitides with small vessel involvement typically include Henoch-Schönlein purpura and cryoglobulinemia. Polyarteritis nodosa and Wegener granulomatosis are small- and medium-sized vessel vasculitides, whereas temporal arteritis and Takayasu arteritis involve large vessels. In this article, the authors provide a review of the neurologic presentations of the major systemic vasculitides.

Neurologic Presentations of Sarcoidosis

Barney J. Stern, Allen Aksamit, David Clifford, and Thomas F. Scott

Neurosarcoidosis is a diagnostic consideration in diverse clinical settings. Efforts should be made to secure pathologic confirmation of systemic sarcoidosis; only rarely is central nervous system (CNS) pathologic confirmation available. CNS infection and malignancy should be reasonably excluded before making a diagnosis of CNS sarcoidosis. Corticosteroid therapy alone may not be sufficient to treat neurosarcoidosis; adjunct immunosuppressive agents are increasingly used to achieve an optimal clinical outcome.

Neurologic Aspects of Drug Abuse

Harold W. Goforth, Reed Murtaugh, and Francisco Fernandez

Neurologic aspects of drug abuse vary. This article explains the general nature of drug abuse, identifies the physiologic effects of certain drugs, and briefly describes the neurobiology of addiction. This article also reviews available treatment options for those addicted to substances of abuse, and clarifies common misconceptions, including the differences between tolerance, abuse, and addiction.

Direct or incidental exposure of the nervous system to therapeutic irradiation carries the risk of symptomatic neurologic injury. Central nervous system toxicity from radiation includes focal cerebral necrosis, neurocognitive deficits, and less commonly cerebrovascular disease, myelopathy, or the occurrence of a radiation-induced neoplasm. Brachial or lumbosacral plexopathy are the most common syndromes of radiation toxicity affecting the peripheral nervous system. This article focuses on the clinical features, diagnosis, and management options for patients with radiation neurotoxicity.

Neurologic complications affect posttransplant recovery of more than 20% of transplant recipients. Etiology is usually related to surgical procedure of transplantation, primary disorders causing failure of transplanted organ, opportunistic infections, and neurotoxicity of immunosuppressive medications. Risk of opportunistic infections and immunosuppressant neurotoxicity is greatest within the first six months, but it persists along with long-term maintenance immunosuppression required to prevent graft rejection. Neurotoxicity may require alteration of immunosuppressive regimen, and prompt therapy of opportunistic infections improves outcomes.

The human immunodeficiency virus (HIV), the cause of AIDS, has infected an estimated 33 million individuals worldwide. HIV is associated with immunodeficiency, neoplasia, and neurologic disease. The continuing evolution of the HIV epidemic has spurred an intense interest in a hitherto neglected area of medicine, neuroinfectious diseases and their consequences. This work has broad applications for the study of central nervous system (CNS) tumors, dementias, neuropathies, and CNS disease in other immunosuppressed individuals. HIV is neuroinvasive (can enter the CNS), neurotrophic (can live in neural tissues), and neurovirulent (causes disease of the nervous system). This article reviews the HIV-associated neurologic syndromes, which can be classified as primary HIV neurologic disease (in which HIV is both necessary and sufficient to cause the illness), secondary or opportunistic neurologic disease (in which HIV interacts with other pathogens, resulting in opportunistic infections and tumors), and treatment-related neurologic disease (such as immune reconstitution inflammatory syndrome).

Only two spirochetal infections are known to cause nervous system infection and damage: neurosyphilis and neuroborreliosis (nervous system Lyme disease). Diagnosis of both generally relies on indirect tools, primarily assessment of the host immune response to the organism. Reliance on these indirect measures poses some challenges, particularly as they are imperfect measures of treatment response. Despite this, both infections are known to be readily curable with straightforward antimicrobial regimens. The challenge is that, untreated, both infections can cause progressive nervous system damage. Although this can be microbiologically cured, the threat of permanent resultant neurologic damage, often severe in neurosyphilis and usually less so in neuroborreliosis, leads to considerable concern and emphasizes the need for prevention or early and accurate diagnosis and treatment.

Fungal infections of the central nervous system (CNS) have a high rate of morbidity and mortality caused by several factors. Most importantly, the last three decades have witnessed a rising prevalence of susceptible hosts from the growing numbers of organ transplants, chemotherapy patients, and intensive care unit hospitalizations. Knowledge of CNS fungal infections including their symptoms and signs, required diagnostic studies, and treatment methods is imperative for all neurologists. This article provides an overview of the clinical features and laboratory findings of the major mycoses affecting the CNS and a focus on their neurologic presentations.

Neurologic complications of bacterial endocarditis have been observed for centuries but its management has remained challenging at all times. The cerebrovascular complications of this disorder are the most feared and difficult to address. The management of mycotic aneurysms, recent ischemic/hemorrhagic strokes with and without brain abscesses, and mechanical valve patients continues as an ongoing challenge. Literature continues to appear, providing new alternatives in treatment and hope for improved therapy.

RELATED INTEREST

Rheumatic Disease Clinics of North America February 2009
Infections and Rheumatic Diseases
Luis R. Espinoza, MD, *Guest Editor*

THE CLINICS ARE NOW AVAILABLE ONLINE!

Access your subscription at:
www.theclinics.com

Preface

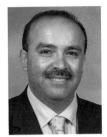

Alireza Minagar, MD, FAAN
Guest Editor

Neurology and internal medicine are two closely connected branches of medical science. In many cases, systemic diseases initially present with neurologic manifestations. Therefore, neurologists should have a thorough understanding of systemic diseases to better diagnose their neurologic complications.

This issue of *Neurologic Clinics* is devoted to the neurologic presentations of systemic disease and evaluates the neurologic problems that complicate a wide range of medical diseases arising from areas outside the central and peripheral nervous system. The issue begins with a detailed article by Yee and Rabinstein delineating the neurologic manifestations of emergent acid-base, electrolyte, and endocrine disorders that pose management challenges to neurologists and internists. Next, Kelley offers a systemic review of neurologic presentations of cardiac disease, examining the intimate relationship between the cardiovascular and nervous systems. This is followed by an article by Dreibelbis and Józefowicz that discusses the relationship between the respiratory and nervous systems and addresses the effects of abnormal ventilation on the nervous system. In the next article, Lacerda and colleagues focus on the neurologic presentations of renal diseases with an extensive discussion of a common and significant syndrome, uremia, and its effects on the human nervous system. The fifth article, by Muscal and Brey, is a balanced review of the neurologic manifestations of systemic lupus erythematosus in children and adults, providing readers with a detailed review of the clinical presentations, pathophysiology, and treatment strategies for neuropsychiatric lupus.

The interface between gastroenterology and neurology is presented in the context of three articles. First, Pfeiffer provides the latest developments in knowledge of neurologic complications of gastrointestinal diseases. This is followed by a comprehensive article by Harris and colleagues, which focuses on the fundamental mechanisms of hepatic encephalopathy and available treatments of this devastating medical disorder. The last article of this section is by Kumar and consists of an extensive review of the neurologic complications of nutritional deficiencies and a discussion of the management of these common disorders.

Neurol Clin 28 (2010) xiii–xiv
doi:10.1016/j.ncl.2009.09.019
0733-8619/09/$ – see front matter © 2010 Elsevier Inc. All rights reserved.

neurologic.theclinics.com

The next article, by Minagar and colleagues, discusses the neurologic presentations and complications of the most common vasculitides and provides readers with the latest findings regarding the pathogenic mechanisms of and treatment strategies for these frequently encountered disorders. This is followed by a remarkable article by Stern and colleagues, an informative review of a great imitator in medicine: sarcoidosis. Sarcoidosis involves the nervous system in up to 26% of affected individuals, and clinicians should be fully aware of its neurologic presentations. In addition, the investigators review diagnostic considerations and, finally, treatment strategies for neurosarcoidosis. This is followed by an article by Goforth and colleagues that focuses on the neurologic aspects of drug abuse and attempts to clarify common misconceptions, including the difference between tolerance, abuse, and addiction. In the next article, Dropcho tackles the issue of neurotoxicity from radiation therapy and discusses the clinical features, diagnosis, and management options. The last article in this section is by Živković and Abdel-Hamid. These investigators discuss the neurologic complications associated with organ transplantation, in particular those stemming from opportunistic infections and immunosuppressive therapies.

The remaining part of this issue of *Neurologic Clinics* is devoted to neurologic disorders and presentations associated with infections. First, Singer and colleagues discuss the neurologic complications of AIDS and discuss the latest developments in this significant area of infectious disease. Next, Halperin discusses the neurologic manifestations of two other increasingly common and controversial infections: neurosyphilis and neuroborreliosis. These two infections, if left untreated, produce devastating neurologic syndromes that leave patients with permanent neurologic disability. The article by Rauchway and colleagues provides an overview of the clinical features and laboratory findings of the major mycoses affecting the central nervous system with a focus on their clinical neurologic presentations. Lastly, Johnson and Johnson examine the neurologic complications of infective endocarditis. This article highlights various neurologic presentations and complications of infective endocarditis with a balanced and comprehensive review of this important subject. Working on this issue was a humbling experience for me because I was able to work with some of the brightest and most knowledgeable neurologists and psychiatrists in the United States and other countries around the globe. Without these wonderful contributors, this issue would never have become a reality. I would also like to acknowledge the effort and assistance of Dr Randolph Evans, Mr Donald Mumford, Ms Annie Calacci and other dedicated and hardworking personnel of Elsevier who aided me in preparing this issue.

In conclusion, I hope that this issue of *Neurologic Clinics* encourages neurologists and neuroscientists to further explore the complex relationships between neurologic and medical diseases.

Alireza Minagar, MD, FAAN
Department of Neurology
Louisiana State University Health Sciences Center
Shreveport
LA 71130, USA

E-mail address:
aminag@lsuhsc.edu

Neurologic Presentations of Acid-Base Imbalance, Electrolyte Abnormalities, and Endocrine Emergencies

Alan H. Yee, DO[a], Alejandro A. Rabinstein, MD[b],*

KEYWORDS

- Neurologic manifestations • Acid-base
- Electrolyte • Endocrine emergencies

ACID-BASE DISEQUILIBRIUM

There are many causes of respiratory and renal system dysfunction that can generate acid-base disarray independently or in combination. Through complex mechanisms, inadequate oxygenation, suboptimal ventilation, and various forms of altered renal physiology (eg, renal tubular acidosis) can disturb nervous system function. All acid-base disturbances—respiratory acidosis, respiratory alkalosis, metabolic acidosis, and metabolic alkalosis—have the potential for producing neurologic manifestations (**Table 1**).

Respiratory Acidosis

Although hypoxemic ischemic nervous system injury is the primary neurologic concern in cases of respiratory failure, prompt recognition of abnormal levels of $Paco_2$ and pH is important. Respiratory acidosis is defined by the presence of acidemia (serum pH <7.36) secondary to elevated $Paco_2$ levels ($Paco_2$ >45 mm Hg). The acuity and severity of hypercarbia and acidosis influence the degree of neurologic involvement, and neurologic symptoms and signs are seen more frequently in cases of respiratory acidosis than with metabolic acidosis because CO_2 diffuses readily across the blood-brain barrier. Asterixis, somnolence, tremor, and cerebral dysfunction are the main signs and worsen as the concentration of blood hydrogen ion content increases along with the $Paco_2$. If left untreated, progressive acidemia may lead to coma.[1] Levels of $Paco_2$ greater than 50 mm Hg can result in changes in cerebral blood

[a] Department of Neurology, Mayo Clinic, 200 First Street SW, Rochester, MN 55905, USA
[b] Division of Critical Care Neurology, Department of Neurology, Mayo Clinic, 200 First Street S.W, Rochester, MN 55905, USA
* Corresponding author.
E-mail address: rabinstein.alejandro@mayo.edu (A.A. Rabinstein).

Neurol Clin 28 (2010) 1–16
doi:10.1016/j.ncl.2009.09.002
0733-8619/09/$ – see front matter © 2010 Elsevier Inc. All rights reserved.

Table 1
Common neurologic symptoms and signs of acidosis and alkalosis

Acidosis	Alkalosis
Central nervous system	Central nervous system
Symptoms	Symptoms
Sleepiness	Lightheadedness
Fatigue	Vertigo
Confusion	Confusion
Headache	Headache
Visual complaints	Tinnitus
Poor sleep architecture	Blurred vision
	Syncope
	Seizure
Signs	Signs
Asterixis	Ataxia
Visual impairment	Chvostek's sign
Encephalopathy	Tremor
Coma	Encephalopathy
Signs of raised intracranial pressure	Coma
(respiratory acidosis)	Seizure manifestations
Increased opening CSF pressure	
Papilledema	
Pupillary light reflex abnormality	
Herniation syndromes	
Peripheral nervous system	Peripheral nervous system
Symptoms/signs	Symptoms
Tremulousness	Circumoral/limb paresthesias
	Cramps
	Tremor
	Signs
	Myoclonus
	Tetany

flow, leading to cerebral vasodilatation and an ensuing rise in intracranial pressure, described in hypoventilation syndromes.[2–4] Symptoms secondary to increased intracranial pressure include headache peaking at night or during the early morning hours, confusion, and visual disturbances, ranging from blurred vision to blindness. Accompanying abnormal signs detected on neurologic examination include papilledema, optic atrophy, elevation of opening cerebrospinal fluid pressure, or, in most severe cases, signs indicative of impending herniation syndromes, such as pupillary changes or upper motor neuron findings.[5,6] Disruption of sleep architecture is frequently encountered in acidotic patients and likely stems from an underlying cause of disordered breathing and disturbed acid-base equilibrium. Many of these clinical features typically improve once ventilatory dysfunction and hypercarbia are corrected. This correction must be gradual, however, because rapid clearance of CO_2 may not allow enough time for excretion of compensatory bicarbonate; the resulting metabolic alkalosis may be complicated by seizures.[7]

Respiratory Alkalosis

Respiratory alkalosis occurs when serum pH is greater than 7.44 primarily due to $Paco_2$ levels (ie, less than 35 mm Hg). This metabolic disturbance can occur from any form of hyperventilation. It leads to a leftward shift of the oxygen disassociation curve, potentially decreasing cerebral blood flow and generating tissue hypoxia.[8] Additional signs may result from secondary decreases in serum calcium and phosphate concentrations.[9] Neurologic diseases affecting the brainstem, such as stroke, malignancies, rhombencephalitis, and Rett syndrome, can lead to hyperventilation-associated alkalosis.[10] Patients typically report lightheadedness, unilateral or bilateral paresthesias of the limbs and perioral area, headache, muscle cramps, vertigo, and, less commonly, tremor, tinnitus, blurred vision, ataxia, confusion, altered level of alertness, and syncope.[9,11] Respiratory alkalosis associated with hyperventilation can lower seizure threshold in susceptible individuals, such as those with absence seizures. Neurologic examination most often yields no specific findings; however, Chvostek's sign is reported in some affected individuals.[9] On electroencephalographic recordings, theta range and other degrees of high amplitude slowing are described without accompanying epileptogenic activity.[8,11]

Metabolic Acidosis

Metabolic acidosis is defined by a depletion of serum bicarbonate or increase in hydrogen ion production, causing acidemia. Two main forms exist, which are typically referred to as anion gap or non–anion gap metabolic acidosis. The importance of making such a distinction is key to determine the underlying mechanism. **Table 2** lists frequently suspected causes of the gap and nongap forms. A meticulous medical history (eg, recent tonic-clonic seizure and elevated lactate) and physical examination (eg, stigmata of renal failure) can often yield the correct diagnosis. When neurologic abnormalities are present in the setting of either form, they are often nonspecific. Headache, lethargy, stupor, and, in most severe cases, coma can result from this metabolic derangement. Additionally, during periods of profound acidosis, cerebral hypoxia may occur secondary to cardiovascular collapse.[12] Signs and symptoms of raised intracranial pressure occur less often when the acidosis is secondary to a metabolic rather than a respiratory cause, as alluded to previously, because the development of respiratory acidosis is often more acute.

Table 2	
Common causes of gap and nongap metabolic acidosis	
Gap Metabolic Acidosis (>12 mEq)	**Nongap Metabolic Acidosis (<12 mEq)**
Toxins	Gastrointestinal
Methanol	Diarrhea
Paraldehyde	Intestinal fistula
Ethylene glycol	Pancreatic shunt/ileostomy
Ammonium chloride	Renal causes
Medications	Renal tubular acidosis
Salicylates	Malignancy
Isoniazid	Multiple myeloma or other causes
Excessive iron	of hyperparaproteinemia
Metformin	Other
Medical conditions	Medications (carbonic anhydrase
Diabetic ketoacidosis	inhibitors)
Lactic acidosis (any cause)	Aggressive saline administration
Alcoholic ketoacidosis	Lithium toxicity
Uremia	

Metabolic Alkalosis

Metabolic alkalosis is defined by the presence of alkalemia (serum >7.45) due to an increased serum bicarbonate concentration (>26 mmol/L); it frequently coexists with elevated $Paco_2$ levels as a compensatory mechanism.[13,14] Metabolic alkalosis commonly occurs in the context of diuretic-associated volume contraction or in cases of recurrent vomiting. The neurologic signs seen with metabolic alkalosis are similar to those seen with other forms of alkalosis and include paresthesias, muscle cramps, and confusion. Concern for seizures may be caused by muscle twitches, limb myoclonus, and transient tetany that are indistinguishable from those observed with severe hypocalcemia.[15–17] Nevertheless, seizures can also occur in severe cases of metabolic alkalosis and should be suspected in profoundly alkalotic patients with an altered or depressed level of consciousness.[18,19] Coma rarely is the presenting manifestation in cases of marked metabolic alkalosis; most often, confusion and disorientation are preceding signs.[20,21]

ELECTROLYTE DISTURBANCES

The brain and nerves are particularly sensitive to environmental chemical and ionic changes. Consequently, many forms of electrolyte imbalance are associated with neurologic manifestations, especially if acute (**Table 3**).

Hyponatremia

A low serum sodium concentration is one of the most frequently encountered electrolyte disturbances in patients with acute neurologic disease. Hyponatremia is defined by a serum sodium concentration below 135 mmol/L. It is caused by an excess in body water in relation to the sodium content and most often associated with serum iso- or hypo-osmolality.[22] Inappropriate secretion of antidiuretic hormone and cerebral salt wasting from excessive secretion of natriuretic peptides are the two most common pathophysiologic mechanisms in neurologic patients. Hyponatremia is

Table 3
Common neurologic features of electrolyte disturbances

Central Nervous System	Peripheral Nervous System
Headache	Limb or acral paresthesias
Visual disturbances	Perioral paresthesias (↓ Ca, ↓ Phos)
Ataxia	Auditory nerve dysfunction (↓ Mg)
Chorea (↓ Ca)	Focal or generalized weakness
Bradykinesia (↑ Ca)	Myalgias
Seizure (↓ Na, ↓ Ca >> ↑ Ca, ↓ Mg)	Paralysis (↑↓ K, ↑↑ Mg, ↓ Phos)
Neuropsychiatric (↑↓ Ca, ↓ Mg, ↓ K)	Muscle atrophy (chronic ↓ K)
Encephalopathy	Fasciculations (↓ Na, ↓ Ca, ↓ Mg)
Cerebral edema (↓ Na)	Tetany/carpopedal spasm (↓ Ca, ↓ K)
Coma	Stridor (↓ Ca)
EEG findings (↓ Na, ↓ Phos, ↑↓ Ca)	Opisthotonus (↓ Ca)
Generalized, focal slowing	Hypertonia (↑ Na)
Triphasic waves	Tremulousness
	Depressed deep tendon reflexes (↑ Mg, ↓ Phos)
	Increased deep tendon reflexes (↑ Na)
	Respiratory depression (↓ K, ↓ Phos)

Abbreviations: Ca, calcium; EEG, electroencephalogram; K, potassium; Mg, magnesium; Na, sodium; Phos, phosphate; ↑, increased; ↓, decreased.

commonly found as a complication from aneurysmal subarachnoid hemorrhage,[23–26] central nervous system malignancy,[27,28] infection,[29,30] and head trauma.[31] It predominantly affects the central more than peripheral nervous system because of the adaptive capacity of the brain to rapid changes in body fluid osmolality. An abrupt decline in serum sodium can lead to rapid fluid shifts causing cerebral edema. Individuals are generally without significant symptoms until serum sodium levels fall below 120 mmol/L, although less pronounced but brisk drops are associated with clinical deterioration.[32,33] In mild cases, generalized fatigue, nausea, headache, dysgeusia, anorexia, and muscle cramps are typical. As levels continue to fall (eg, 120 to 130 mmol/L), worsening of the aforementioned symptoms can be accompanied by vomiting, fasciculations, tremulousness, and progressive deterioration in mental alertness and orientation.[34] Life-threatening levels of hyponatremia (ie, <115 mmol/L) that develop acutely are known to cause focal and generalized seizures and may cause coma.[35,36] If left untreated, progressive cerebral edema may lead to brain herniation.[37] Extreme care must be taken when treating this electrolyte abnormality as overzealous correction may lead to central (pontine or extrapontine) myelinolysis. This neurologic complication typically presents with altered cognition and decreased alertness; however, localizing features, such as ataxia, hemiparesis, and upper motor neuron signs, may occur.[38–40] An EEG often reveals varying degrees of nonspecific slowing; triphasic waves, high-voltage rhythmic delta, and periodic lateralized epileptiform discharges also are described in more severe cases.[41]

Hypernatremia

Hypernatremia is defined by a serum sodium concentration greater than 145 mEq/L and is caused by the presence of excess sodium in relation to body water. Diabetes insipidus and iatrogenic causes predominate in neurologic patients. Hypernatremic patients are often irritable and complain of thirst when they have an intact sensorium; however, with progressive worsening of the electrolyte disturbance, varying degrees of depressed mental alertness, ranging from sleepiness to coma, may occur. Abnormal neuromuscular signs of muscle irritation such as increased tone and tendon stretch reflexes are frequently seen in the context of volume depletion and hypernatremia.[42] Unlike hyponatremia, hypernatremia does not lead to seizures but may result from them due to lactate-induced intracellular osmolality gradient shifts.[41] Catastrophic hemorrhage from tearing of bridging cerebral veins is possible in the most severe cases of brain shrinking.[43]

Potassium Disturbances

The cardiac complications from disturbances in serum potassium concentrations are well known; however, the associated neurologic manifestations are less frequently recognized. Hypokalemia-related neuromuscular symptoms typically manifest after serum potassium levels fall below 2.5 mEq/L.[34] The neurologic manifestations of hypokalemia have been best studied in familial forms of paralysis.[44] Muscular weakness is the main clinical feature with predominating involvement of proximal lower limb muscles. Cranial nerve innervated muscles are rarely involved and deep tendon reflexes are often spared.[34,44] When severe, respiratory depression can occur as a result of diaphragmatic and accessory muscle weakness.[45] The more commonly encountered symptoms include muscle cramps, paresthesias, lethargy, irritability, and drowsiness. Tetany can occur independently of low serum calcium levels[46] or after unmasking of coexisting hypocalcemia during potassium replacement.[34,47] Elevation of muscle enzymes[48] has been reported and muscle biopsy can at times reveal muscle atrophy and necrosis.[49,50]

Hyperkalemia is less commonly associated with neurologic manifestations. Nonspecific generalized weakness may be present. Rarely, complete or near complete reversible paralysis has been reported after correction of elevated serum potassium levels.[51–53] Subjective paresthesias along with long track sensory signs may occasionally accompany this electrolyte abnormality.[34]

Calcium Abnormalities and Parathyroid Disease

Disturbances in serum calcium homeostasis often result in neurologic symptoms and signs. This is not surprising particularly because myocyte and neuronal cell membranes are sensitive to fluctuations in serum calcium concentration as this ion is a stabilizer of electrically excitable tissue. Primary and secondary forms of parathyroid disorders induce changes in serum calcium ion concentrations—hyperparathyroidism leading to hypercalcemia and hypoparathyroidism to hypocalcemia—along with altered phosphate levels. Parathyroid adenomas are one of the most common causes of primary hyperparathyroidism whereas secondary disease is often related to longstanding renal failure. When clinical manifestations of low parathyroid levels are evident, they typically occur as a result of parathyroidectomy.

Hypo- and hypercalcemia can cause alterations in cognition and alertness. Serum calcium levels greater than 14 mg/dL are more frequently associated with deeper suppression of consciousness. When severe, progression to coma can be anticipated.[34,38] Nevertheless, the majority of hypercalcemic patients tend to have only a mild to moderate elevation in serum calcium concentration and the usual neurologic manifestations consist of headache, lethargy, proximal leg muscular fatigue, confusion, and myalgias, which may be severe. Electromyography can reveal myopathic changes and muscle biopsy may show focal type II fiber muscle atrophy along with inflammatory cellular infiltration.[54] Neuropsychiatric manifestations are common and include paranoia, delirium, excessive agitation, and hallucinations.[34,55,56] Occasionally, symptoms and signs consistent with motor neuron disease can develop in the context of hypercalcemia and primary hyperparathyroidism; however, there is lack of supportive evidence to suggest a causal link.[57,58] Adequate treatment of the hyperparathyroidism may not result in improvement of these abnormalities.[57,58] Additional clinical features may include hyperkinetic movement disorders, such as chorea or choreoathetosis, with hypocalcemia, and bradykinetic manifestations that are suggestive of parkinsonism, with hypercalcemia.[59–63] These clinical findings might be related to basal ganglia calcifications often seen in cases of chronic hypoparathyroidism[34,64,65] and rarely hyperparathyroidism,[66] but this association is not solidly established.

Seizures occur infrequently with abnormally elevated serum calcium concentrations[67] but are relatively common with hypocalcemia. Generalized, focal, and prolonged seizure activity due to hypocalcemia has been reported.[41,68,69] Additional EEG features that may occur at either end of the spectrum of calcium derangements include progressive generalized or focal slowing and other findings consistent with metabolic encephalopathy, such as triphasic waves,[41,70] all of which gradually resolve once serum calcium concentrations normalize.

Tetany is one of the best-known neuromuscular signs attributed to hypocalcemia. This cardinal manifestation occurs as a result of increased axonal excitability and increased spontaneous firing of action potentials. Early symptoms include tingling or burning paresthesias involving the fingers, lips, and tongue. The typical motor findings—cramps, fasciculations, and the classic spasms themselves—follow.[34] As the name implies, carpopedal spasms involve contractures of the hands and feet. Provocative maneuvers, such as occluding extremity arterial blood flow with a pressure cuff

(Trousseau's test) or tapping over the facial nerve (Chvostek's sign), can reproduce distal limb and facial spasms, respectively. When hypocalcemia is severe, laryngeal stridor and opisthotonos may be striking clinical manifestations.

Magnesium Disturbances

Neurologic signs and symptoms seen as a result of abnormal serum magnesium levels are similar to those observed with disturbances in serum calcium concentration. Hypomagnesemia is frequently accompanied by hypokalemia and hypocalcemia, making it difficult to determine the underlying metabolic cause for the neurologic manifestations. Progressive personality changes, confusion, ataxia, and head and limb tremors[71,72] can occur when serum levels were allowed to fall below 1 mEq/L. Additional complaints of headache, blurred vision, and generalized weakness are not uncommon. Auditory changes also are speculated as resulting from magnesium deficiency.[73] Neuromuscular features later become evident and consist of fasciculations with EMG evidence of myopathic-like changes. Chvostek's sign and an abnormal Trousseau's test may be present in patients with coexistent hypocalcemia. Tonic-clonic generalized convulsions and recurrent seizures also are described.[71]

In this current era of readily available laboratory monitoring, clinically apparent manifestations from hypermagnesemia are infrequently encountered. Abnormally elevated levels are found most commonly in patients with underlying renal failure. Dramatic rises in serum magnesium (>15 mEq/L) may produce depressed levels of consciousness and even coma. The presence of depressed tendon stretch reflexes can be a warning sign that impending motor paralysis will ensue.[34]

Phosphate Abnormalities

Disruption of phosphate homeostasis often occurs in association with other metabolic derangements (eg, hypocalcemia). Neurologic features are only encountered when serum phosphate levels become markedly abnormal. Hyperphosphatemia alone does not lead to any clinically significant manifestations, but its effects on calcium metabolism may lead to symptomatic hypocalcemia.[74–76] Instead, hypophosphatemia is associated with significant cognitive, sensory, and neuromuscular symptoms that can be anticipated when serum levels fall below 1 mg/dL.[77,78] Circumoral paresthesias develop early and are followed by ptosis, dysphagia, and significant limb weakness that can progress to complete paralysis. Many additional clinical manifestations, such as ataxia, tremor, asterixis, depressed reflexes, and EEG background slowing, are described.[77,79] Similar to profound disturbances in calcium, potassium, and sodium serum concentrations, markedly decreased serum phosphorus levels may also lead to severe encephalopathy and coma. In debilitated individuals, hypophosphatemia can compromise diaphragmatic function.[80,81]

ENDOCRINE EMERGENCIES
Hyperglycemic Emergencies

The two main diabetic emergencies, hyperglycemic hyperosmolar state (HHS) and diabetic ketoacidosis (DKA), can have devastating neurologic outcomes when left untreated. Both can occur in either type 1 or 2 diabetes mellitus (DM); however, HHS is more often associated with type 2 DM whereas DKA classically develops in those with type 1 DM. The key differentiating features between the two entities are that patients with HHS tend to have minimal or no ketoacidosis present, a greater degree of intravascular volume depletion, and likely a higher level of counter-regulatory hormones that ultimately decrease glucose uptake and use, hence leading to more profound hyperglycemia (often >600 mg/dL) when compared with DKA.[82] Nevertheless, both have otherwise similar pathophysiologic mechanisms and neurologic manifestations. A common presentation in both disorders is that individuals have some degree of altered mental status. As the hyperglycemia progresses to alarming levels, coma can ensue in both forms. A key historical feature that may distinguish DKA from HHS is that the latter frequently develops insidiously whereas the former can manifest abruptly only hours after an inciting event (eg, myocardial infarction or infection).[82] Coma develops in nearly 30% of HHS cases and usually results from a serum osmolarity exceeding 340 mOsm/L with accompanying severe hyperglycemia rather than from the generation of ketoacidosis.[83,84] In DKA, coma occurs in cases of severe acidemia and worsening hyperosmolality.[85]

Additional neurologic and brain imaging findings more often seen with HHS include: seizure; transient focal deficits, such as hemiparesis; extensor plantar responses; chorea-ballismus; and reversible subcortical white matter changes visualized on MRI.[86–89] Cerebral edema is most often seen in DKA during the treatment phase.[90–92] Although the precise mechanism is not fully understood, proposed theories revolve around the accumulation of undefined osmotically active molecules[93] within the brain and activation of a Na^+/H^+ ionic pump,[92] both of which can potentially lead to cerebral edema during rapid correction of serum hyperglycemia despite the presence of biochemical and clinical improvement. Rapid evolution to coma with signs of brain herniation can be expected if the edema is not detected and treated early.

Hypoglycemia

Hypoglycemia is most often seen in the context of insulin use in diabetic and hospitalized nondiabetic patients. The neurologic manifestations can be protean and at times mimic primary nervous system diseases (eg, stroke). Altered sensorium with behavioral changes, visual disturbances, convulsions, and transient focal motor and speech deficits can be seen.[94–97] Focal deficits can last up to several hours. Patients who become stuporous or comatose often improve promptly after glucose administration; however, they may remain poorly responsive if postictal after a seizure or if the hypoglycemic episode was severe and prolonged. Permanent sequelae may occur (eg, vegetative state).[98] Diagnostic studies can reveal variable changes. Electroencephalographic abnormalities may range from focal slowing to epileptiform activity.[99,100] MRI scans may show cortical and subcortical (hippocampus, basal ganglia) abnormalities on diffusion-weighted sequences.[101–103]

Acute Adrenal Insufficiency

Addison's disease, or adrenal insufficiency, is a deficiency in adrenocorticosteroid hormones (eg, cortisol, aldosterone, and adrenal androgens) from primary adrenal glandular deficiency or secondary pituitary failure.[104] Acute adrenal insufficiency can be striking and is often seen in patients with known Addison's disease who abruptly discontinue steroid supplementation or take insufficient doses of steroids during times of physiologic stress (eg, infection or surgery). Direct adrenal injury from other causes can also lead to identical clinical manifestations.[104] Systemic manifestations, such as nausea with vomiting, hyponatremia, hyperkalemia, and hypovolemic shock, often coexist with the characteristic generalized fatigue, malaise, and musculoskeletal weakness. The neurologic examination confirms diffuse motor weakness and, when most severe, quadraparesis with muscle atrophy or a Guillain-Barré–like syndrome.[105,106] Electromyography usually confirms a predominantly motor pathologic process.[106,107] Hypoglycemic and febrile seizures can be the initial manifestations of this disorder in children[108,109] along with progressive

Table 4
Common neurologic features of endocrine emergencies

Disorder	Central Nervous System	Peripheral Nervous System
Parathyroid disease		
Hyperparathyroidism (causes hypercalcemia)	Headache Encephalopathy (moderate-severe) Neuropsychiatric (manifestations) Bradykinesia	Proximal muscular fatigue Myalgia
Hypoparathyroidism (causes hypocalcemia)	Encephalopathy (generally mild) Hyperkinesia Basal ganglia calcification Seizures	Acral, lips, tongue paresthesias Cramps/fasciculations Tetany/carpopedal spasms Opisthotonos (with severe hypocalcemia)
Hyperglycemia		
Hyperglycemic hyperosmolar state	Encephalopathy (insidious onset) Seizure Transient focal deficits Coma Reversible white matter MRI changes	
Diabetic ketoacidosis	Encephalopathy (acute onset) Cerebral edema	
Hypoglycemia	Encephalopathy (acute onset) Behavioral change Visual disturbance Seizure Focal motor/speech deficits	
Acute adrenal insufficiency	Encephalopathy (insidious) Seizure (from secondary hypoglycemia) Coma (rare)	Generalized muscular weakness Limb paralysis (rare)
Pituitary apoplexy	Thunderclap headache (retro-orbital) Cranial nerve palsies (III, IV, VI) Optic nerve dysfunction (ie, bitemporal hemianopsia)	
Thyroid disease		
Myxedema	Encephalopathy Myoclonus Seizures Coma	Hyporeflexia-areflexia
Thyroid storm	Encephalopathy Seizure Upper motor neuron signs Coma	Tremulous Hyperreflexia

encephalopathy.[110] Coma rarely is reported and typically occurs in the context of severe metabolic disturbances from corticosteroid or aldosterone deficiency, such as hypoglycemia or hyponatremia.[111]

Pituitary Apoplexy

Acute hemorrhage or infarction of the pituitary gland may cause pituitary apoplexy. Its occurrence is often described in patients with associated pituitary adenomas; however, the presence of tumor is not obligatory. Although the presentation may be similar to that of abrupt adrenal insufficiency, a classic retro-orbital thunderclap headache is frequently the sentinel neurologic symptom. Accompanying clinical features that may evolve over the ensuing several hours to days point to the focal structural pathology and include palsies of cranial nerves confined to the cavernous sinus— oculomotor, abducens, and trochlear nerve—and visual field deficits from pressure on the optic chiasm. Patients typically complain of a reduction in their visual field or acuity, monocular blindness, photophobia, or diplopia. Clinical examination usually confirms the presence of ocular cranial nerve abnormalities and bitemporal hemianopsia.[112–114] Mental status changes can be variable and range from lethargy to coma. Prolonged periods of postoperative coma can be seen in patients who had undergone emergent surgical decompression.[112,115]

Severe Thyroid Disease (Myxedema Coma and Thyroid Storm)

Myxedema results from markedly depressed levels of thyroxine (T4), as a result of thyroid or pituitary gland failure. Patients with myxedema often present with variable degrees of encephalopathy. The disturbed cognitive function is typically associated with hypothyroid features: limb, face, and periorbital nonpitting edema; cardiovascular collapse; poor ventilation; hyponatremia; and hypothermia.[116] Seizures[117] are reported in greater than 20% of cases along with the more usual physical manifestations of metabolic encephalopathies, such as myoclonus. Neurologic examination frequently reveals hypo- or areflexia but localizing signs are characteristically absent.[62] A delayed relaxation phase of the tendon stretch reflex (Woltman's sign) can be suggestive of marked hypothyroidism.

A marked elevation in serum-free thyroid concentration can lead to a rare and severe form of thyrotoxicosis, thyroid storm, which can produce dire central and peripheral nervous system consequences. The development of seizure, severe hyperthermia, and eventually coma are seen in lethal cases of thyroid storm.[118] Initially mild neuromuscular features, such as tremulousness and hyperreflexia,[119] can progress to profound flaccid areflexic quadraparesis with electrodiagnostic evidence of a mixed axonal and demyelinating sensory-motor neuropathy.[120] Signs of cortical spinal tract dysfunction can be detected on physical examination and they resolve after the initiation of appropriate therapy.[62]

Table 4 summarizes the frequently encountered neurologic manifestations of the acute endocrinopathies discussed in this article.

REFERENCES

1. Kilburn KH. Neurologic manifestations of respiratory failure. Arch Intern Med 1965;116:409–15.
2. Jennum P, Borgesen SE. Intracranial pressure and obstructive sleep apnea. Chest 1989;95(2):279–83.

3. Kirkpatrick PJ, Meyer T, Sarkies N, et al. Papilloedema and visual failure in a patient with nocturnal hypoventilation. J Neurol Neurosurg Psychiatr 1994; 57(12):1546–7.
4. Reeve P, Harvey G, Seaton D. Papilloedema and respiratory failure. Br Med J (Clin Res Ed) 1985;291(6491):331–2.
5. Varelas PN, Spanaki MV, Rathi S, et al. Papilledema unresponsive to therapy in Pickwickian syndrome: another presentation of pseudotumor cerebri? Am J Med 2000;109(1):80–1.
6. Pitt B, Sweet R, Stein M. Respiratory failure with focal neurological sings. Arch Intern Med 1965;115:14–7.
7. Faden A. Encephalopathy following treatment of chronic pulmonary failure. Neurology 1976;26(4):337–9.
8. Gotoh F, Meyer JS, Takagi Y. Cerebral effects of hyperventilation in man. Arch Neurol 1965;12:410–23.
9. Saltzman HA, Heyman A, Sieker HO. Correlation of clinical and physiologic manifestations of sustained hyperventilation. N Engl J Med 1963;268: 1431–6.
10. Evans RW. Neurologic aspects of hyperventilation syndrome. Semin Neurol 1995;15(2):115–25.
11. Perkin GD, Joseph R. Neurological manifestations of the hyperventilation syndrome. J R Soc Med 1986;79(8):448–50.
12. Wijdicks E. Acid-base, electrolyte, and endocrine disorders. Neurology of critical illness. Philadelphia: F.A. Davis Company; 1995. p. 104–6.
13. DuBose TD. Acidosis and alkalosis. In: Braunwald E, Fauci A, Kasper D, et al, editors. Harrison's principles of internal medicine. 15th edition. New York: McGraw-Hill Companies; 2001. p. 283–91.
14. Haber RJ. A practical approach to acid-base disorders. West J Med 1991; 155(2):146–51.
15. Ishiguchi T, Mikita N, Iwata T, et al. Myoclonus and metabolic alkalosis from licorice in antacid. Intern Med 2004;43(1):59–62.
16. Okada K, Kono N, Kobayashi S, et al. Metabolic alkalosis and myoclonus from antacid ingestion. Intern Med 1996;35(6):515–6.
17. Simons P, Nadra I, McNally PG. Metabolic alkalosis and myoclonus. Postgrad Med J 2003;79(933):414–5.
18. Kilburn KH. Shock, seizures, and coma with alkalosis during mechanical ventilation. Ann Intern Med 1966;65(5):977–84.
19. Rotheram EB Jr, Safar P, Robin E. Cns disorder during mechanical ventilation in chronic pulmonary disease. JAMA 1964;189:993–6.
20. Fraley DS, Adler S, Bruns F. Life-threatening metabolic alkalosis in a comatose patient. Southampt Med J 1979;72(8):1024–5.
21. Lubash GD, Cohen BD, Young CW, et al. Severe metabolic alkalosis with neurologic abnormalities; report of a case. N Engl J Med 1958;258(21): 1050–2.
22. Adrogue HJ, Madias NE. Hyponatremia. N Engl J Med 2000;342(21):1581–9.
23. Isotani E, Suzuki R, Tomita K, et al. Alterations in plasma concentrations of natriuretic peptides and antidiuretic hormone after subarachnoid hemorrhage. Stroke 1994;25(11):2198–203.
24. McGirt MJ, Blessing R, Nimjee SM, et al. Correlation of serum brain natriuretic peptide with hyponatremia and delayed ischemic neurological deficits after subarachnoid hemorrhage. Neurosurgery 2004;54(6):1369–73 [discussion: 1373–4].

25. Wijdicks EF, Vermeulen M, Hijdra A, et al. Hyponatremia and cerebral infarction in patients with ruptured intracranial aneurysms: is fluid restriction harmful? Ann Neurol 1985;17(2):137–40.

26. Wijdicks EF, Vermeulen M, ten Haaf JA, et al. Volume depletion and natriuresis in patients with a ruptured intracranial aneurysm. Ann Neurol 1985;18(2):211–6.

27. Kim JH, Kang JK, Lee SA. Hydrocephalus and hyponatremia as the presenting manifestations of primary CNS lymphoma. Eur Neurol 2006;55(1): 39–41.

28. Poon WS, Lolin YI, Yeung TF, et al. Water and sodium disorders following surgical excision of pituitary region tumours. Acta Neurochir (Wien) 1996; 138(8):921–7.

29. Moller K, Larsen FS, Bie P, et al. The syndrome of inappropriate secretion of antidiuretic hormone and fluid restriction in meningitis—how strong is the evidence? Scand J Infect Dis 2001;33(1):13–26.

30. Narotam PK, Kemp M, Buck R, et al. Hyponatremic natriuretic syndrome in tuberculous meningitis: the probable role of atrial natriuretic peptide. Neurosurgery 1994;34(6):982–8 [discussion: 988].

31. Moro N, Katayama Y, Igarashi T, et al. Hyponatremia in patients with traumatic brain injury: incidence, mechanism, and response to sodium supplementation or retention therapy with hydrocortisone. Surg Neurol 2007;68(4):387–93.

32. Arieff AI, Llach F, Massry SG. Neurological manifestations and morbidity of hyponatremia: correlation with brain water and electrolytes. Medicine (Baltimore) 1976;55(2):121–9.

33. Rabinstein AA, Wijdicks EF. Hyponatremia in critically ill neurological patients. Neurologist 2003;9(6):290–300.

34. Weiner M, Epstein FH. Signs and symptoms of electrolyte disorders. Yale J Biol Med 1970;43(2):76–109.

35. Arieff AI. Hyponatremia, convulsions, respiratory arrest, and permanent brain damage after elective surgery in healthy women. N Engl J Med 1986;314(24): 1529–35.

36. Wijdicks EF, Sharbrough FW. New-onset seizures in critically ill patients. Neurology 1993;43(5):1042–4.

37. Mulloy AL, Caruana RJ. Hyponatremic emergencies. Med Clin North Am 1995; 79(1):155–68.

38. Riggs JE. Neurologic manifestations of electrolyte disturbances. Neurol Clin 2002;20(1):227–39, vii.

39. Schwartz E, Fogel RL, Chokas WV, et al. Unstable osmolar homeostasis with and without renal sodium wastage. Am J Med 1962;33:39–53.

40. Schwartz WB, Bennett W, Curelop S, et al. A syndrome of renal sodium loss and hyponatremia probably resulting from inappropriate secretion of antidiuretic hormone. Am J Med 1957;23(4):529–42.

41. Castilla-Guerra L, del Carmen Fernandez-Moreno M, Lopez-Chozas JM, et al. Electrolytes disturbances and seizures. Epilepsia 2006;47(12):1990–8.

42. Arieff AI, Guisado R. Effects on the central nervous system of hypernatremic and hyponatremic states. Kidney Int 1976;10(1):104–16.

43. Adrogue HJ, Madias NE. Hypernatremia. N Engl J Med 2000;342(20):1493–9.

44. Buruma OJ, Bots GT, Went LN. Familial hypokalemic periodic paralysis. 50-year follow-up of a large family. Arch Neurol 1985;42(1):28–31.

45. Stedwell RE, Allen KM, Binder LS. Hypokalemic paralyses: a review of the etiologies, pathophysiology, presentation, and therapy. Am J Emerg Med 1992; 10(2):143–8.

46. Ault MJ, Geiderman J. Hypokalemia as a cause of tetany. West J Med 1992; 157(1):65–7.
47. Engel FL, Martin SP, Taylor H. On the relation of potassium to the neurological manifestations of hypocalcemic tetany. Bull Johns Hopkins Hosp 1949;84(4): 285–301.
48. Van Horn G, Drori JB, Schwartz FD. Hypokalemic myopathy and elevation of serum enzymes. Arch Neurol 1970;22(4):335–41.
49. Finsterer J, Hess B, Jarius C, et al. Malnutrition-induced hypokalemic myopathy in chronic alcoholism. J Toxicol Clin Toxicol 1998;36(4):369–73.
50. Martin JB, Craig JW, Eckel RE, et al. Hypokalemic myopathy in chronic alcoholism. Neurology 1971;21(11):1160–8.
51. Maury E, Lemant J, Dussaule JC, et al. A reversible paralysis. Lancet 2002; 360(9346):1660.
52. McCarty M, Jagoda A, Fairweather P. Hyperkalemic ascending paralysis. Ann Emerg Med 1998;32(1):104–7.
53. Tapiawala S, Badve SV, More N, et al. Severe muscle weakness due to hyperkalemia. J Assoc Physicians India 2004;52:505–6.
54. Patten BM, Bilezikian JP, Mallette LE, et al. Neuromuscular disease in primary hyperparathyroidism. Ann Intern Med 1974;80(2):182–93.
55. Brown SW, Vyas BV, Spiegel DR. Mania in a case of hyperparathyroidism. Psychosomatics 2007;48(3):265–8.
56. Chiba Y, Satoh K, Ueda S, et al. Marked improvement of psychiatric symptoms after parathyroidectomy in elderly primary hyperparathyroidism. Endocrinol Jpn 2007;54(3):379–83.
57. Jackson CE, Amato AA, Bryan WW, et al. Primary hyperparathyroidism and ALS: is there a relation? Neurology 1998;50(6):1795–9.
58. Patten BM, Pages M. Severe neurological disease associated with hyperparathyroidism. Ann Neurol 1984;15(5):453–6.
59. Fernandez R, Ashraf A, Dure LS. Nutritional vitamin D deficiency presenting as hemichorea. J Child Neurol 2007;22(1):74–6.
60. Hirooka Y, Yuasa K, Hibi K, et al. Hyperparathyroidism associated with parkinsonism. Intern Med 1992;31(7):904–7.
61. Kovacs CS, Howse DC, Yendt ER. Reversible parkinsonism induced by hypercalcemia and primary hyperparathyroidism. Arch Intern Med 1993;153(9): 1134–6.
62. Tonner DR, Schlechte JA. Neurologic complications of thyroid and parathyroid disease. Med Clin North Am 1993;77(1):251–63.
63. Topakian R, Stieglbauer K, Rotaru J, et al. Hypocalcemic choreoathetosis and tetany after bisphosphonate treatment. Mov Disord 2006;21(11):2026–7.
64. Cheek JC, Riggs JE, Lilly RL. Extensive brain calcification and progressive dysarthria and dysphagia associated with chronic hypoparathyroidism. Arch Neurol 1990;47(9):1038–9.
65. Levin P, Kunin AS, Donaghy RM, et al. Intracranial calcification and hypoparathyroidism. Neurology 1961;11:1076–80.
66. Margolin D, Hammerstad J, Orwoll E, et al. Intracranial calcification in hyperparathyroidism associated with gait apraxia and parkinsonism. Neurology 1980;30(9):1005–7.
67. Chen TH, Huang CC, Chang YY, et al. Vasoconstriction as the etiology of hypercalcemia-induced seizures. Epilepsia 2004;45(5):551–4.
68. Kline CA, Esekogwu VI, Henderson SO, et al. Non-convulsive status epilepticus in a patient with hypocalcemia. J Emerg Med 1998;16(5):715–8.

69. Mrowka M, Knake S, Klinge H, et al. Hypocalcemic generalised seizures as a manifestation of iatrogenic hypoparathyroidism months to years after thyroid surgery. Epileptic Disord 2004;6(2):85–7.

70. Kossoff EH, Silvia MT, Maret A, et al. Neonatal hypocalcemic seizures: case report and literature review. J Child Neurol 2002;17(3):236–9.

71. Langley WF, Mann D. Central nervous system magnesium deficiency. Arch Intern Med 1991;151(3):593–6.

72. Shils ME. Experimental human magnesium depletion. I. Clinical observations and blood chemistry alterations. Am J Clin Nutr 1964;15:133–43.

73. Cevette MJ, Vormann J, Franz K. Magnesium and hearing. J Am Acad Audiol 2003;14(4):202–12.

74. Escalante CP, Weiser MA, Finkel K. Hyperphosphatemia associated with phosphorus-containing laxatives in a patient with chronic renal insufficiency. Southampt Med J 1997;90(2):240–2.

75. Hsu HJ, Wu MS. Extreme hyperphosphatemia and hypocalcemic coma associated with phosphate enema. Intern Med 2008;47(7):643–6.

76. Marraffa JM, Hui A, Stork CM. Severe hyperphosphatemia and hypocalcemia following the rectal administration of a phosphate-containing Fleet pediatric enema. Pediatr Emerg Care 2004;20(7):453–6.

77. Knochel JP. The pathophysiology and clinical characteristics of severe hypophosphatemia. Arch Intern Med 1977;137(2):203–20.

78. Knochel JP. Neuromuscular manifestations of electrolyte disorders. Am J Med 1982;72(3):521–35.

79. Chudley AE, Ninan A, Young GB. Neurologic signs and hypophosphatemia with total parenteral nutrition. Can Med Assoc J 1981;125(6):604–7.

80. Aubier M, Murciano D, Lecocguic Y, et al. Effect of hypophosphatemia on diaphragmatic contractility in patients with acute respiratory failure. N Engl J Med 1985;313(7):420–4.

81. Rie MA. Hypophosphatemia and diaphragmatic contractility. N Engl J Med 1986;314(8):519–20.

82. Kitabchi AE, Nyenwe EA. Hyperglycemic crises in diabetes mellitus: diabetic ketoacidosis and hyperglycemic hyperosmolar state. Endocrinol Metab Clin North Am 2006;35(4):725–51, viii.

83. Carroll P, Matz R. Uncontrolled diabetes mellitus in adults: experience in treating diabetic ketoacidosis and hyperosmolar nonketotic coma with low-dose insulin and a uniform treatment regimen. Diabetes Care 1983;6(6):579–85.

84. Umpierrez GE, Kelly JP, Navarrete JE, et al. Hyperglycemic crises in urban blacks. Arch Intern Med 1997;157(6):669–75.

85. Kitabchi AE, Wall BM. Diabetic ketoacidosis. Med Clin North Am 1995;79(1):9–37.

86. Chu K, Kang DW, Kim DE, et al. Diffusion-weighted and gradient echo magnetic resonance findings of hemichorea-hemiballismus associated with diabetic hyperglycemia: a hyperviscosity syndrome? Arch Neurol 2002;59(3):448–52.

87. Lai PH, Tien RD, Chang MH, et al. Chorea-ballismus with nonketotic hyperglycemia in primary diabetes mellitus. AJNR Am J Neuroradiol 1996;17(6):1057–64.

88. Raghavendra S, Ashalatha R, Thomas SV, et al. Focal neuronal loss, reversible subcortical focal T2 hypointensity in seizures with a nonketotic hyperglycemic hyperosmolar state. Neuroradiology 2007;49(4):299–305.

89. Singh BM, Strobos RJ. Epilepsia partialis continua associated with nonketotic hyperglycemia: clinical and biochemical profile of 21 patients. Ann Neurol 1980;8(2):155–60.
90. Arieff AI. Cerebral edema complicating nonketotic hyperosmolar coma. Miner Electrolyte Metab 1986;12(5–6):383–9.
91. Arieff AI, Kleeman CR. Studies on mechanisms of cerebral edema in diabetic comas. Effects of hyperglycemia and rapid lowering of plasma glucose in normal rabbits. J Clin Invest 1973;52(3):571–83.
92. Van der Meulen JA, Klip A, Grinstein S. Possible mechanism for cerebral oedema in diabetic ketoacidosis. Lancet 1987;2(8554):306–8.
93. Arieff AI, Kleeman CR. Studies on mechanisms of cerebral edema in diabetic comas: effects of hyperglycemia and rapid lowering of plasma glucose in normal rabbits (J Clin Invest 52:571–83, 1973). J Am Soc Nephrol 2000;11(9): 1776–88.
94. Pocecco M, Ronfani L. Transient focal neurologic deficits associated with hypoglycaemia in children with insulin-dependent diabetes mellitus. Italian Collaborative Paediatric Diabetologic Group. Acta Paediatr 1998;87(5):542–4.
95. Montgomery BM, Pinner CA. Transient hypoglycemic hemiplegia. Arch Intern Med 1964;114:680–4.
96. Malouf R, Brust JC. Hypoglycemia: causes, neurological manifestations, and outcome. Ann Neurol 1985;17(5):421–30.
97. Foster JW, Hart RG. Hypoglycemic hemiplegia: two cases and a clinical review. Stroke 1987;18(5):944–6.
98. Agardh CD, Rosen I, Ryding E. Persistent vegetative state with high cerebral blood flow following profound hypoglycemia. Ann Neurol 1983;14(4):482–6.
99. Tamburrano G, Lala A, Locuratolo N, et al. Electroencephalography and visually evoked potentials during moderate hypoglycemia. J Clin Endocrinol Metab 1988;66(6):1301–6.
100. Soltesz G, Acsadi G. Association between diabetes, severe hypoglycaemia, and electroencephalographic abnormalities. Arch Dis Child 1989;64(7):992–6.
101. Maruya J, Endoh H, Watanabe H, et al. Rapid improvement of diffusion-weighted imaging abnormalities after glucose infusion in hypoglycaemic coma. J Neurol Neurosurg Psychiatr 2007;78(1):102–3.
102. Lo L, Tan AC, Umapathi T, et al. Diffusion-weighted MR imaging in early diagnosis and prognosis of hypoglycemia. AJNR Am J Neuroradiol 2006;27(6): 1222–4.
103. Finelli PF. Diffusion-weighted MR in hypoglycemic coma. Neurology 2001;57(5): 933.
104. Bouillon R. Acute adrenal insufficiency. Endocrinol Metab Clin North Am 2006; 35(4):767–75, ix.
105. Calabrese LH, White CS. Musculoskeletal manifestations of Addison's disease. Arthritis Rheum 1979;22(5):558.
106. Abbas DH, Schlagenhauff RE, Strong HE. Polyradiculoneuropathy in Addison's disease. Case report and review of literature. Neurology 1977;27(5):494–5.
107. Mor F, Green P, Wysenbeek AJ. Myopathy in Addison's disease. Ann Rheum Dis 1987;46(1):81–3.
108. Bremer AA, Ranadive S, Conrad SC, et al. Isolated adrenocorticotropic hormone deficiency presenting as an acute neurologic emergency in a peripubertal girl. J Pediatr Endocrinol Metab 2008;21(8):799–803.
109. Arlt W, Allolio B. Adrenal insufficiency. Lancet 2003;361(9372):1881–93.

110. Shulman DI, Palmert MR, Kemp SF. Adrenal insufficiency: still a cause of morbidity and death in childhood. Pediatrics 2007;119(2):e484–94.
111. Devendra D, Walker A, MacFarlane IA, et al. Confusion after visiting the radiology department. Lancet 1997;350(9080):780.
112. Randeva HS, Schoebel J, Byrne J, et al. Classical pituitary apoplexy: clinical features, management and outcome. Clin Endocrinol (Oxf) 1999;51(2):181–8.
113. Noel NE, Ruthman JC. Pituitary apoplexy presenting as monocular blindness. Ann Emerg Med 1989;18(4):414–7.
114. Bonicki W, Kasperlik-Zaluska A, Koszewski W, et al. Pituitary apoplexy: endocrine, surgical and oncological emergency. Incidence, clinical course and treatment with reference to 799 cases of pituitary adenomas. Acta Neurochir (Wien) 1993;120(3–4):118–22.
115. Vidal E, Cevallos R, Vidal J, et al. Twelve cases of pituitary apoplexy. Arch Intern Med 1992;152(9):1893–9.
116. Wartofsky L. Myxedema coma. Endocrinol Metab Clin North Am 2006;35(4): 687–98, vii–viii.
117. Jansen HJ, Doebe SR, Louwerse ES, et al. Status epilepticus caused by a myxoedema coma. Neth J Med 2006;64(6):202–5.
118. Burch HB, Wartofsky L. Life-threatening thyrotoxicosis. Thyroid storm. Endocrinol Metab Clin North Am 1993;22(2):263–77.
119. Nayak B, Burman K. Thyrotoxicosis and thyroid storm. Endocrinol Metab Clin North Am 2006;35(4):663–86, vii.
120. Pandit L, Shankar SK, Gayathri N, et al. Acute thyrotoxic neuropathy—Basedow's paraplegia revisited. J Neurol Sci 1998;155(2):211–4.

Neurologic Presentations of Cardiac Disease

Roger E. Kelley, MD

KEYWORDS

• Syncope • Cardioembolic stroke • Cardiac arrest
• Atrial fibrillation • Valvular heart disease • Heart failure

Cardiac disease is intimately involved with neurologic disorders. The relationship between cardiac disease and embolic stroke (ie, cardioembolic stroke) is usually thought of as the primary relationship. Syncope, however, which is a not uncommon referral to the neurologist, is most likely on a cardiac basis. Furthermore, it is not unexpected that the neurologist be consulted for hypoxic encephalopathy when it follows cardiac arrest. Neurologists still have to keep the possibility of either infectious or marantic endocarditis in the differential diagnosis of patients presenting with cerebral embolus who are at particular risk including valvular heart disease, history of rheumatic fever, intravenous drug abuse, or malignancy. Cardiac rhythm disturbances are of particular importance in view of their ability to either promote severely impaired cardiac output or thromboembolism. Atrial fibrillation (AF) is increasingly more common as patients age, and risk stratification for this arrhythmia is a very important aspect of present management. Sick sinus syndrome can present with unexplained nonspecific neurologic symptoms, such as episodic lightheadedness with or without gait instability. The presentation often involves the vertebrobasilar circulation. Acute myocardial infarction (MI) can be complicated by stroke especially with large transmural wall anterior infarctions. There can be immediate cerebrovascular sequelae in up to 1% to 2% of patients or a more insidious process with development of mural wall thrombus and impaired ejection fraction (EF). Cardiac-related procedures are also an important aspect. Cardiac catheterization every so often prompts neurologic consultation for cardioembolic complication. Coronary artery bypass surgery is also a potential cause of cardioembolic complication and hypoperfusion, during the procedure, can lead to variable degrees of encephalopathy. There are also cardiac tumors to consider, with atrial myxoma the one that comes most frequently to mind. There is also the potential tie-in with illicit drug use. The drug abuser whose choice is a sympathomimetic agent, such as cocaine, can suffer cardiac consequences and

Department of Neurology, LSU Health Sciences Center-Shreveport, 1501 Kings Highway, Shreveport, LA 71103, USA
E-mail address: rkelly@lsuhsc.edu

Neurol Clin 28 (2010) 17–36
doi:10.1016/j.ncl.2009.09.014
0733-8619/09/$ – see front matter © 2010 Elsevier Inc. All rights reserved.
neurologic.theclinics.com

cerebrovascular complications related to impaired heart function. Neurologists are often called in to address effects of cardiac disease on the central nervous system.

SYNCOPE

This is sudden loss of consciousness, although the terminology is often obscured with the term "presyncope." There is often an overlap with "lightheadedness" or "dizziness" or "black-out spells." Despite the apparent nonspecificity of the presentation, the implications can be quite serious. It is very important to address the circumstance of the presentation. For example, this can be the initial manifestation of pregnancy and probably reflects altered body hemodynamics. Certain medications, especially certain antihypertensives and tizanidine, can result in a sudden precipitous drop in blood pressure, which can lead to cerebral hypoperfusion and syncope. In such an instance, the heart is probably not the primary determinant of the effect, but may well play some role. Orthostasis is a very common phenomenon and can be exacerbated by a number of medications including antihypertensives; tricyclic antidepressants; and medications prescribed for Parkinsonapos;s disease, such as levodopa, amantadine, and dopamine agonists.

Probably the most relevant cardiac explanation for syncope is the so-called "neurocardiogenic syncope," which was commonly attributed to "a vasovagal reaction" in the past. This was often the explanation for a "faint" during a wedding or a military march where the activity overstimulated the vagus nerve resulting in slowing of the heart to the point that the person passed out.

Box 1 outlines potential cardiac-related causes of syncope. Neurocardiogenic syncope, also known as "vasovagal," is viewed as having neurally mediated cerebral perfusion either through hypotension or bradycardia. This mechanism is also involved with carotid sinus stimulation and syncope associated with cough, micturition, swallowing, or defecation. Neurocardiogenic syncope can be set off in susceptible individuals by such activities as emotional excitement, overexertion, excessive heat exposure, or severe pain. Premonitory symptoms, reflecting presyncope, can include lightheadedness, sense of weakness, anxiety, diaphoresis, and headache.

Evaluation, outside of a careful history, including family history and examination, includes a standard 12-lead EKG. One is looking for rhythm disturbance, QT interval prolongation, bundle branch block, and possible evidence of ischemia.

Echocardiography to evaluate for possible valvular heart disease, especially if a heart murmur is detected, and possible severely impaired EF, as a possible

---

Box 1
Potential cardiac-related causes of syncope

1. Neurocardiogenic (vasovagal)
2. Atrial myxoma
3. Aortic stenosis
4. Cardiac asystole
5. Sick sinus syndrome
6. Ventricular flutter/fibrillation
7. Severely impaired cardiac EF
8. Cardiogenic cerebral embolus

explanation for cardiovascular collapse, is typically part of the work-up. Heart monitoring, either by inpatient EKG telemetry, 24-hour Holter monitoring, or more extended monitoring with a "capture" device, is often indicated in the patient presenting with unexplained syncope believed to be of cardiac origin.

The tilt-table test, which is associated with sudden change in body position, to assess for hypotension or bradycardia, with reproduction of symptoms, is viewed as the most reliable test for neurocardiogenic syncope.[1] If the symptoms persist, however, despite a negative or equivocal tilt study, then an implantable loop recorder of electrocardiographic information may be helpful. This device can store up to 45 minutes of retrospective recording and can be set to record automatically or can be activated by the patient to record the syncopal episode.[2]

Treatment of neurocardiogenic syncope can include avoidance of activities associated with its occurrence for a particular patient. Presyncopal symptoms should lead to a reclining position as effectively as possible. Methods to increase skeletal muscle tone with secondary improvement in venous tone have been proposed. This has been supported by a study in which susceptible patients had a significant elevation of mean systolic blood pressure with leg crossing combined with muscle tensing.[3]

Despite the lack of a Food and Drug Administration approved medication for neurocardiogenic syncope, β-blockers are commonly used with some degree of success.[4] They have been hypothesized to blunt left ventricular mechanoreceptor activation in an effort to block their contribution to withdrawal of sympathetic tone and suppression of the increase in the levels of epinephrine that can precede syncope. Although observational and uncontrolled studies have supported efficacy for β-blocker therapy in this disorder, this has not been reported in controlled trials.[5]

Other therapies reported to have some potential in preventing neurocardiogenic syncope include fludrocortisone,[6] the direct α_1-receptor antagonist midodrine,[7] and selective serotonin-reuptake inhibitors, which impact on regulation of sympathetic tone.[8] In intractable cases, implantation of a dual-chamber cardiac pacemaker may have some value in delaying the onset of syncope in the presyncope phase, which may allow greater protection against falling out.[9] Potential management approaches for neurocardiogenic syncope are summarized in **Box 2**.

From a neurologic perspective, there can be convulsive-type activity associated with neurocardiogenic syncope, which is important to sort out from a differential diagnosis standpoint and from a treatment perspective. Vertebrobasilar insufficiency can also result in syncope, but there are typically associated symptoms of posterior circulation involvement. In addition, one can see syncope as the aura of migraine or as part

---

Box 2
Potential preventive approaches to neurocardiogenic syncope

1. Avoidance of activities that precipitate events
2. Assumption of a reclining position during the presyncope phase
3. Muscle tension maneuvers to improve venous return and raise the blood pressure
4. β-blockers
5. Fludrocortisone acetate
6. Midodrine hydrochloride
7. Selective serotonin-reuptake inhibitors
8. Dual-chamber cardiac pacemaker implantation

of the clinical picture, which has been termed "complicated migraine" or vertebrobasilar migraine. Typically, in such a presentation there is a significant vascular-type headache, which is temporally related to the event.

INFECTIVE ENDOCARDITIS

It is always important to consider the possibility of infective endocarditis in the acute stroke patient with any of the following features: (1) fever, (2) new or changing cardiac murmur, (3) history of rheumatic fever or other explanations for valvular heart disease, (4) intravenous drug abuse, (5) HIV-1 infection, (6) patients with stroke and unexplained markedly elevated erythrocyte sedimentation rate, and (7) "shower" of cerebral emboli in different vascular territories with no obvious explanation. *Staphylococcus aureus* is the most common pathogen and accounts for roughly one third of cases with stroke as a complication in 16.9%.[10] Involvement of either the mitral valve or the aortic valve is the most common location for vegetations with fairly equivalent representation for these two valves, which account for roughly 80% of all cases.

Rapid assessment with blood cultures and echocardiographic evaluation for valvular vegetations remains the standard approach along with timely institution of the appropriate antibiotic, usually with empiric therapy until the blood culture results are available. Prognosis tends to be negatively impacted by any of the following: (1) prosthetic valve involvement, (2) increasing age, (3) pulmonary edema, (4) *S aureus* or coagulase-negative staphylococcal infection, (5) vegetations on the mitral valve, and (6) paravalvular complications.[10]

Despite a clinical presentation of cerebral embolus, septic emboli from infective endocarditis are not believed to be effectively and safely managed with anticoagulant therapy because of the reported risk of enhanced intracerebral bleeding as a complication.[11] The risks versus benefits might be of particular concern when there is a coexistent cardiac arrhythmia, such as AF. Despite the absence of a controlled clinical trial, observational studies warrant against full-dose anticoagulant therapy in such a clinical setting.

MARANTIC (NONBACTERIAL THROMBOTIC) ENDOCARDITIS

This disorder is characterized by platelet fibrin thrombi that are deposited most commonly on either the aortic or mitral valve and have been termed "verrucous vegetations." There is a clear association with hypercoagulable conditions and advanced malignancy. It often presents with arterial cerebral embolism. This risk of the disorder is roughly 1% of all cancer patients,[12] but it accounts for up to 20% to 30% of stroke in patients with cancer.[13,14] Characteristics of this uncommon disorder are listed in **Box 3**.

The identification of associated conditions, such as advanced malignancy or hypercoagulable condition, in a patient with stroke should lead to investigation for possible noninfectious valvular vegetations on the left side of the heart. The most sensitive study in this regard is transesophageal echocardiography (TEE), with one study reporting a yield of 18% in cancer patients with cerebral ischemia.[13] If such vegetations are detected in a stroke patient with negative blood cultures and no obvious associated condition then evaluation for occult malignancy or clotting disorder, such as disseminated intravascular coagulation, is indicated.[15] There is a tendency to use anticoagulant therapy in such a clinical setting, especially when there is clearly established thrombotic coagulopathy, although controlled clinical studies are lacking and there is concern over the potential for hemorrhagic complications.[16]

Box 3
Characteristics of marantic (nonbacterial thrombotic) endocarditis

1. Associated with sterile platelet-fibrin thrombi on heart valves

2. Most commonly affects the aortic and mitral valves

3. Associated with advanced malignancies and hypercoagulable states

4. Seen in approximately 1% of malignancies and most commonly associated with adenocarcinoma of either the pancreas, lungs, or stomach

5. Accounts for up to 20% to 30% of stroke in cancer patients

6. Often associated with other manifestations of hypercoagulation, such as venous thrombosis and disseminated intravascular coagulation

7. Transesophageal echocardiography is the most sensitive imaging device for detection of the verrucous vegetations on affected heart valves

8. Evaluation for malignancy or a hypercoagulable state is indicated when such vegetations are detected if such a condition has not already been found

9. Anticoagulant therapy may have some benefit for the associated hypercoagulable condition, but effective treatment of the underlying condition has the greatest potential for longer-lasting benefit

---

LIBMAN-SACKS ENDOCARDITIS

This is a verrucous valvulopathy associated with systemic lupus erythematosus. It is associated with disease duration; level of activity of the disease; and associated factors, such as thrombocytopenia, presence of anticardiolipin antibodies including antiphospholipid antibody syndrome, and thromboses including stroke.[17] It is reported that up to 10% of patients with systemic lupus erythematosus have such vegetations.[17] Because of the risk of thrombotic complications, it is recommended that the association of Libman-Sacks endocarditis and antiphospholipid antibodies be treated with anticoagulant therapy.[18]

PROSTHETIC HEART VALVES

Mechanical heart valve replacement is well recognized as a source for cardioembolic stroke. This risk translates into the general recommendation that all patients with mechanical heart valve replacement be placed on lifelong anticoagulant therapy. It is reported that stroke accounts for up to 70% to 90% of thromboembolic complications of such prosthetic heart valves.[19] In a recently reported prospective study of the etiology of stroke, however, in 89 subjects with mechanical heart valve replacement,[19] hemorrhagic strokes accounted for 77.5%, lacunar-type infarctions were seen in 8%, and embolic were seen in 17% with roughly half of the embolic group having their event attributed to carotid atherothrombotic disease. Furthermore, the stroke mechanisms observed did not correlate with the intensity of the oral anticoagulation.

Mechanical valves tend to be preferred over bioprosthetic heart valves for patients who will live longer and want to avoid valve reoperation. In a study of 73 children and adolescents under the age of 18 years with mechanical versus biologic prosthetic heart valves for rheumatic valvular heart disease,[20] the overall mortality rate over the 9 years of the study was 8.2%. For the 71 survivors (52 in the mechanical valve group and 19 in the bioprosthesis group), mortality rate was 3.8% for those with mechanical heart valves and 10.5% for those with bioprosthetic valves. The severe hemorrhage rate was 3.8% and the stroke rate was 5.8% in those with the mechanical valves. The reoperation rate was 3.8% for the mechanical heart valve group and 21% for the bioprosthetic group. The authors concluded that the bioprosthetic valves are an option when the risks of anticoagulation are substantial.

A major recently addressed issue has been the level of intensity of anticoagulant therapy in patients with mechanical heart valves. Dentali and colleagues[21] reported a low risk of subtherapeutic international normalization ratio (INR) with only one patient (0.3%) out of 254 studied over a 90-day observation period having a thromboembolic event. Akhtar and colleagues[22] reported that INR levels of 2 to 2.5 are generally acceptable for both risk of hemorrhage and thromboembolic events. In a study of low-intensity anticoagulation with the St Jude Medical valve,[23] patients were randomly assigned to INRs of 3 to 4.5, 2.5 to 4, and 2 to 3.5. Thromboembolism was observed less frequently with aortic valve replacement (0.53% per patient year) compared with mitral valve replacement (1.64% per patient year). Although the bleeding complication rate was reported at 24.8% per patient year, most were minor events (22.2% per patient year). Of particular note, bleeding complications and moderate and severe thromboembolic events were not significantly different in the three INR groups.

Antiplatelet therapy combined with an anticoagulant is a consideration in higher-risk patients for thromboembolic events especially those who are symptomatic on a dose of warfarin, which results in an acceptable INR. According to a 2003 Cochrane Review,[24] there is a benefit to the addition of either low-dose aspirin or dipyridamole to oral anticoagulation for protection against thromboembolism, but with an increased risk of bleeding complications. The efficacy and safety of lower-dose aspirin (100 mg/day) was similar to either higher-dose aspirin or dipyridamole.

A potentially serious complication of prosthetic heart valves is hemolysis. This is usually a complication of structural deterioration of the heart valve or paravalvular leak. Severe hemolysis is more effectively accomplished with surgical repair or replacement of the prosthetic valve, whereas less serious hemolysis may be amenable to pharmacologic agents, such as erythropoietin or pentoxifylline, or with endovascular closure of a paravalvular leak with devices, such as coils.[25]

ATRIAL MYXOMA

Myxomas are histologically benign cardiac tumors and comprise roughly one half of cardiac benign tumors. Most tend to be calcified and they are composed of spindle or stellate myxoma cells. Roughly 10% are hereditary and the most common location is the left atrium. They can arise from the ventricles. The potential manifestations are protean (**Box 4**). The classic triad of left atrial myxoma is (1) symptoms of mitral valve obstruction; (2) symptoms of embolism; and (3) constitutional symptoms, which can include fever, weight loss, and manifestations suggestive of a connective tissue disorder.[26] In one study, cardiac symptoms were the most prominent in 66.6% of 81 patients, with an age range of 1 month to 80 years, with cerebrovascular disease most prominent in 24.7%.[27] Right atrial myxomas are often associated with nonspecific constitutional symptoms, but can include syncope, pulmonary embolism with secondary pulmonary hypertension, secondary infection of the tumor, myocardial tamponade, and possible blocking of the atrioventricular ostium resulting in a Budd-Chiari syndrome with acute abdominal pain.[28] Imaging for detection is usually either transthoracic or transesopheal echocardiography. The nature and characteristics of the lesion can be better demonstrated with either CT or MRI scan.[29] The prognosis with surgical resection of the tumor tends to be excellent with a low recurrence rate

---

Box 4
Potential manifestations of atrial myxoma

1. Cardioembolic stroke

2. Syncope

3. Fever of unknown origin

4. Cardiac arrhythmia

5. Acute or chronic congestive heart failure

6. Heart murmur

7. Weight loss

8. Anemia

9. Elevated sedimentation rate

10. Elevated gamma globulin

11. Thrombocytopenia

12. Leukocystosis

---

of 5%.[26] An interesting example of a presentation of left atrial myxoma is seen in **Fig. 1.**

PATENT FORAMEN OVALE

A patent foramen ovale (PFO) is not an uncommon incidental finding in the general population. It is generally a benign anomaly, but it has the potential to serve as a conduit for a peripheral embolus to travel from the right side to left side of the heart and lead to embolic stroke often referred to as "paradoxical cerebral embolism." It has been particularly cited as a potential mechanism for stroke in the young. There is reported to be a modest increased risk of recurrent stroke in the young attributed to this mechanism.[30] Factors that may impact on risk of such a phenomenon include coexistent atrial septal aneurysm and size of the PFO, degree of shunting, and concomitant hypercoagulable state.[31] The presence of a peripheral thrombotic source, such as deep venous thrombosis of the leg, is expected to enhance the risk of a paradoxical embolus. Newer methods for detection of such a thromboembolic source, such as pelvic magnetic resonance venography and more sensitive methods for cardiac predisposition, such as aerated ultrasound contrast, TEE, and the potential for transcranial Doppler ultrasound to detect cerebral emboli, have the potential to significantly enhance diagnostic yield for such a mechanism.[30] Cumulative information collected as a Practice Parameter of the American Academy of Neurology in 2004[32] reported that among patients with cryptogenic stroke and PFO or atrial septal aneurysm, there was no significant difference in stroke or rate of death in patients treated with either warfarin or aspirin. They concluded that there was not an increased risk of subsequent stroke or death among medically treated PFO patients with cryptogenic stroke. They cited the possibility of an increased risk of subsequent stroke, but not death, however, in medically treated patients less than 55 years of age. They were unable to determine, at least at this time, whether PFO closure with interventional techniques was of any benefit. Alsheikh-Ali and colleagues,[33] based on a review of 23 case-control studies of cryptogenic stroke with or without coexistent PFO, reported that PFO was likely incidental in roughly one third of patients. At least in this subgroup, they did not believe that PFO is beneficial.

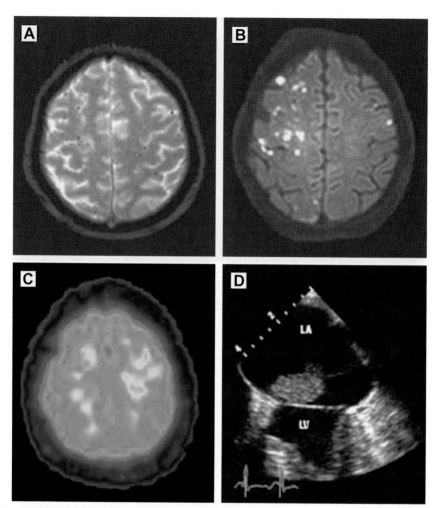

Fig. 1. MRIs, distribution volume ratio image of positron emission tomography, and an echocardiogram. Gradient-echo MRI shows numerous microhemorrhages in the fronto-occipital lobes and basal ganglia (*A*), some of which are diffusion restricted (*B*). (*C*) Distribution volume ratio images of carbon 11-labeled Pittsburgh Compound B positron emission tomography exclude an increase ß-amyloid burden. (*D*) An echocardiogram reveals left atrial myxoma. LA, left atrium; LV, left ventricle. (*From* Vanacker P, Nelissen N, Van Laere K, et al. Scattered cerebral microbleeds due to cardiac myxoma. Arch Neurol 2009;66:796; with permission. Copyright © 2009 American Medical Association. All rights reserved.)

There is also literature to suggest a relationship between PFO and migraine with aura.[34] It is theorized that right-to-left cardiac shunting might play a role in the mechanism. The literature has been somewhat conflicting, however, with some studies suggesting a potential benefit of PFO closure[35] and other studies reporting no benefit.[36] Vigna and colleagues[35] reported an improvement in migraineurs with a large PFO and subclinical brain lesions who underwent PFO closure. The prospective, randomized, double-blind MIST trial,[36] however, despite confirming the high prevalence of right-to-left shunts in migraine patients with aura, found no significant benefit to PFO closure when compared with sham procedure controls.

CORONARY ISCHEMIA

It is well recognized that acute MI can be complicated by embolic stroke.[37,38] Factors associated with such a phenomenon include transmural anterior wall infarction with or without mural wall thrombus formation.[39,40] Coexistent factors, such as heart failure or AF, can enhance the risk of stroke.[41] There is an interplay among contributing factors. For example, impairment of left ventricular systolic function can lead to impaired left atrial function, development of left atrial filling associated with left atrial appendage thrombus formation, and subsequent development of AF.[42,43]

In terms of risk stratification for stroke in patients with documented coronary artery disease, left ventricular hypertrophy[44] and left ventricular diastolic dysfunction[45] are associated with enhanced risk of stroke, whereas a left atrial diameter greater than 40 mm in nonvalvular AF (NVAF)[46] and mitral regurgitation may be protective.[47] In a recent study of non–ST elevation acute coronary syndromes,[48] patient low-risk stratification included absence of ST deviation and absence of other risk factors, and this correlated with freedom from vascular events including stroke. In a study of a low-molecular-weight heparin in acute MI presenting with ST-segment elevation or new left bundle branch block,[49] there was a significant reduction in 30-day mortality compared with placebo. The 30-day risk of stroke was 0.8% in the heparinoid group and 1% in the placebo group, which provides a reasonable estimate of risk of stroke complicating acute MI with modern day interventional therapy.

CHRONIC HEART FAILURE

There is a relationship between impaired cardiac EF and cardioembolic events. EF is the proportion of left ventricular volume emptied during systole. EF reflects left ventricular systolic function and can be noninvasively assessed with echocardiography. Typically, a normal EF is 50% to 70%. Heart failure is characterized by reduced cardiac output and elevated left ventricular filling pressure.[50] A reduced EF does not strictly correlate with risk of heart failure because one can see a normal EF in certain patients with heart failure related to impairment of left ventricular diastolic relaxation secondary to hypertrophic cardiomyopathy. In terms of cardiomyopathy, one can see either dilated cardiomyopathy, in which the diastolic dimension of the left ventricle is enlarged, or hypertrophic when the left ventricular wall thickness is increased. Ischemic cardiomyopathy typically corresponds to the patient having long-standing, often poorly controlled, risk factors for ischemia, such as diabetes mellitus, hypertension, smoking, and those genetically prone to atherosclerosis. Nonischemic cardiomyopathy can be related to metabolic myocardial cell structure disturbance, seen in certain genetic disorders, and related to toxin exposure or viral-induced.[51]

It is well established that certain agents can prolong survival in heart failure despite apparent divergent effects on reduced cardiac output and elevated left ventricular filling pressure. For example, β-blockers have the potential to initially worsen the symptoms of heart failure, but are associated with longer-term survival.[52] Vasodilators have the potential to positively affect hemodynamic mechanisms and improve congestion in heart failure, with the most marked response, in terms of survival, being with either angiotensin-converting enzyme inhibitors[53] or angiotensin-receptor blockers.[54] The fixed dose combination of isosorbide dinitrate–hydralazine is associated with a vasodilatory effect and enhancement of nitric oxide bioavailability and has translated into a 37% improvement in event-free survival and a 39% reduced risk of first hospitalization in the African-American Heart Failure Trial.[50]

The risk of cardioembolism in heart failure is typically cumulative in nature. For example, the coexistence of NVAF with either moderately or severely impaired left ventricular systolic function or heart failure identifies patients who are in a higher-risk category of cardioembolism and who would be most likely to benefit from long-term anticoagulant therapy.[55] The major issue still unresolved, however, is the optimal treatment for patients with an EF less than 35% without coexistent cardiac arrthymia. In the WASH trial of warfarin versus aspirin therapy versus placebo in patients with chronic heart failure,[56] there was no difference in the primary outcome of death, nonfatal MI, or nonfatal stroke between the three arms of the study. Significantly more of the patients assigned to aspirin were hospitalized for cardiovascular reasons, however, especially worsening of their heart failure.

The Warfarin and Antiplatelet Therapy in Chronic Heart Failure trial had an open-label warfarin arm, with a target INR of 2.5 to 3, versus double-blind aspirin (162 mg/day) or clopidogrel (75 mg/day).[57] The study was based on patients with symptomatic heart failure of at least 3 months, a left ventricular EF of less than or equal to 35%, who were in normal sinus rhythm. The primary end points were first occurrence of death, nonfatal MI, or nonfatal stroke. Warfarin was associated with fewer nonfatal strokes than either aspirin or clopidogrel. Hospitalization for worsening heart failure occurred in 22.2% treated with aspirin, 18.5% treated with clopidogrel, and 16.5% for warfarin (*P* value 0.02 warfarin over aspirin). The authors concluded that there was not a clear superiority of warfarin over either aspirin or clopidogrel in the primary outcome measures. Protection against decompensation of heart failure, however, is quite possible. Despite the post hoc analysis of the Studies of Left Ventricular Dysfunction trial,[58] which demonstrated morbidity and mortality rates with warfarin, more recent studies have indicated a potential benefit in terms of protection against heart failure decompensation, but not necessarily cardioembolism. It is hoped that the Warfarin Versus Aspirin in Reduced Cardiac Ejection Fraction study will be more definitive in resolving these somewhat conflicting reports.[51]

Another aspect of congestive heart failure (CHF) is the potential effect on cognition. There is reported to be a prominent correlation between CHF and cognitive disturbance.[59] Some reports cite the relationship between cerebral hypoperfusion and impaired cerebral reactivity with specific areas of deficit in the cognitive domain, such as attention and verbal memory. In one study,[60] cognitive impairment was found in 26% of patients with heart failure. Specifically, systolic hypotension was associated with clinically significant impaired cognition in elderly patients with CHF. The degree of deficit tends to correlate with the severity of the heart failure based on studies of patients eligible for heart transplantation.[61,62] It has been theorized, however, that at least some of the cognitive impairment in CHF is related to cardioembolic disease[63] in view of the not uncommon association of ventricular thrombus formation seen in roughly 12% of patients with cardiomyopathy.[64] Features of heart failure are summarized in **Box 5**.

NVAF

AF affects up to 1% of the population with an increasing prevalence with age with up to 10% of persons 80 years of age or older having AF.[65] The risk of stroke with AF is very much reflective of coexistent disease and the patient's age. For example, patients less than 65 years or age with a structurally normal heart and no risk factors, such as hypertension, diabetes mellitus, or prior embolism, have a stroke risk similar to an age-matched control without AF. This has been termed "lone atrial fibrillation." AF in combination with rheumatic valvular heart disease, however, is associated with up to a 17-fold increased risk of cardioembolic events. In a systemic review of independent predictors of stroke in AF,[66] the most consistent independent risk factors were

---

Box 5
Features of chronic heart failure

1. Characterized by reduced cardiac output and elevated left ventricular filling

2. Can be associated with a dilated cardiomyopathy, in which the diastolic dimension of the left ventricle is enlarged or hypertrophic where the left ventricular wall thickness is increased

3. Ischemic cardiomyopathy is often associated with risk factors for ischemia, such as hypertension, diabetes mellitus, and so forth

4. Nonischemic cardiomyopathy can be associated with metabolic disturbance and toxic or viral exposure

5. Survival in heart failure can be prolonged with either angiotension-converting enzyme inhibitors, angiotensin-receptor blockers, β-blockers, or the combination of isosorbide dinitrate–hydralazine

6. There is a clear relationship between the degree of heart failure and cognitive impairment with potential mechanisms including cardioembolic stroke and cerebral hypoperfusion

---

prior stroke or transient ischemic attack (TIA), advancing age, hypertension, and diabetes. The most reliable risk factor, conferring a stroke risk of approximately 10% per year, was prior stroke or TIA.

Other risk factors cited have included heart failure or significant left ventricular systolic dysfunction by echocardiography. This is more of a relative issue, however, and is dependent on the impaired level of the EF and whether or not there is associated left ventricular thrombus formation. There has also been some information identifying female gender and age greater than 75 years as enhancing the risk of stroke with AF. Coronary artery disease and AF that is paroxysmal, however, have not been identified as particularly important contributors to higher risk stratification in AF. Risk stratification is very important in terms of the decision about whether to initiate long-term anticoagulation versus antiplatelet therapy, usually with aspirin, in patients at higher risk of stroke with AF (**Box 6**).

With recognition that duration and severity of associated risk factors most likely play a role in the level of contribution to the risk.

In the Practice Parameter of the American Academy of Neurology,[67] published in 1998, three categories were identified: (1) high-risk with a stroke risk with aspirin of approximately 8% or greater per year, (2) moderate-risk with a stroke rate of approximately 3.5% per year with aspirin, and (3) low-risk with a stroke rate of approximately 1% per year with aspirin. Higher-risk patients are those with hypertension, diabetes mellitus, and coronary artery disease, but as mentioned previously, cumulative information raises questions about the contribution of coronary artery disease. Furthermore, when citing either hypertension or diabetes mellitus as contributing factors to risk, one should also include duration and level of control. They cite an EF less than or equal to 25% and recent decompensation of CHF and the recognized prior stroke or TIA to help identify higher risk. Mention is also made of women greater than 75 years of age. Moderate risk includes age greater than or equal to 65 years with either no higher-risk features or with a history of hypertension. Low risk is lone AF in patients less than 65 years of age. Higher-risk patients should be assigned to warfarin therapy with an INR range of 2 to 3 and INR target of around 2.5 being perhaps optimal for younger higher-risk patients and closer to 2 for patients greater than 75 years of age because of the enhanced risk of bleeding complications.

Box 6
Risk Stratification for NVAF

Low risk of stroke (roughly 1% risk per year of stroke without therapy)

Age <65 years with structurally normal heart

No other risk factors for stroke

Moderate risk of stroke (roughly 2% risk per year of stroke without therapy)

Patients ≥65 years of age with no high-risk coexistent disease

High risk (roughly 6% or greater per year risk of stroke without therapy)

History of hypertension

History of diabetes mellitus

Prior embolic event or TIA

Women >75 years of age

Recent, less than 3 months, decompensation of CHF or cardiac EF ≤25% or presence of mural wall thrombus

Data from Report of the Quality Standards Subcommittee of the American Academy of Neurology. Practice parameter: stroke prevention in patients with nonvalvular atrial fibrillation. Neurology 1998;51:671–3.

Some have advocated an INR range of 1.5 to 2.1 for older patients at considerable risk for bleeding complications.[68] Hylek and colleagues,[69] however, reported a greater risk of stroke and a greater severity and increased risk of death from stroke with an INR less than 2 in a study of 13,559 patients with NVAF treated either with warfarin, aspirin, or untreated. In a meta-analysis of oral anticoagulants versus aspirin in NVAF,[70] the authors reported that treating 1000 patients with AF with oral anticoagulant instead of aspirin, for 1 year, prevents 23 ischemic strokes, but causes nine additional major bleeds. In an updated meta-analysis,[71] the relative risk reduction for stroke in NVAF was 64% with vitamin K antagonists and 22% with antiplatelet therapy. This reinforces the selection process as recently outlined by American College of Chest Physicians Evidence-Based Clinical Practice Guidelines for Antithrombotic Therapy in Atrial Fibrillation.[55] They recommend aspirin at a dose of 75 to 325 mg per day for patients less than or equal to 75 years of age with NVAF, but no other risk factors. With higher-risk patients, warfarin is generally recommended both for AF and atrial flutter as long as the risk of bleeding is judged acceptable on clinical grounds.

Combination therapy, either combining an oral anticoagulant with an antiplatelet agent, or combining two antiplatelet agents, has also been addressed to some degree. In the Stroke Prevention in Atrial Fibrillation III study,[72] which looked at the combination of low-intensity fixed-dose warfarin (mean INR, 1.3) plus 325 mg of aspirin per day versus adjusted dose warfarin with a mean INR of 2.4. This study did not find that the combination of low-intensity warfarin with aspirin provided adequate stroke prevention in patients with NVAF who were at higher risk for thromboembolism. It is recognized, however, that some AF patients have symptoms of stroke while taking warfarin with the INR in a desirable range or who are believed have a need for both warfarin and an antiplatelet agent for coronary artery disease. Shireman and colleagues[73] looked at such a combination in elderly patients with AF. They reported that antiplatelet agents increased major bleeding rates from 1.3% to 1.9% with factors associated with an enhanced risk of bleeding in the multivariate analysis reported to be age, anemia, and history of bleeding along with concurrent therapy. In a randomized study of clopidogrel or placebo added to aspirin at 75 to 100 mg a day for patients with AF who were not believed to be suitable for anticoagulant therapy,[74] the risk of stroke was 2.4% per year in the clopidogrel group compared with 3.3% per year with placebo. This was a relative risk reduction of 0.72 (P <0.001). There was a trade off, however, because major bleeding was 2% per year in patients receiving clopidogrel and 1.3% per year in patients receiving placebo (relative risk, 1.57; P <0.001). Careful patient selection for such an approach is mandatory.

MANAGEMENT OF ACUTE CARDIOEMBOLIC STROKE

It is now fairly well recognized that heparin or heparinoid therapy in acute stroke has little effect on outcome, but there is some role for subcutaneous therapy to protect against the development of deep venous thrombosis for patients who are immobilized by the nature of their presentation.[75] In patients with an ongoing cardiogenic source of embolism, the major concern is the potential for recurrent thromboembolism. This tends to be reflective of the risk stratification of the underlying cardiogenic process. For example, few would argue with consideration of acute anticoagulant therapy in a patient presenting with a TIA who has valvular AF and a negative CT brain scan. Some have advocated the use of unfractionated intravenous heparin for patients with acute ischemic stroke who have "high risk" for early recurrent ischemic events, such as patients with AF or those with acute MI associated with large mural thrombi,[76] but such an approach has been questioned based on review of individual studies that have tried to address this issue.[77]

Camerlingo and colleagues[78] re-evaluated the use of intravenous heparin within the first 3 hours of presentation of acute nonlacunar hemispheric cerebral infarction. They reported better recovery and fewer deaths in the treated group versus placebo, but more symptomatic brain hemorrhages. They attributed their positive results to the relatively high percentage of cardioembolic infarcts in their study, and the cited tendency for a more aggressive dose of anticoagulant therapy to have a beneficial effect on outcome.[69] In a study of the low-molecular-weight heparin tinzaparin, Bath and colleagues[79] tested this agent versus 300 mg of aspirin per day with treatment started within 48 hours of onset of acute ischemic stroke and continued for 10 days. No benefit was observed even with those patients with a presumptive cardioembolic mechanism. In another study of low-molecular heparin versus aspirin in patients who had acute ischemic stroke and AF,[80] no benefit was seen with one therapy over the other. Acute treatment of acute cardioembolic (ischemic) stroke with intravenous unfractionated heparin, low-molecular-weight-heparin, and heparinoids have not been consistently found to be beneficial. Intravenous recombinant tissue plasminogen activator is an accepted choice for patients presenting, and capable of being evaluated, within 3 hours of onset. Such an approach is not necessarily dependent on the ischemic stroke mechanism as long as the patient's degree of neurologic deficit and acknowledgement of the potential risks and exclusion of well-recognized contraindications makes this a plausible choice.

Sooner or later, anticoagulant therapy needs to be considered for the patient presenting with acute cardioembolic stroke if there is an ongoing cardiogenic source of embolism. The major concern, in terms of timing, is the potential for hemorrhagic transformation of the infarction (**Fig. 2**), which can occur spontaneously in up to 30% of patients by serial CT brain scan.[81] This can be exacerbated by full-dose intravenous heparin, especially if there is an initial bolus of heparin. With a presentation of a high-risk patient for recurrent cerebral embolism, with minor or resolved neurologic deficit on serial examination, and little or no manifestations of early infarction by CT

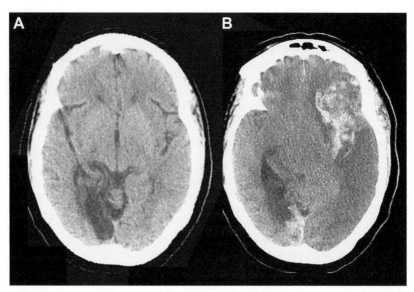

Fig. 2. Noncontrast CT brain scan within 1 hour of acute onset of aphasia and right-sided weakness (*A*), which demonstrates an old right posterior cerebral artery territory infarct, and 24 hours later, after thrombolytic therapy (*B*), demonstrating dramatic hemorrhage transformation of the cerebral infarct.

brain scan, intravenous heparin remains a reasonable choice for protection against further embolic cerebral infarction. For patients with moderate or greater neurologic deficits, and a clear infarction pattern on initial CT brain scan, however, it is generally prudent to defer intravenous anticoagulant therapy for at least up to several days. Assuming the patient is stable, one can repeat the noncontrast CT brain scan and, if there is no evidence of hemorrhagic transformation, then judicious initiation of intravenous heparin with avoidance of a bolus and a too prolonged partial thromboplastin time is a reasonable approach. Factors that tend to be associated with hemorrhagic transformation include the size of the infarct, advancing age, and elevated blood pressure.

In a recent study of anticoagulation after cardioembolic stroke,[82] a bimodal pattern of hemorrhagic transformation was observed with an early, generally benign transformation according to the report, and a later transformation that tended to be symptomatic. Of interest, in this study they found that bridging of anticoagulant therapy with either intravenous heparin or full-dose enoxaparin, a low-molecular-weight heparin, was associated with an enhanced risk of hemorrhagic transformation compared with early initiation of warfarin alone. Of particular importance, the risk of recurrent stroke was quite low, as has been reported in other studies, and only affected 2 (1%) of their 204 patients. This low recurrence rate was not affected by anticoagulant therapy and underscores that there seems to be little need for immediate anticoagulant therapy in most patients with cardioembolic stroke.

Once one commits to the use of anticoagulant therapy for protection against recurrent cardiogenic cerebral embolism, it is generally a good idea to avoid further brain imaging unless warranted by a change in the patient's neurologic status. Despite the established benefit of anticoagulant therapy for prevention of recurrent cerebral embolism with a cardiogenic source, there can be a sense of unease that develops when a follow-up CT brain scan, or more likely an MRI brain scan, indicates some degree of hemorrhagic transformation that is not at all unexpected and is probably of very questionable clinical significance unless indicated by the clinical picture.

SUMMARY

Cardiac evaluation as part of the assessment of neurologic presentations is very much reflective of the diligence in the pursuit of the mechanism. For example, syncope is potentially a very devastating symptom. It can result in head trauma, motor vehicle accidents, and drowning. It restricts driving and other aspects of employability and quality of life. The expeditious determination of the explanation, and how to prevent recurrence, is of utmost importance. Similarly, rapid evaluation of a possible cardiogenic source of cerebral embolus can have a great impact on management and can make a big difference in terms of outcome. Newer and more aggressive techniques as part of the evaluation process can enhance the diagnostic yield. Detection of a cardiac arrhythmia, which can be paroxysmal, such as sick sinus syndrome or AF, can be enhanced by so-called "capture" cardiac monitoring over a more prolonged period of time as opposed to the traditional 24-hour Holter monitor or shorter term EKG telemetry while hospitalized. In a study of Mobile Cardiac Outpatient Telemetry for up to 21 days in 56 patients with either cryptogenic stroke or TIA,[83] the detection rate of AF was 23%. In terms of enhanced heart imaging, Hur and colleagues[84] reported on the diagnostic yield of two-phase 64-slice cardiac tomographic angiography for the detection of potential sources of cardiogenic embolism in stroke patients. For the 137 patients studied, TEE detected a total of 47 high-risk sources, whereas cardiac tomographic angiography detected 44 lesions. The yield was actually better for TEE, although the less invasive nature of cardiac tomographic angiography may provide some usefulness. This illustrates that the detection and management of cardioembolic disease remains an evolutionary process. In this regard, the WATCHMAN device[85] is designed to occlude the left atrial appendage to prevent migration of in situ thrombi in patients with AF. Based on a recent study that demonstrated that this device was noninferior to warfarin for stroke prevention in AF, this device could soon become an option for patients.

REFERENCES

1. Grubb BP, Kosinski D. Tilt table testing: concepts and limitations. Pacing Clin Electrophysiol 1997;20:781–7.
2. Krahn AD, Klein GJ, Yee R, et al. Randomized assessment of syncope trial: conventional testing versus prolonged monitoring strategy. Circulation 2001;104:45–61.
3. Kredict CT, van Dijk N, Linzer M, et al. Management of vasovagal syncope: controlling or aborting faints by leg crossing and muscle tensing. Circulation 2002;106:1684–9.
4. Brignole M. Randomized clinical trials of neurally mediated syncope. J Cardiovasc Electophysiol 2003;14(Suppl):S64–9.
5. Grubb BP. Neurocardiogenic syncope. N Engl J Med 2005;352:1004–10.
6. Scott WA, Pangiglion G, Bromberg BI, et al. Randomized comparison of atenolol and fludrocortisone acetate in the treatment of pediatric neurally mediated syncope. Am J Cardiol 1995;76:400–2.
7. Ward CR, Gray JC, Gilroy JJ, et al. Midodrine: a role in the management of neurocardiogenic syncope. Heart 1988;79:45–9.
8. Di Girolamo E,, Di Iorio C, Sabatini P, et al. Effects of paroxetine hydrochloride, a selective serotonin reuptake inhibitor, on refractory vasovagal

syncope: a randomized, double-blind, placebo-controlled study. J Am Coll Cardiol 1999;33:1227–30.

9. Sutton R. Has cardiac pacing a role in vasovagal syncope? J Interv Card Electrophysiol 2003;9:145–9.

10. Murdoch DR, Corey GR, Hoen B, et al. Clinical presentation, etiology, and outcome of infective endocarditis in the 21st century: the International Collaboration on Endocarditis-Prospective Cohort Study. Arch Intern Med 2009;169(5):463–73.

11. Hart RG, Kagan-Hallet K, Joerns SE. Mechanisms of intracranial hemorrhage in infective endocarditis. Stroke 1987;18:1048–56.

12. Lopez JA, Ross RS, Fishbein MC, et al. Nonbacterial thrombotic endocarditis: a review. Am Heart J 1987;113(3):773–8.

13. Macdonnell RA, Kalnis RM, Donnan GA. Non-bacterial thrombotic endocarditis and stroke. Clin Exp Neurol 1986;22:123–32.

14. Dutta T, Karas MG, Segal AZ, et al. Yield of transesophageal echocardiography for nonbacterial thrombotic endocarditis and other cardiac sources of embolism in cancer patients with cerebral ischemia. Am J Cardiol 2006;97(6):894–8.

15. Graus F, Rogers JB. Cerebrovascular complications in patients with cancer. Medicine (Baltimore) 1985;64(1):16–35.

16. Rogers LR. Cerebrovascular complications in cancer patients. Neurol Clin 2003; 21(1):167–92.

17. Moyssakis I, Tektonidou MG, Vasilliou VA, et al. Libman-Sacks endocarditis in systemic lupus erythematosus: prevalence, associations, and evolution. Am J Med 2007;120(7):636–42.

18. Lonnebakken MT, Gerdts E. Libman-Sacks endocarditis and cerebral embolization in antiphospholipid antibody syndrome. Eur J Echocardiogr 2008;9(1):192–3.

19. Piper C, Hering D, Langer C, et al. Etiology of stroke after mechanical heart valve replacement: results from a ten-year prospective study. J Heart Valve Dis 2008; 17(4):413–7.

20. Travancas PR, Dorigo AH, Simoes LC, et al. Comparison of mechanical and biological prostheses when used to replace heart valves in children and adolescents with rheumatic fever. Cardiol Young 2009;19(2):192–7.

21. Dentali F, Riva N, Malato A, et al. Incidence of thromboembolic complications in patients with mechanical heart valves with a subtherapeutic international normalization ratio. J Thorac Cardiovasc Surg 2009;137(1):91–3.

22. Akhtar RP, Abid AR, Zafar H, et al. Anticoagulation in patients following prosthetic heart valve replacement. Ann Thorac Cardiovasc Surg 2009;15(1):10–7.

23. Hering D, Piper C, Bergemann R, et al. Thromboembolic and bleeding complications following St. Jude Medical valve replacement: results of the German Experience with Low-Intensity Anticoagulation Study. Chest 2005; 127(1):53–9.

24. Little SH, Massel DR. Antiplatelet and anticoagulation for patients with prosthetic heart valves. Cochrane Database Syst Rev 2003;(4):CD003464.

25. Shapira Y, Vaturi M, Sagie A. Hemolysis associated with prosthetic heart valves: a review. Cardiol Rev 2009;17(3):121–4.

26. Pineda L, Duhaut P, Loire R. Clinical presentation of left atrial cardiac myxoma: a series of 112 consecutive cases. Medicine (Baltimore) 2001;80(3):159–72.

27. Jelic J, Milicic D,, Alfirevic I, et al. Cardiac myxoma: diagnostic approach, surgical treatment and follow-up: a twenty years experience. J Cardiovasc Surg 1996;37(6 Suppl 1):113–7.

28. Kuon E, Kreplin M, Weiss W, et al. The challenge presented by right atrial myxoma. Herz 2004;29(7):702–9.

29. Grebenc ML, Rosado-de-Christenson ML, Green CE, et al. Cardiac myxoma: imaging features in 83 patients. Radiographics 2002;22(3):673–89.
30. Saver JL. Cryptogenic stroke in patients with patent foramen ovale. Curr Atheroscler Rep 2007;9(4):319–25.
31. Thaler DE, Saver JL. Cryptogenic stroke and patent foramen ovale. Curr Opin Cardiol 2008;23(6):537–44.
32. Messe SR, Sliverman IE, Kizer Homma S, et al. Quality Standards Subcommittee of the American Academy of Neurology. Practice parameter: recurrent stroke with patent foramen ovale and atrial septal aneurysm: report of the Quality Standards Subcommittee of the American Academy of Neurology. Neurology 2004;62(7): 1042–50.
33. Alsheikh-Ali AA, Thaler DE, Kent DM. Patent foramen ovale in cryptogenic stroke. Incidental or Pathogenic? Stroke 2009;40:2289–93.
34. Tepper SJ, Cleves C, Taylor FR. Patent foramen ovale and migraine: association, causation, and implications of clinical trials. Curr Pain Headache Rep 2009;13(3): 221–6.
35. Vigna C, Marchese N, Inchingolo V, et al. Improvement of migraine after patent foramen ovale percutaneous closure in patients with subclinical brain lesions: a case-control study. JACC Cardiovasc Interv 2009;2(2):107–13.
36. Dowson A, Mullen MJ, Peatfield R, et al. Migraine intervention with STARFlex Technology (MIST) trial. A prospective, multicenter, double-blind, sham-controlled trial to evaluate the effectiveness of patent foramen ovale closure with STARFlex septal repair implant to resolve refractory migraine headache. Circulation 2008;117:1397–404.
37. Maggioni AP, Franzosi MG, Santoro E, et al. The risk of stroke in patients with acute myocardial infarction after thrombolytic therapy and antithrombotic treatment. N Engl J Med 1992;327:1–6.
38. Kannel WB, Wolf PA, Verter J. Manifestations of coronary artery disease predisposing to stroke. The Framingham Study. JAMA 1983;250:2942–6.
39. Loh E, Sutton MS, Wun CC, et al. Ventricular dysfunction and the risk of stroke after myocardial infarction. N Engl J Med 1997;336:251–7.
40. Cerebral Embolism Task Force. Cardiogenic brain embolism. Arch Neurol 1986; 43:71–84.
41. Palmiero P, Maiello M, Passantino A. Coronary artery disease, left ventricular hypertrophy and diastolic dysfunction are associated with stroke in patients affected by persistent non-valvular atrial fibrillation: a case-control study. Int Heart J 2009;3:4–7.
42. Okura H, Inoue H, Tomon M, et al. Is the left atrium the only embolic source in ischemic stroke patients with atrial fibrillation? Am J Cardiol 1999;84: 1259–61.
43. Cemri M, Timurkaynak T, Ozdemir M, et al. Effects of left ventricular systolic dysfunction on left atrial appendage and left atrial functions in patients with chronic atrial fibrillation. Acta Cardiol 2002;57:101–5.
44. Dahlo FB, Devereux RB, Kjeldsen SE, et al. Cardiovascular morbidity and mortality in the Losartan Intervention For Endpoint reduction in hypertension study (LIFE): a randomized trial against atenolol. Lancet 2002;359:995–1003.
45. Poulsen SH. Clinical aspects of left ventricular diastolic function assessed by Doppler echocardiography following acute myocardial infarction. Dan Med Bull 2001;48(4):199–210.
46. Labovitz AJ, Bransford TL. Evolving role of echocardiography in the management of atrial fibrillation. Am Heart J 2001;141:518–27.

47. Diwan A, McCulloch M, Lawrie GM, et al. Doppler estimation of left ventricular filling pressures in patients with mitral valve disease. Circulation 2005;111:3281–9.
48. Brieger D, Fox KA, Fitzgerald G, et al. Predicting freedom from clinical events in non-ST-elevation acute coronary syndromes. The Global Registry of Acute Coronary Events. Heart 2009;95(11):888–94.
49. The CREATE Trial Group Investigators. Effects of reviparin, a low molecular-weight heparin on mortality, reinfarction and strokes in patients with acute myocardial infarction presenting with ST-segment elevation. JAMA 2005;293:427–36.
50. Taylor AE, Ziesche S, Yancey CW, et al, on behalf of the African-American Heart Failure Study. Early and sustained benefit of event-free survival and heart failure hospitalization from fixed-dose combination of isorbide dinitrate/hydrazaline. Circulation 2007;115:1747–53.
51. Pullicino PM, Halperin JL, Thompson JLP. Stroke in patients with heart failure and reduced left ventricular ejection fraction. Neurology 2000;54:288–94.
52. Packer M, Coats AJS, Fowler M, et al. Effect of carvedilol on survival in severe chronic heart failure. N Engl J Med 2001;344:1651–8.
53. Garg R, Yusuf S, for the Collaborative Group on ACE Inhibitor Trials. Overview of randomized trials of angiotensin-converting enzyme inhibitors on mortality and morbidity in patients with heart failure. JAMA 1995;273:1450–6.
54. Cohn JN, Tognoni, for the Valsartan Heart Failure Trial Investigators G. A randomized trial of the angiotensin-receptor blocker valsartan in chronic heart failure. N Engl J Med 2001;345:1667–75.
55. Singer DE, Albers GW, Dalen JE, et al. Antithrombotic therapy in atrial fibrillation. American College of Chest Physicians Evidence-Based Clinical Practice Guidelines. Chest 2008;133(Suppl 6):593S–629S.
56. Cleland JG, Findlay I, Jafri S, et al. The Warfarin/Aspirin Study in Heart failure (WASH): a randomized trial comparing antithrombotic strategies for patients with heart failure. Am Heart J 2004;148(1):157–64.
57. Massie BM, Collins JF, Ammon SE, et al. Randomized trial of warfarin, aspirin, and clopidogrel in patients with chronic heart failure. The Warfarin and Antiplatelet Therapy in Chronic Heart Failure (WATCH) Trial. Circulation 2009;119:1616–24.
58. Al-Khandra AS, Salem DN, Udelson JE, et al. Warfarin anticoagulation and survival: a cohort analysis from the Studies of Left Ventricular Dysfunction. J Am Coll Cardiol 1998;31:749–53.
59. Cohen MB, Mather PJ. A review of the association between congestive heart failure and cognitive impairment. Am J Geriatr Cardiol 2008;16(3):171–4.
60. Zuccala G, Onder G, Pedone C, et al, for the GIFA-ONLUS Study Group. Hypotension and cognitive impairment: selective association in patients with heart failure. Neurology 2001;57:1986–92.
61. Bornstein RA, Starling RC, Myerowitz PD, et al. Neuropsychological function in patients with end-stage heart failure before and after cardiac transplantation. Acta Neurol Scand 1995;91:260–5.
62. Schall RR, Petrucci RJ, Brozena SC, et al. Cognitive function in patients with symptomatic dilated cardiomyopathy before and after cardiac transplantation. J Am Coll Cardiol 1989;14:1666–72.
63. Pullucino PM, Hart J. Cognitive impairment in congestive heart failure? Embolism vs hypoperfusion? Neurology 2001;57:1945–6.
64. Kalaria VG, Passannante MR, Shah T, et al. Effect of mitral regurgitation on left ventricular thrombus in dilated cardiomyopathy. Am Heart J 1998;135:215–20.

65. Go AS, Hylek EM, Phillips KA, et al. Prevalence of diagnosed atrial fibrillation in adults: national implications for rhythm management and stroke prevention: the AnTicoagulation and Risk Factors in Atrial Fibrillation (ATRIA) Study. JAMA 2001;285:2370–5.
66. The Stroke Risk in Atrial Fibrillation Working Group. Independent predictors of stroke in patients with atrial fibrillation: a systematic review. Neurology 2007;69: 546–54.
67. Report of the Quality Standards Subcommittee of the American Academy of Neurology. Practice parameter: stroke prevention in patients with nonvalvular atrial fibrillation. Neurology 1998;51:671–3.
68. Yamaguchi, for Japanese Nonvalvular Atrial Fibrillation-Embolism Secondary Prevention Cooperative Study Group T. Optimal intensity of warfarin therapy for stroke prevention in patient with nonvalvular atrial fibrillation: a multicenter, prospective, randomized trial. Stroke 2000;31:817–21.
69. Hylek EM, Go AS, Chang Y, et al. Effect of intensity of oral anticoagulation on stroke severity and mortality in atrial fibrillation. N Engl J Med 2003;349:1019–26.
70. van Walraven C, Hart RG, Singer DE, et al. Oral anticoagulants vs aspirin in non-valvular atrial fibrillation: an individual patient meta-analysis. JAMA 2002;288: 2441–8.
71. Hart RG, Pearce LA, Aguilar MI. Meta-analysis: antithrombotic therapy to prevent stroke in patients who have nonvalvular atrial fibrillation. Ann Intern Med 2007; 146:857–67.
72. Stroke Prevention in Atrial Fibrillation Investigators. Adjusted-dose warfarin versus low-intensity, fixed-dose warfarin plus aspirin for high-risk patients with atrial fibrillation: Stroke Prevention in Atrial Fibrillation III randomised clinical trial. Lancet 1996;348:633–8.
73. Shireman TI, Howard PA, Kresowik TF, et al. Combined anticoagulant-antiplatelet use and major bleeding events in elderly atrial fibrillation patients. Stroke 2004; 35:2362–7.
74. The ACTIVE Investigators. Effect of clopidogrel added to aspirin in patients with atrial fibrillation. N Engl J Med 2009;360:2066–78.
75. Bath PMW, Iddenden R, Bath FJ. Low-molecular-weight heparins and heparin-oids in acute ischemic stroke: a meta-analysis of randomized controlled trials. Stroke 2000;31:1770–8.
76. Moonis M, Fisher M. Considering the role of heparin and low-molecular-weight heparins in acute ischemic stroke. Stroke 2002;33:1927–33.
77. Adams HP Jr. Emergent use of anticoagulation for treatment of patients with ischemic stroke. Stroke 2002;33:856–61.
78. Camerlingo M, Salvi P, Bellone G, et al. Intravenous heparin started within the first 3 hours after onset of symptoms as a treatment for acute nonlacunar hemispheric infarctions. Stroke 2005;36:2415–20.
79. Bath PMW, Lindenstrom E, De Deyn G, et al, for the TAIST Investigators. Tinzapar-in in acute ischemic stroke (TAIST): a randomized aspirin-controlled trial. Lancet 2001;358:702–10.
80. Berge E, Abdelnoor M, Nakstad PH, et al, on behalf of the HAEST Study Group. Low-molecular-weight heparin versus aspirin in patients with acute ischaemic stroke and atrial fibrillation: a double-blind study. Lancet 2000;355:1205–10.
81. Weisberg LA. Nonseptic cardiogenic cerebral embolic stroke: clinical-CT correlations. Neurology 1985;35(6):896–9.
82. Hallevi H, Albright KC, Martin-Schild S, et al. Anticoagulation after cardioembolic stroke: to bridge or not to bridge? Arch Neurol 2008;65(9):1169–73.

83. Tayal AH, Tian M, Kelly KM, et al. Atrial fibrillation detected by mobile cardiac outpatient telemetry in cryptogenic stroke. Neurology 2008;71:1696–701.

84. Hur J, Kim YJ, Lee H-J, et al. Cardiac computed tomographic angiography for detection of cardiac sources of embolism in stroke patients. Stroke 2009;40: 2073–8.

85. Mobius-Winkler S, Schuler GC, Sick PB. Interventional treatments for stroke prevention in atrial fibrillation with emphasis on the WATCHMAN device. Curr Opin Neurol 2008;21(1):64–9.

Neurologic Complications of Respiratory Disease

Joy E. Dreibelbis, MD, Ralph F. Józefowicz, MD*

KEYWORDS

- Hypoxia • Respiratory failure • Altitude sickness
- Sleep apnea • Hypoventilation • Hyperventilation

The respiratory and central nervous system (CNS) are intimately connected through strict control of ventilation by central mechanisms. The exquisite sensitivity of central chemoreceptors and cerebral blood vessels to changes in CNS oxygenation mandate this type of control to maintain proper brain function. When diseases of the lung and respiratory system interfere with this fine balance, neurologic symptoms, sometimes severe, may develop. This article deals with the effects of abnormal ventilation on the nervous system.

BASIC PHYSIOLOGY

The CNS regulates ventilation through peripheral and central chemoreceptors. These receptors are sensitive to changes in the Po_2, Pco_2, and blood pH. Their function is to provide feedback to the brainstem respiratory centers, which in turn drive respiratory rhythms.[1] The carotid bodies are particularly responsive to changes in arterial Po_2 and relay information to the nucleus tractus solitarius, which then provides information to the ventral medulla where respiratory rhythms are generated. In the ventral medulla, there are additional chemoreceptive neurons that respond to local CO_2 and H^+ concentrations. In the presence of hypoxia or hypercarbia, cerebral blood vessels dilate, causing increased cerebral blood flow.[2] When these compensatory mechanisms are not adequate in the face of respiratory failure, a variety of neurologic symptoms can result.

ACUTE HYPOXIA
Acute Respiratory Failure

The cardinal features of respiratory failure are dyspnea, hypoxia, and hypercarbia. Hypoxia can be caused by a variety of medical conditions including pulmonary,

Department of Neurology, University of Rochester School of Medicine and Dentistry, 601 Elmwood Avenue, Box 673, Rochester, NY 14642, USA
* Corresponding author.
E-mail address: Ralph_Jozefowicz@urmc.rochester.edu (R.F. Józefowicz).

Neurol Clin 28 (2010) 37–43
doi:10.1016/j.ncl.2009.09.005
0733-8619/09/$ – see front matter © 2010 Elsevier Inc. All rights reserved.

neurologic.theclinics.com

cardiac, and hematologic disorders, and environmental changes such as high altitude. In acute respiratory failure, which is defined by a drop in Po_2 below 60 mm Hg or a rise of pCO_2 above 50 mm Hg, neurologic dysfunction may occur abruptly. The neurologic sequelae depend upon the rate of onset, duration, and severity of the hypoxia. The possible symptoms are diverse and include delirium, somnolence, anxiety, tremor, myoclonus, headaches, and ultimately, if ventilatory support is not provided, loss of consciousness or coma. If oxygenation is restored promptly, the patient may regain consciousness without neurologic residua.[2] Prolonged CNS hypoxia, on the other hand, especially in the presence of pre-existing cerebrovascular disease, may lead to hypoxic-ischemic encephalopathy (HIE). This condition is commonly seen as a complication of cardiac or pulmonary arrest. The prolonged anoxia causes neuronal death, usually in sensitive areas such as the cortex, hippocampus, and Purkinje cells of the cerebellum.[2] Convulsions, pupillary dilation, and upper motor neuron signs may result if anoxia is complete.

Acute pulmonary encephalopathy, or HIE, was described by Kilburn[3] in the mid-1960s as a syndrome of "disorientation, confusion, incoherence, somnolence, bewilderment, obstreperousness, and combativeness." The study correlated the occurrence of neurologic symptoms with arterial blood gas parameters. The most common symptoms in these patients were cerebral dysfunction, asterixis, and tremors. The severity of neurologic symptoms most closely correlated with the degree of acidosis rather than the arterial Po_2. Consequently, it was found that reducing the pCO_2 ameliorated symptoms, but raising the Po_2 did not.

In acute respiratory failure with neurologic injury, prognosis cannot be judged immediately after providing ventilator support and restoring oxygenation. Depending upon the length of the hypoxic event and the neurologic examination postarrest on days 3, 7, and 14, prognosis is estimated based on the algorithm generated by Levy and colleagues.[4] In this landmark study of 210 patients with respiratory arrest, absent pupillary reflexes on the initial examination predicted low probability of regaining consciousness. In patients who regain consciousness after a prolonged hypoxic event, subtle cognitive or motor deficits may persist. Only 13% of the patients in this study regained functional independence in 1 year. A typical constellation of symptoms after cardiac arrest includes subtle memory and executive deficits.[5]

The mainstay of treating acute respiratory failure is ventilatory support. Identification and treatment of the underlying cause of the acute event is paramount, whether it is pneumonia, sepsis, chronic obstructive pulmonary disease (COPD), heart failure, or another cause. Prompt initiation of supportive ventilation during this time is key to preserving CNS function and preventing complications such as HIE.

Altitude Sickness

Another cause of acute hypoxia is exposure to high altitude, where the Po_2 is lower. High-altitude sickness, or acute mountain sickness (AMS), is defined as the abrupt onset, in a nonacclimatized person at 2500 m or higher, of headache plus one of the following: nausea, vomiting, anorexia, insomnia, dizziness, somnolence, or fatigue. The development of this condition depends greatly on the rate of ascent, the absolute altitude, the sleeping altitude, and the individual's physiologic response. AMS tends to be more common in younger (<50 years old) individuals and this has been theorized to be due to a greater propensity toward cerebral edema and raised intracranial pressure related to the amount of brain tissue and relative lack of atrophy in the young.[6] This has been labeled the tight-fit hypothesis. A study of actual intracerebral pressure (ICP) measurements at high altitude was performed in 1985 by a neurosurgeon, Brian Cummings, the data having been recently recovered and published.[7] In this study, three subjects on a Himalayan expedition had ICP monitors implanted before their ascent. Among the subjects in whom ICP was monitored were the researcher himself and one subject with a ventriculoperitoneal shunt. In an adjunctive study, CT scans were performed on all members of the expedition at baseline, and team members were surveyed for signs and symptoms of AMS or headache during the ascent. The researchers found no change in ICP at any altitude, but did find a reverse correlation between ventricular size and AMS symptoms. Although a small and imperfect study, it lends support to the tight-fit hypothesis.

When AMS progresses without any intervention, symptoms of high-altitude cerebral edema can develop. This serious condition is diagnosed clinically when a patient has AMS or high-altitude pulmonary edema, and then develops ataxia and altered mental status. Other neurologic symptoms may develop such as papilledema, cranial nerve palsies, retinal hemorrhages, and somnolence. If left untreated, coma and death result from brainstem herniation. The physiology behind this is thought to be dilatation of cerebral vessels and vasogenic edema causing raised intracranial pressure. The treatment for AMS or high-altitude cerebral edema involves descent to a lower altitude (at least 500–1000 m), supplemental oxygen, hyperbaric chambers, and medical therapies such as acetazolamide or dexamethasone.[6]

CHRONIC HYPOXIA
Chronic Respiratory Failure

Chronically reduced Po_2 may be seen in both respiratory and systemic diseases, but is most commonly seen in COPD. It is estimated that at least 14 million Americans have COPD, which includes chronic bronchitis and emphysema.[8] Early in the disease, dyspnea on exertion may be the main symptom. However, in the late stages, chronic hypoxia and hypercarbia may cause headache, abnormal movements, and mental status changes. These patients may function normally with a pCO_2 in the 55 to 60 mm Hg range as long as this level was achieved slowly over time. An acute rise to this level in another individual would cause stupor.[2] When chronic pulmonary encephalopathy becomes symptomatic, it is usually heralded by the insidious onset of dull headache, drowsiness, and in some, papilledema. Seizures and focal neurologic signs are rare.[2] When treating these patients, giving high concentrations of inspired oxygen will reduce the stimulus to the carotid body and, therefore, decrease the ventilatory drive. This will increase hypercarbia and make symptoms worse.[8] For this reason, treatment of chronic hypoxia is typically restricted to low-flow oxygen. In an acute situation where high-flow oxygen is necessary, it can be given as long as ventilator support is provided. Medical therapies such as bronchodilators, steroids, and smoking cessation when appropriate are all key parts of treating this disease.

DISORDERS OF HYPOVENTILATION

Control of ventilation is strictly maintained based on pH and pCO_2, and to a lesser extent, Po_2.[1,8] Hypoventilation can occur as a result of toxic or metabolic insults, central dysregulation, or peripheral and mechanical causes. The term Ondine curse has been used in the medical literature to refer to a variety of hypoventilatory syndromes including central hypoventilation syndrome, sleep apnea, or any failure of autonomic respiration.[9] This term is based on the story of a mythological water nymph named Ondine fabled to have placed a curse on a mortal robbing him of his automatic functions, including breathing, for being unfaithful to her.[9] Although this is a misinterpretation of the original fable, it has become commonplace in the medical literature. This term may have originally been coined in patients with bulbar poliomyelitis, but now is often used to refer to various brainstem conditions affecting respiration such as infarctions or tumors.

The obesity-hypoventilation syndrome, first termed the pickwickian syndrome, is becoming more prevalent as obesity increases in the United States. Recent statistics from the National Health and Nutrition Examination Survey (NHANES) found the prevalence of obesity to be 33.3% in men and 35.3% in women.[10] The syndrome is defined as chronic hypercapnia and obesity (body mass index at least 30) with symptoms of dyspnea and, in the later stages, cor pulmonale.[8] The main neurologic symptoms are daytime sleepiness and cognitive changes. In this condition, alveolar hypoventilation occurs because of blunted respiratory drive and mechanical pressure on the chest from obesity. There has been some recent work showing that the hormone leptin is elevated in the obese and is postulated to cause the blunted respiratory drive, possibly through central resistance.[11] Voluntary hyperventilation can improve the symptoms of obesity-hypoventilation syndrome. The main treatment is weight loss although respiratory stimulants such as theophylline, acetazolamide, or medroxyprogesterone are sometimes used.

Sleep Disordered Breathing

One of the most common causes of hypoventilation in the United States is sleep-disordered breathing related to obesity. In the Wisconsin Sleep Cohort Study, the prevalence of OSA was 9% in females and 24% in males ages 30–60 years.[12] Sleep disordered breathing, or sleep apnea, is defined by episodic cessation of breathing for at least 10 seconds (apnea) or a decrease in airflow with a drop in hemoglobin saturation of at least 4% (hypopnea). Sleep apneas are divided into categories of obstructive, central, and mixed. Obstructive sleep apnea (OSA), the most common form, is caused by upper airway blockage due to anatomic abnormalities or mechanical force from obesity narrowing the airway during sleep when pharyngeal tone is low. It can be exacerbated by alcohol, sedatives, or upper respiratory infections and allergies. Sleep apnea, and the sleep fragmentation that accompanies it, have neurologic effects that extend into the waking hours. The main daytime neurologic symptoms are headaches, memory loss, mood and personality changes and fatigue.[13] The functions of the frontal and prefrontal cortex seem to be preferentially affected, causing decreased attention, mental speed of processing, and poor performance on mental tasks.[13] There has been some recent work suggesting OSA could be linked to another neurologic disease—idiopathic intracranial hypertension. In a retrospective study, Wall and colleagues[14] found a relationship between men with OSA and idiopathic intracranial hypertension, although it was unclear whether the relationship is causal or if the syndromes are independently related to obesity. The proposed mechanism for the relationship is that nocturnal hypoxemia and hypercarbia cause chronic cerebral vasodilatation, which leads to raised intracranial pressure.

The gold standard for diagnosis of sleep apneas is the polysomnogram. During this test, an electroencephalogram is recorded along with electromyography of the anterior tibialis muscle, oxygen saturation, respiratory effort, cardiac rhythm, airflow, and video if needed. Sleep laboratories often set their own criteria, but, in general, five or more apneic or hypopneic episodes per hour are considered diagnostic.[13]

When there is an absence of ventilatory effort once an apneic episode has begun, central sleep apnea (CSA) is diagnosed. CSAs are most commonly due to medullary lesions, either ischemic, structural, or otherwise, but have also been linked to genetic and paraneoplastic disorders.[15,16] In a rare disorder called congenital central hypoventilation syndrome (CCHS), patients have a blunted response to hypercapnia, which results in decreased ventilation during sleep and autonomic dysfunction.[13] The genetic defect in CCHS is due to mutations in PHOX2B, a gene responsible for maturation of the neural crest and formation of facial structures.[16,17] There is an association of CCHS with ganglioblastomas and Hirschsprung disease.[18] A recent study of CCHS patients used diffusion tensor imaging to highlight areas of injury to the myelin. In these patients, there was evidence of injury in the lateral medulla, dorsal midbrain, periaqueductal gray, raphe nuclei, and the cerebellum, indicating that these areas are important in the disease.[19]

There may be an association between paraneoplastic disorders and CSA. In a recent retrospective study of patients with Hu-antibody syndromes, the investigators identified a subset of 14 patients who were Hu-antibody positive and had features of central hypoventilation in addition to other brainstem findings. Three of these patients presented with CSA and, in one of these patients, an autopsy showed inflammation in the medulla.[15]

Mixed sleep apnea is diagnosed when the polysomnogram shows features of both obstructive and central apneas. There is some evidence that patients with neuromuscular conditions may be more prone to both OSA and CSA, or the mixed form. In one study, patients with Charcot-Marie-Tooth disease, particularly Type 1A, were more likely to have OSA, which the authors hypothesize is due to pharyngeal muscle weakness and low muscle tone.[20] Other neuromuscular conditions that are frequently associated with pulmonary complications and sleep disordered breathing include amyotrophic lateral sclerosis, postpolio syndrome, myotonic dystrophy, myasthenia gravis, Duchenne muscular dystrophy, and acid maltase deficiency.[21] In these conditions, diaphragmatic weakness predisposes to hypoventilation, combined with upper airway resistance from bulbar weakness, respiratory muscle weakness, and possibly impaired chemosensitivity. These patients are especially prone to sleep disordered breathing and the neurologic sequelae that result.

Treatment for the various sleep apneas involves nighttime ventilatory support. This is typically achieved with continuous positive airway pressure or bilevel positive airway pressure machines, or surgical interventions, to open the upper airway.

DISORDERS OF HYPERVENTILATION

Hyperventilation, or an increase in alveolar ventilation sufficient to produce hypocapnia, is a common and underrecognized cause of neurologic symptoms. This can be caused by a myriad of conditions including pain, fever, sepsis, pregnancy, pulmonary or cardiac disease, CNS tumors, anxiety, metabolic changes, and medications.[22] In a clinical evaluation of patients complaining of dizziness, hyperventilation was the cause in 24%.[23] In the early 1990s, Evans[24] evaluated a group of medical students who were asked to hyperventilate and then describe their symptoms. Bilateral paresthesias developed in 84% of the subjects; in 16%, the paresthesias were unilateral. Blurred vision and diplopia were also common complaints. Acute hyperventilation may also cause distal and perioral paresthesias, carpopedal spasm, and even tetany. The pathophysiology behind the association of hyperventilation and neurologic symptoms is believed to be due to a decrease in the pCO_2 leading to respiratory alkalosis. This causes a decrease in plasma calcium leading to tetany, and decreased oxygen delivery to tissues because of the Bohr effect.

Chronic hyperventilation can be more difficult to recognize because breathing does not necessarily appear to be rapid and, since it may be intermittent, spot measurements of pCO_2 will be normal. Chronic hyperventilation causes nonspecific neurologic symptoms such as fatigue, dizziness, lightheadedness, and anxiety, or even symptoms referable to more than one organ system. The diagnosis is made when other medical conditions have been ruled out and the symptoms are reproduced with observed hyperventilation. The hyperventilation test is easily and safely performed with most patients, provided they do not have the following conditions in which it is contraindicated: heart disease, cerebrovascular disease, pulmonary disease, sickle cell anemia, or hyperviscosity states.[25] The patient is asked to increase ventilation to 60 breaths per minute or do deep breathing for 3 minutes.[26] The test is considered positive if it provokes recurrence of the symptoms. Treatment involves addressing the underlying cause of the hyperventilation, but if medical conditions have been excluded and anxiety is felt to be the cause, treatment with beta blockers, benzodiazepines, or antidepressants may be helpful.

SUMMARY

Regardless of the cause, respiratory compromise of any sort can have profound effects on the nervous system. These effects are mostly mediated by an increase in pCO_2, rather than low Po_2. Given the prevalence of chronic conditions such as COPD and OSA, respiratory diseases have become a common cause of neurologic diseases. Neurologic symptoms resulting from impaired respiration include headaches, dizziness, delirium, visual changes, abnormal movements, and even coma. The mainstay of treating any of these disorders is providing ventilatory support to prevent permanent neurologic sequelae.

REFERENCES

1. Eldridge F. Central nervous system and chemoreceptor factors in control of breathing. Chest 1978;73(Suppl 2):256–8.
2. Posner JB. Plum and Posner's diagnosis of stupor and coma. New York: Oxford University Press; 2007.
3. Kilburn KH. Neurologic manifestations of respiratory failure. Arch Intern Med 1965;116:409–15.
4. Levy DE, Caronna JJ, Singer BH, et al. Predicting outcome from hypoxic-ischemic coma. JAMA 1985;253(10):1420–6.
5. Lim C, Alexander MP, LaFleche G, et al. The neurological and cognitive sequelae of cardiac arrest. Neurology 2004;63(10):1774–8.
6. Hackett PH, Roach RC. Current concepts: high altitude sickness. N Engl J Med 2001;345(2):107–14.
7. Wilson MH, Milledge J. Direct measurement of intracranial pressure at high altitude and correlation of ventricular size with acute mountain sickness: Brian Cummins' results from the 1985 Kishtwar expedition. Neurosurgery 2008;63(5):970–5.
8. Piper AJ, Grunstein RR. Current perspectives on the obesity hypoventilation syndrome. Curr Opin Pulm Med 2007;13(6):490–6.
9. Nannapaneni R, Behari S, Todd NV, et al. Retracing "Ondine's curse". Neurosurgery 2005;57(2):354–63.
10. Ogden CL, Carroll MD, McDowell MA, et al. Obesity among adults in the United States: no change since 2003–4. NCHS data brief. No. 1. Hyattsville (MD): National Center for Health Statistics; 2007.
11. Phipps PR, Starritt E, Caterson I, et al. Association of serum leptin with hypoventilation in human obesity. Thorax 2002;57:75–6.
12. Finn L, Young T, Palta M, et al. Sleep-disordered breathing and self-reported general health status in the Wisconsin Sleep Cohort Study. Sleep 1998;21(7):701–6.

13. Broderick M, Guilleminault C. Neurological aspects of obstructive sleep apnea. Ann N Y Acad Sci 2008;1142:44–57.
14. Wall M, Purvin V. Idiopathic intracranial hypertension in men and the relationship to sleep apnea. Neurology 2009;72(4):300–1.
15. Gomez-Choco MJ, Zarranz JJ, Saiz A, et al. Central hypoventilation as the presenting symptom in Hu associated paraneoplastic encephalomyelitis. J Neurol Neurosurg Psychiatry 2007;78(10):1143–5.
16. Sasaki A, Kanai M, Kijima K, et al. Molecular analysis of congenital central hypoventilation syndrome. Hum Genet 2003;114:22–6.
17. Weese-Mayer DE, Berry-Kravis EM, Zhou L, et al. Idiopathic congenital central hypoventilation syndrome: analysis of genes pertinent to early autonomic nervous system embryologic development and identification of mutations in PHOX2b. Am J Med Genet 2003;123A:267–78.
18. Guilleminault C, Brassiri AG. Obstructive and nonobstructive sleep apnea: the neurological perspective. In: Culebras A, editor. Sleep disorders and neurological disease. New York: Marcel Dekker Inc; 1999. p. 275–87.
19. Kumar R, Macey PM, Woo MA, et al. Diffusion tensor imaging demonstrates brainstem and cerebellar abnormalities in congenital central hypoventilation syndrome. Pediatr Res 2008;64(3):275–80.
20. Dziewas R, Waldmann N, Bontert M, et al. Increased prevalence of obstructive sleep apnea in patients with Charcot-Marie-Tooth disease: a case control study. J Neurol Neurosurg Psychiatry 2008;79(7):829–31.
21. Upinder KD, Rajiv D. Sleep disorders in neuromuscular diseases. Curr Opin Pulm Med 2006;12(6):402–8.
22. Laffey JG, Kavanagh BI. Medical progress: hypocapnia. N Engl J Med 2002;347(1):43–53.
23. Drachman DA, Hart CW. An approach to the dizzy patient. Neurology 1972;22:233–4.
24. Evans RW. Neurologic aspects of hyperventilation syndrome. Semin Neurol 1995;15(2):115–25.
25. Brashear RE. Hyperventilation syndrome. Lung 1983;161:257–73.
26. Lum LC. Hyperventilation syndromes in medicine and psychiatry: a review. J R Soc Med 1987;80:229–31.

Neurologic Presentations of Renal Diseases

Glenda Lacerda, MD[a,b], Thierry Krummel, MD[c],
Edouard Hirsch, MD[d,e],*

KEYWORDS

- Renal diseases • Neurologic presentations
- Uremic encephalopathy • Peripheral nervous system disorders
- Dialysis • Renal transplantation

Renal diseases characterized by glomerular, tubular, and parenchymal disturbances lead to metabolic abnormalities known as uremia. Uremia is linked to accumulation of toxins, anemia, increased inflammatory, and oxidative stress, producing reactive nitrogen species, disturbances in intermediate metabolism with impaired $Na+/K+$ ATPase activity, and accumulation of intracellular $Ca2+$, parathormone (PTH) and other hormones.[1–3] Such processes are more intense in end-stage renal disease (ESRD) and promote central and peripheral nervous system disorders. Moreover, specific renal diseases may disclose with nervous system syndromes. ESRD treatment with hemodialysis (HD), peritoneal dialysis (PD), or renal transplantation (RT) may provoke neurologic disorders.

CNS DISORDERS CAUSED BY UREMIA
Uremic Encephalopathy Syndrome

Uremic encephalopathy syndrome develops in hours to days with fatigue, apathy, emotional instability, sleep disorders, forgetfulness, neuroendocrine dysregulation, perceptual errors, agitation, and impaired cognition with aggravation to delirium, delusions, hallucinations, frontal release phenomena, tremor, asterixis, and multifocal myoclonus, generalized tonic-clonic seizures, and coma.[2,4] In chronic uremia, less obvious cognitive abnormalities take place that are frequently overlooked and regard

---

[a] Serviço de Neurologia, Hospital Universitário Antônio Pedro, Universidade Federal Fluminense, Rua Marquês do Paraná 303, Centro, Niterói, Rio de Janeiro, Brazil
[b] Electroencephalography Unit, Hospital São Vicente de Paulo, Rio de Janeiro, Brazil
[c] Service de Néphrologie, Hémodialyse et Transplantation Rénale, 1 Place de Íhôpital, Hôpitaux Universitaires de Strasbourg, Strasbourg 67091, France
[d] Service de Neurologie, 1 Place de Íhôpital, Strasbourg 67091, France
[e] CTRS Fondation IDEE, LINC CNRS, HUS Strasbourg, France
* Corresponding author. Service de Neurologie, 1 Place de Íhôpital, Strasbourg, France.
E-mail address: edouard.hirsch@chru-strasbourg.fr (E. Hirsch).

Neurol Clin 28 (2010) 45–59
doi:10.1016/j.ncl.2009.09.003
0733-8619/09/$ – see front matter
neurologic.theclinics.com

psychomotor slowing and attention deficit.[4–6] The Wechsler battery of neuropsychologic tests applied to chronic renal failure (CRF) patients under HD showed a significant score decline in Trail Making tests, parts A and B, replacing symbols for algorithms, and a modified copying symbols tests in patients when compared with controls. The mini mental state examination did not show a significant score difference between them. Trails Making part B test measures of executive functions were more affected in all patients when HD was delayed for 24 hours.[4] Psychometric deficits without obvious cognitive, behavioral, or affective abnormalities may accompany cerebral atrophy.[7] There are abnormal somatosensory and cognitive-related evoked potentials (increase in P latency and decrease in P3 amplitude).[2,7] Electroencephalograms may be initially normal, but slowing of background activity ensues with increasing theta and delta rhythms, culminating with irregular, low-voltage, slow, arreactive rhythms. Predominantly frontal triphasic waves, spikes and sharp waves, discharges or prolonged bursts of bilateral synchronous, mixed slow and sharp activity, and photoparoxysmal responses can be found. Sleep records may show increased vertex waves, lack of spindles in stage 2 sleep, and prolonged high-voltage, slow bursts on awakening.[8–10] There are abnormal somatosensory and cognitive-related evoked potentials (increase in P latency and decrease in P3 amplitude).[2,7]

Seizures

One third of patients with uremic encephalopathy shows various types of seizures—myoclonic, simple partial motor (including epilepsia partialis continua), partial complex, absence, and generalized tonic-clonic seizures. Convulsive and nonconvulsive (absence or partial complex) status epilepticus are frequent.[11–13] Causes are accumulation of organic acids and uremic complications as malignant hypertension, subdural and intracranial hemorrhage due to clotting defects, sepsis, dysglycemia, hyponatremia, hypomagnesemia or hypocalcemia, and acid-base disorders.[11,14] Guanidino compounds activate aspartate receptors and inhibit GABAergic neurotransmission.[7] Reversible posterior leukoencephalopathy syndrome, consequent to renal disease, hypertension, malignancy, or transplantation, comprises seizures, headache, clouding of sensorium, and visual disturbances.[15–17] Infections treatment with β-lactam penicilins, cephalosporins, carbapenems, and quinolone antibiotics (ABs) may generate convulsive and nonconvulsive status epilepticus in renal patients as toxic organic acids inhibit active transport of ABs from cerebrospinal fluid (CSF) to blood, leading to CSF neurotoxic concentrations. β-Lactams structurally resemble bicuculline, an epileptogenic γ-aminobutyric acid antagonist.[3,18–20]

Movement Disorders

Uremia, medication, cerebral vascular, neoplastic, or infectious lesions may be accompanied by asterixis or "flapping," a sudden cortical-related loss of tonus. Spontaneous and stimulus-sensitive myoclonia are also seen related to water-electrolyte imbalance or to ischemia or degeneration in lower brain stem and reticular formation. The twitch-convulsive syndrome comprises intense asterixis, myoclonus, muscle twitches, fasciculations, and seizures. Thiamine deficiency, hypoperfusion, a selective basal ganglia vulnerability to hypoxia, uremic toxins and diabetes cause chorea, dysarthria, masked facies, bradykinesia, rigidity, small-stepped gait, tremor, stooped posture, frequent falls, and myoclonus. CT scan shows decreased density in basal ganglia bilaterally. MRI shows decreased T1- and increased T2-weighted images signals. positron emission tomography scan reveals significant reduction in glucose metabolism in the bilateral basal ganglia and in the frontal and occipital cortices when compared with controls. Histology reveals reactive astrocytosis with plump astrocytes and edema, consistent with metabolic failure.[7,21] Basal ganglia cells may be compromised by long-term diabetes mellitus through microangiopathy, energy utilization failure, and uremic toxins. Acute symptoms and imaging lesions usually regress, but derangement could persist.[22] Uremic acute chorea improve with increasing HD frequency.[23,24]

Stroke

Chronic kidney disease (CKD) increases cardiovascular (CV) disease risk, including transient ischemic attacks (TIA) and stroke. ESRD is associated with a 10- to 20-fold larger rate of CV mortality and advanced carotid atherosclerosis compared with the general population.[25,26] In the British Regional Heart Study a serum creatinine level over 1.3 mg/dL significantly increased the risk of stroke, even after adjustment for several CV risk factors.[27] Among patients with isolated systolic hypertension, higher creatinine levels increased the odds-ratio (OR) for stroke.[28] Diminished creatinine clearance worsens CV risk even when serum creatinine levels are normal[29] and CKD was associated with a significant OR for stroke.[30] Lacunar silent brain infarcts correlate independently to estimated declining glomerular filtration rates (GFR).[31] A glance at less advanced renal dysfunction in selected patients with chronic heart disease followed-up for incidental ischemic stroke or TIA over years showed that those with CKD (ie eGFR<60 mL/min/1.73 m2) had a 1.54-fold OR (CI 95%:1.13 to 2.09) of incident ischemic stroke and TIA. A decreasing risk was observed with increasing estimated GFR, even when this was over 60 mL/mim/1.73m2. Cumulative ischemic stroke or TIA-free curves decline by increasing serum creatinine levels.[26] Increased CV risk is explained by anemia,[32] oxidative stress, hypercalcemia, hyperphosphatemia and secondary hyperparathyroidism,[33] increased homocysteine, inflammation, atherosclerosis, endothelial dysfunction, and coagulation promotion; this last one most associated with nephrotic syndrome.[26,34] Nephrotic syndrome is characterized by heavy proteinuria (> 3 g/d), hypoalbuminemia (<3 g/dL), edema and hyperlipidemia, resulting from primary or secondary glomerular diseases.[34,35] Venous sinus thrombosis in pediatric patients with nephrotic syndrome present with headache, vomiting, coma, or seizures.[34,36] This usually occurs during relapse in steroid-resistant nephrotic syndrome due to hepatic coagulation inhibitors synthesis increase and abrupt urinary antithrombin loss.[34,36] Serum protein C and protein S levels were reported to be increased in steroid-resistant nephrotic children.[37,38] Prudent use of diuretics, avoidance of infection, and maintenance of albumin levels are useful preventive measures.[38] Prophylactic anticoagulation is recommended when plasma albumin is below 3 g/dL.[39–41] Intracerebral, subdural, and subarachnoid hemorrhage (SAH) yield a mortality index of up to 60% in CKD. It is related to platelet dysfunction, altered platelet-vessel wall interaction, arterial hypertension, head trauma, polycystic kidney disease, use of anticoagulants, and platelet antiaggregants. Subdural hematomas may clinically resemble encephalopathy. Management includes minimal or heparin-free HD, switch from HD to PD (not requiring anticoagulation), and surgery.[7,42]

Sleep Disorders

Two studies addressing patients on HD showed 80% prevalence of sleep disorders.[43,44] Insomnia (69%), obstructive sleep apnea syndrome (OSAS 24%), restless legs syndrome (RLS) (18%), and excessive daytime sleepiness (12%) were most often present.[43] Age, alcohol intake, cigarette smoking, and morning dialysis (with extracellular fluid accumulation during night) may significantly relate to them, although dialysis schedule effect is arguable.[43,44] CRF increases ventilatory effort secondary to acidemia, contributing to upper airway collapse and to OSAS, characterized by choking during sleep, recurrent awakenings, nonrefreshing sleep, morning headache, daytime fatigue, and impaired concentration.[45] RLS refers to an imperative need to move the legs (and the arms) due to paresthesias that worsen in night inactivity. Iron deficiency, uremic toxins, a central dopaminergic disturbance, and the existence of polyneuropathy contribute to its pathogenesis. HD does not improve it, but use of cool dialysate fluid brings relief. Substantial improvement occurs after renal transplantation.[7,44] Also reported are periodic limb movements, nightmares, sleepwalking, REM behavior disorder, and narcolepsy.[43,44]

PERIPHERAL NERVOUS SYSTEM DISORDERS CAUSED BY UREMIA
Polyneuropathy

Polyneuropathy (PN) is the most common CRF neurologic complication, with prevalence rates of 60% to100%.[14] This is an insidious chronic length-dependent distal sensorimotor PN with greater lower than upper limb involvement.[46–48] It may either be painless or begin with burning dysesthesia of the feet or creeping, crawling, and itching sensations, impaired temperature sensibility, paradoxical heat sensation, ascending hypesthesia to pinprick or touch, and pruritus. Large fiber involvement causes paresthesias, deep hyperreflexia, impaired vibration sense, muscle wasting, cramps, and weakness. Autonomic features, like postural and intradialytic hypotension, impaired sweating, esophageal dysfunction, diarrhea, constipation, hyperhidrosis, incontinence, or impotence may occur. Cranial nerves involvement (optic, trigeminal, facial, vestibulocochlear) was described.[7,14,48] All types of CKD may give rise to PN, but diabetes produces the most severe ones.[47,48] Duration and severity of CKD correlate with PN development, usually with GFR under 12 mL/min.[48] Symptoms usually arise with GFR under 6 mL/min. Pathology reveals axonal degeneration, loss of large distal fibers, cell bodies chromatolysis and sparing of proximal segments and roots.[14,47] Sympathetic and parasympathetic dysfunction occurs, as shown by impaired heart rate variability, with improvement after HD.[49] CSF increased protein concentrations may simulate Guillain-Barré albuminocytogenic dissociation.[48] Retained middle molecular range toxins (eg, PTH, β2-microglobulin, myo-inositol) have been suggested to cause PN, but no definite culprit has been identified.[14] Predialysis measurements of recovery cycles of sensory or motor nerve excitability in uremic patients show prolonged refractory periods, decreased superexcitability, and late subexcitability periods, indicating an axonal depolarized state before HD. HD restores resting membrane potential.[48] Depolarization degree correlates with serum K+ levels (which may be just within high normal levels), leading to depolarization and reverse operation of the Na+/Ca2+ exchange pump, increased intracellular Ca2+, and axonal damage. Maintenance of serum K+ levels between HD sessions by means of intake control and exchange resins should reduce the burden of PN. Predialysis depolarization was also related to PTH serum levels.[48,50,51] RT can recover sensory and motor functions in days, unless axonal loss is marked, while autonomic symptoms respond less well.[52] Treatments include erythropoietin, biotin, pyridoxine, cobalamine, and thiamine supplements. Tricyclic antidepressants and anticonvulsants relieve pain.[7,48,53] With electroneuromyography, the most sensitive signs of PN are sural nerve amplitude and conduction velocity reduction, followed by prolongation of tibial F-wave minimum latency and H-reflex, diminished peroneal motor nerve conduction velocities, diminished sensory amplitudes, and prolongation of other sensory and motor nerves conduction velocities. There are increased vibratory perception thresholds and somatosensory-evoked potential delays. Sympathetic dysfunction is marked by reduced low-frequency heart rate power in supine position and failure to increase diastolic blood pressure with handgrip. Parasympathetic failure is most often recognized by reduced heart rate variation between quiet and deep breathing.[48–50]

Mononeuropathies

Mononeuropathies (MN) result from compression susceptibility, β2-microglobulin-related amyloidosis, local ischemia, uremic tumoral calcinosis, and HD. Carpal tunnel syndrome (CTS) consists of entrapment of the median nerve in the carpal tunnel formed by the flexor retinaculum and the carpal bones. This causes burning pain and paresthesias in the ventral surface of the hand, the first three fingers, the medial surface of the fourth finger, and thenar muscle atrophy. Renal transplantation relieves symptoms but does not reverse amyloidosis. Use of highly permeable biocompatible HD membranes, convective techniques, pure HD water, and β2-microglobulin adsorption columns may prevent it.[54] Ulnar neuropathy at the wrist due to uremic tumoral calcinosis in Guyon canal causes motor dysfunction of intrinsic hand muscles and sensory loss to the hypothenar eminence, the small finger, and lateral part of ring finger. Treatment includes surgical decompression, local corticosteroids injections, splinting, antiinflammatories, tricyclic antidepressants, and anticonvulsants.[55,56]

Myopathy

Myopathy appears with GFR less than 25 mL/min and its progression parallels decline in renal function. Its prevalence goes up to 50% in HD patients.[57] Signs and symptoms include proximal limb weakness, muscle wasting, limited endurance, exercise limitation, and easy fatigability. Muscle biopsy shows predominant type II fibers atrophy. Cardiomyopathy is sometimes present. Putative pathogenetic mechanisms are toxins accumulation, abnormalities in vitamin D metabolism, serum PTH increase, insulin resistance, carnitine deficiency, protein deficiency, anemia, and alterations in mitochondria oxygen handling. Hypermagnesemia, hypo- or hypercalcemia, hypo- or hyperkalemia mimic myopathy. Other causes are steroid-induced and ischemic myopathy. Use of high-flux HD membranes, aerobic exercises, prevention of secondary hyperparathyroidism, dietary correction, and treatment of anemia with recombinant human erythropoietin are recommended.[7] L-carnitine supplementation usefulness is uncertain.[58] RT reduces symptoms within few months, but does not fully restore strength.[7]

SPECIFIC RENAL DISEASES PRESENTING WITH NEUROLOGIC SYNDROMES
Inherited Renal Diseases

Glomerular disorders
Alport syndrome is a dominant X-linked or recessive autosomal transmitted condition wherein changes in collagen type IV chains cause damage to glomerular and tubular basal membranes, to the eye, and the cochlea. A progressive symmetric sensorineural hearing loss is often its first sign. About 2% to 3% of patients will need HD or RT.[59,60] Fabry disease is due to α-galactosidase A deficiency and is characterized by angiokeratomas, corneal opacities, conjunctival, retinal, and systemic vascular involvement. Casts, red blood cells, and lipid inclusions with birefringent Maltese cross configurations are found in urinary sediment. Proteinuria and isosthenuria mark renal deterioration. Acroparesthesia and intense neuropathic pain, either paroxystic or chronic, may be the first symptom and correspond to globotriasosylceramide storage in dorsal root ganglia, sympathetic ganglia, and temperature-dependent vasa nervorum constriction. Dolichoectasia and increased leucocyte adhesion molecules

expression lead to CV disease, mainly lacunar infarcts, producing hemiparesis, vertigo, diplopia, dysarthria, ataxia, nystagmus, and headache. Sensorineural hearing loss, vascular dementia, aseptic meningitis, and cramp-fasciculation syndrome without PN are also seen. MRI T1-hypointensity and low N-acetylaspartate/creatine ratio in pulvinar nuclei are characteristic. Intravenous recombinant algasidase-α may slow disease progression.[61–63]

Proximal tubular disorders

Deficient tubular basolateral membrane Na+/H+ exchange or carbonic anhydrase activity accelerate loss of bicarbonate and K+ causing a hypochloremic, hypokalemic metabolic acidosis with normally acidic urine and high bicarbonate wasting after plasma bicarbonate normalization. This (proximal) type II renal tubular acidosis most often accompanies Fanconi syndrome, a multiple proximal tubular dysfunction with glucosuria, aminoaciduria, phosphaturia, and uricosuria. Besides osteomalacia, rickets, nausea, vomiting, and growth failure, a paroxystic muscle weakness following low plasma K+ levels ensues.[64] It may be associated to Wilson disease, and respond to D-penicillamine,[64–66] or to Lowe syndrome, the oculocerebrorenal syndrome, caused by a mutation in the OCRL 1 gene at Xq26.1, coding for the enzyme phosphatidylinositol (4,5) biphosphate 5 phosphate in the trans-Golgi network. Manifestations include neonatal hypotonia and areflexia, suction and respiratory difficulties, psychomotor delay with stereotypic behavior, aggressiveness, and obsessive-compulsive disorder. Over 50% of adult patients have seizures and up to 9% of patients have febrile convulsions. Aphakia and retinal degeneration probably cause nystagmus. Cataracts, glaucoma, corneal, and conjunctival cheloids are seen.[67] Brain MRI shows light ventriculomegaly, periventricular cysts and diffuse foci of white matter T2 signal increase sparing commissural fibers, pyramidal tracts, and cerebellum.[67,68] Axonal PN has been reported.[68] Autosomal recessive transmitted Hartnup disease, linked to mutations in SLCGA19 and SLCGA 18 neutral amino acid transporter family, causes enhanced tryptophan loss and thus deficient nicotinamide production. Consequences are cerebellar ataxia, psychiatric disturbances, and photosensitive pellagra-like skin rash.[69,70]

Loop of Henle disorders

Bartter syndrome is a disorder of K+, Ca2+, and Mg2+ reabsorption by the thick ascending loop of Henle caused by mutations in the renal bumetanide-sensitive Na+-K+2Cl-cotransporter (NKCC2) gene or the ATP-sensitive inwardly rectifying K+ channel (ROMK) (neonatal form) or the renal Cl-channel(C1C-Kb) (classic form). Hypokalemia leads to muscle weakness, growth failure, and polyuria. Hypocalcemia leads to tetany and appearance of Trousseau and Chvostek signs. Treatment includes K+ and Mg2+ repletion, prostaglandin inhibitors (aspirin, indomethacin), captopril, and K+-sparing diuretics.[64,71]

Distal tubular disorders

Gitelman syndrome is due to mutations at the distal convoluted tubule thiazide-sensitive Na+-Cl- cotransporter causing hypocalciuria, hypokalemia, hypomagnesemia, and metabolic alkalosis. Symptoms range from aches, fatigue, weakness, dizziness, nocturia, and polydipsia to severe hypokalemic paralysis, tetany, carpopedal spasm, and rhabdomyolysis. Oral magnesium supplementation is needed.[64,71–73] Distal (type 1) renal tubular acidosis is a distal nephron acidification defect due to insufficient proton-secreting pumps or to an acid back leak across the luminal membrane leading to periodic hypokalemic paralysis. It may be linked to autoimmune diseases (eg, Sjögren syndrome). Inherited autosomal dominant and recessive forms

are described, the latter being often associated with an irreversible bilateral sensorineural hearing loss.[74,75]

Parenchymal disorders

Autosomal dominant polycystic kidney disease, related to PKD1 and PKD2 (chromosomes 16 and 4) gene mutations account for a 4- to 10-fold increase in risk of saccular cerebral aneurisms, which tend to rupture at smaller sizes and in individuals 10 years younger than in the general population, leading to SAH recognized by severe headaches, seizures, altered sensorium, and death. Usually silent intact aneurysms can present with headache and focal deficits such as III, IV, VI, V cranial nerves paresis. Giant intracavernous aneurysms can be treated by endoscopic coil occlusion.[76] Von Hippel-Lindau disease is an autosomal dominant inherited disorder due to mutations in VHL tumor suppressor gene located at 3p25-p26, marked by retinal and other CNS hemangioblastomas, renal cysts, and renal cell carcinoma. Visual loss, appendicular ataxia from cerebellar involvement, syringobulbia, and syringomyelia may arise.[77] In autosomally recessive Joubert syndrome, renal cysts, and CRF accompany psychomotor delay, hypotonia, nystagmus, and ataxia linked to cerebellar vermian hypoplasia with thickened superior cerebellar peduncles and interpeduncular fossa.[78]

ACQUIRED DISEASES WITH CONCOMITANT RENAL AND NEUROLOGIC IMPAIRMENT
Poststreptococcal Glomerulonephritis

Poststreptococcal glomerulonephritis (GNP) occurring after pharyngitis or impetigo, may lead to acute disseminated encephalomyelitis. Angiography may show vasculitis in caudate and putamen nuclei topography.[79]

Renal Cancer

Paraneoplastic syndromes may announce a renal cell carcinoma. Reports include opsoclonus-myoclonus syndrome (conjugated chaotic saccades, head and appendicular myoclonus, truncal ataxia, vertigo, and nausea),[80,81] lower motor neuron disease with weakness, and fasciculations improving after nephrectomy[82] or causing neuromyotonia (continuous muscular activity with cramps, muscle rippling, and weakness) probably related to tumoral anti-K+ channels antibodies,[83] limbic encephalitis, cerebellar ataxia, drug-resistant ballistic-choreic movements, severe chronic axonal sensory-motor or acute demyelinating PN, and myopathy.[84–88] Renal cell carcinoma cerebral and cerebellar metastasis affect cognition, behavior, strength, coordination, and language. Pituitary metastasis may cause intraventricular hemorrhage. Large tumors are prone to bleeding.[89–92] Other reports describe spinal cord relapse 31 years after primary tumor ressection,[93] papillary cell carcinoma intradural spinal metastasis with cauda equina infiltration, causing low back pain irradiating to both legs, vesical incontinence and paraparesis.[94] A sciatica disclosed an endoneurial relapse of renal cell carcinoma.[95] Non-Hodgkin lymphoma kidney infiltration may produce tubular compression and necrosis, renal tubular acidosis with hypokalemic acute onset flaccid tetraparesis.[96]

Primary Vasculitis

Polyarteritis nodosa is a necrotizing vasculitis of medium and small vessels causing renal failure, hypertension, painful PN, mononeuropathy multiplex (MM), SAH, and seizures. Churg-Strauss angiitis is an eosinophilic necrotizing vasculitis of medium and small vessels with infrequent renal involvement causing MM, encephalopathy, SAH, and chorea. Wegener granulomatosis is a necrotizing granulomatous vasculitis

affecting the upper and lower respiratory tract and the kidneys, causing cranial neuropathies, MM, PN, and stroke.[77]

Vasculitis in Connective Tissue Disease

Rheumatoid arthritis rarely causes GNP and is associated with PN, MM, and cervical cord lesions due to atlanto-axial subluxation. Lupus erythematosus systemicus causes GNP, nephritic, and nephrotic syndrome through immune complex deposition and produces encephalopathy, psychosis, seizures, stroke, chorea, transverse myelitis, PN including chronic inflammatory demyelinating polyneuropathy (CIDP). Sjögren syndrome causes interstitial nephropathy, tubular disorders, failure of urine acidification and PN, dorsal ganglionopathy, cranial neuropathy, autonomic PN, psychosis, and multiple sclerosis-like CNS lesions.[97]

Plasma Cell Dyscrasias

Multiple myeloma leads to plasma cell tissue infiltration and antibodies binding, nephrotic syndrome, and renal failure, in addition to nerve root, spinal cord, and intracranial compression and axonal PN. In POEMS syndrome (PN, organomegaly, endocrinopathy, M protein, and skin changes), there may be kidney hemangioma and CIDP. Waldenström macroglobulinemia causes proliferation of tissue plasma cells and lymphocytes. Nephrotic syndrome and renal failure ensue, in addition to sensorimotor PN, encephalopathy, myelopathy, stroke, and SAH.[77]

NEUROLOGIC DISORDERS CAUSED BY RENAL REPLACEMENT THERAPY
HD

Dialysis disequilibrium syndrome comprises headache, irritability, blurred vision, nausea, emesis, muscle cramps and twitching, delirium, and seizures. It is self-limited and related to the start of HD or of highly effective HD in severely hyperazotemic patients, because increased osmotic gradient and brain edema as urea is cleared more rapidly from blood than from brain.[7,11,14] Focal neurologic deficit (limb monoplegia, facial palsy) has also been reported.[98] Wernicke encephalopathy comprises confusion, ophthalmoplegia, and ataxia described in HD or PD patients with acute precipitating events like sepsis or CV disease. Relapses are common in survivors of a first episode.[99–102] Risk factors are exposure to organophosphate compounds, low thiamine intake, and accelerated thiamine loss through HD.[7,101] Other symptoms are nausea, anorexia, fatigue and abulia, slurred speech, poor language and word-searching, mental clouding, gait, and fine-hand movements disturbances. EEG shows diffuse slowing. MRI may show bilateral symmetric basal ganglia T2 hyperintensity and T1 hypointensity with oedematous reaction.[101] Resolution evolves over weeks to months of thiamine supplementation.[99,101] Dialysis dementia is marked by dysarthria, dysphasia, dysgraphia, dyspraxia, ataxia, apathy, depression, myoclonus, seizures, paranoid delusions, and eventual immobilization and mutism. It was common before 1980 owing to intoxication by aluminum contaminating the dialysate and used to bind the dietary phosphate. Nowadays, dialysate aluminum concentration below 20 ug/L and use of aluminum-free phosphate binders prevent it.[77,103] Subdural hematoma is caused by rapid ultrafiltration and use of hypertonic dialysate.[7] Sudden visual loss is a rare complication of HD associated to anemia, dehydration, and hypotension resulting in ischemic optic neuropathy. In anterior ischemic optic neuropathy, ophthalmoscopy shows pale optic disks with blurred margins and retinal hemorrhage. Fluorescein may show peripapillary leakage. Posterior ischemic optic neuropathy shows normal optic disk at onset, with pallor appearing within 4 to 8 weeks.[104–106]

Mononeuropathies, particularly CTS, are due to β2-microglobulin amyloidosis in long term HD patients. It's due to abolished renal clearance of β2-microglobulin and chronic inflammation (bioincompatibility, contaminate dialysate, catheter use).[107] Wrist arteriovenous fistula are also risk factors for developing a homolateral CTS.[108]

PD

Rare instances of acute sensorimotor PN mainly in diabetic patients treated by PD have been reported.[47] Osmotic icodextrin used in PD may mask hypoglycemia, predisposing to hypoglycemic coma.[109] PD high glucose content may contribute to hyperosmolar coma in diabetic patients.[11,110]

RT

Encephalopathy, seizures and movement disorders combining cerebellar and extrapyramidal signs may derive from direct immunosuppressant neurotoxicity and disruption of blood-brain barrier causing axonal swelling, extracellular edema, demyelination due to inflammation or to thrombotic microangiopathy, ultimately leading to reversible posterior leukoencephalopathy.[111–113] Neoplasms are relatively common in RT patients exposed to immunosuppressants, especially malignant meningioma and primary central nervous system lymphoma. Most of these are of B-cell origin and contain Epstein-Barr virus antigens. Ceasing immunosuppressant, radiotherapy, surgery, acyclovir, and monoclonal antilymphoma immunotherapy are useful. Incidence of brain metastatic cancer is increased.[20,77,114,115] Opportunistic infections caused by bacteria and mycobacteria such as *Nocardia asteroids*, *Listeria monocytogenes*, *Mycobacterium tuberculosis*, or fungi such as *Cryptococcus neoformans*, *Aspergillus fumigatus*, or *Paracoccidioides* cause meningitis, encephalitis, myelitis, or brain abscess.[7,19] Protozoa infection by *Toxoplasma gondii* and *Trypanosoma cruzi* (Chagas disease) may cause meningoencephalitis.[116,117] JC virus causes progressive multifocal leukoencephalopathy (dementia, ataxia, visual and focal deficits, and maybe vegetative state).[118] Immunosuppressants enhance immune-related atherosclerosis.[7] Acute femoral neuropathy presents in 2% of RT patients as thigh weakness and pain or sensory deficit on thigh and inner calf, due to peroperative compression by retractors or to nerve ischemia.[7,46]

SUMMARY

Renal disease may cause nervous system involvement through several mechanisms including toxic metabolic accumulation, hyperkalemia, hypercoagulability, immunologic disturbances, and tubular acido-basic disequilibrium, among others. Clinical symptoms usually indicate severe renal dysfunction, but subtle abnormalities may occur. Judiciously tailored renal replacement therapy may avoid these complications, whereas others may emerge from these very therapies, with overlapping clinical pictures. This makes an already complex management of renal patients even more difficult and asks for tight collaboration between nephrologists and neurologists.

REFERENCES

1. Himmelfarb J, Hakim RM. Oxidative stress in uremia. Curr Opin Nephrol Hypertens 2003;12:593–8.
2. Deng G, Vaziri ND, Jabbari B, et al. Increased tyrosine nitration in the brain in chronic renal insufficiency: reversal by antioxidant therapy and angiotensin-converting enzyme inhibitors. J Am Soc Nephrol 2001;12:1892–9.

3. Fukagawa M. Cell biology of parathyroid hyperplasia in uremia. Am J Med Sci 1999;317(6):377–82.
4. Figueiredo WM, Oliveira-Souza RO, Figueiredo RB, et al. Cognitive and psychomotor slowing in chronic hemodialysis patients. Arq Neuropsiquiatr 2007; 65(3-B):875–9.
5. Murray AM, Tupper DE, Knopman DS, et al. Cognitive impairment in hemodialysis patients is common. Neurology 2006;67:216–23.
6. Kurella M, Mapes DL, Port FK, et al. Correlates and outcomes of dementia among dialysis patients: the Dialysis Outcome and Practice Patterns Study. Nephrol Dial Transplant 2006;21(9):2543–8.
7. Brouns R, Deyn PP. Neurological complications in renal failure: a review. Clin Neurol Neurosurg 2004;107:1–16.
8. Aminoff MJ. Electroencephalography: general principles and clinical applications. In: Aminoff MJ, editor. Electrodiagnosis in clinical neurology. 4th edition. Chapter 3. Churchill Livingstone; 1999. p. 71–2.
9. Niedermeyer E. Metabolic central nervous system disorders. In: Niedermeyer E, Lopes da Silva F, editors. Electroencephalography: basic principles, clinical applications and related fields. 4th edition. Chapter 23. Williams & Wilkins; 1999. p. 420–1.
10. Young GB, Bolton CF. Electrophysiologic evaluation of patients in the intensive care unit. In: Aminoff MJ, editor. Electrodiagnosis in clinical neurology. 4th edition. Chapter 30. Churchill Livingstone; 1999. p. 655–6.
11. Aminoff MJ, Parent JM. Comorbidity in adults. In: Engel, Jr J, Pedley TA, editors. Epilepsy: a comprehensive textbook. Philadelphia-Lippincott-Raven Publishers; 1997. p. 1957–9, 184.
12. Danlami ZT, Obeid T, Awada A, et al. Absence status: an overlooked cause of acute confusion in hemodialysis patients. J Nephrol 1998;11:146–7.
13. Palmer CA. Neurologic manifestations of renal disease. Neurol Clin 2002;20: 23–34.
14. Victor M, Ropper A. The acquired metabolic disorders of the nervous system. In: Ropper AH, Brown RJ, editors. Adams and Victor's principles of neurology. 7th edition. New York: McGraw-Hill; 2001. p. 1184–90.
15. Hernandez CM, Núñez FA, Mesa LT, et al. Reversible posterior leukoencephalopathy syndrome in patients with immunosuppressive treatment: report of four cases. Rev Med Chil 2008;136(1):93–8.
16. Martínez-Rodríguez JE, Barriga FJ, Santamaria J, et al. Nonconvulsive status epilepticus associated with cephalosporins in patients with renal failure. Am J Med 2001;111:115–9.
17. Alpay H, Altun O, Biyikh NK. Cefepime-induced non-convulsive status epilepticus in a peritoneal dialysis patient. Pediatr Nephrol 2004;19:445–7.
18. Tattevin P, Messiaen T, Pras V, et al. Confusion and general seizures following ciprofloxacin administration. Nephrol Dial Transplant 1998;13:2712–3.
19. Nampoory MRN, Khan ZU, Johny KV, et al. Nocardiosis in renal transplant recipients in Kuwait. Nephrol Dial Transplant 1996;11:1134–8.
20. Lacerda G, Krummel T, Sabourdy C, et al. Optimizing therapy of seizures in renal and hepatic dysfunction. Neurology 2006;67(Suppl 4):S28–33.
21. Wang HC, Hsu JL, Shen YY. Acute bilateral basal ganglia lesions in patients with diabetic uremia: an FDG-PET study. Clin Nucl Med 2004;29:475–8.
22. Li JY, Yong TY, Sebben R, et al. Bilateral basal ganglia lesions in patients with end-stage diabetic nephropathy. Nephrology (Carlton) 2008;13(1): 68–72.

23. Park JH, Kim HJ, Kim SM. Acute chorea with bilateral basal ganglia lesions in diabetic uremia. Can J Neurol Sci 2007;34:248–50.
24. Stripoli GF, Montinaro V, Manno C, et al. Chorea in hemodialysis: is chorea just a neurological syndrome or is it related to uremia or dialysis? G Ital Nefrol 2002; 19(5):575–84.
25. Go AS, Chertow GM, Fan D, et al. Chronic kidney disease and the risks of death, cardiovascular events, and hospitalization. N Engl J Med 2004;351:1296–305.
26. Koren-Morag N, Goldbourt U, Tanne D. Renal dysfunction and risk of ischemic stroke or TIA in patients with cardiovascular disease. Neurology 2006;67:224–8.
27. Wanamethee SG, Shaper AG, Perry IJ. Serum creatinine concentrationand risk of cardiovascular disease: a possible marker for increased risk of stroke. Stroke 1997;28:557–63.
28. De Leeuw PW, Thijs L, Birhenhäger WH, et al. Systolic hypertension in Europe(syst-eur)trial investigation. Prognostic significance of renal function in elderly patients with isolated systolic hypertension: results from the syst-eur trial. J Am Soc Nephrol 2002;13:2213–22.
29. Zamora E, Lupón J, Urrutia A, et al. Prognostic significance of creatinine clearance rate in patients with heart failure and normal serum creatinine. Rev Esp Cardiol 2007;60(12):1315–8.
30. Weiner DE, Tighiouart H, Amin MG, et al. Chronic kidney disease as a risk factor for cardiovascular disease and all-cause mortality: a pooled analysis of community-based studies. J Am Soc Nephrol 2004;15:1307–15.
31. Kobayashi M, Hirawa N, Yatsu K, et al. Relationship between silent brain infarction and chronic kidney disease. Nephrol Dial Transplant 2009;24(1):201–7.
32. Vlagopoulos PT, Tighiouart H, Weiner DE, et al. Anemia as a risk factor for cardiovascular disease and all-cause mortality in diabetes: the impact of chronic kidney disease. J Am Soc Nephrol 2005;16(11):3403–10.
33. Block GA, Klassen PS, Lazarus JM, et al. Mineral metabolism, mortality, and morbidity in maintenance hemodyalisis. J Am Soc Nephrol 2004;15:2208–18.
34. Papachistou FT, Petridou SH, Pritza NG, et al. Superior sagittal sinus thrombosis in steroid-resistant nephrotic syndrome. Pediatr Neurol 2005;32:282–4.
35. Falk RJ, Jennette JC, Nachman PH. Primary glomerular disease. In: Brenner BM, editor. The kidney. 6th edition. Saunders; 2000. p. 1266–71.
36. Chong Lin C, Chung Lui C, Tain YL. Thalamic stroke secondary to straight sinus thrombosis in a nephrotic child. Pediatr Nephrol 2002;17:184–6.
37. André E, Voisin P, André JL, et al. Hemorrheological and hemostatic parameters in children with nephrotic syndrome undergoing steroid therapy. Nephron 1994; 68(2):184–91.
38. Lilora MI, Velkovski JG, Topalov IB. Thromboembolic complications in children with nephrotic syndrome in Bulgaria (1979–1996). Pediatr Nephrol 2000;15:74–8.
39. Eddy AA, Symous JM. Nephrotic syndrome in childhood. Lancet 2003;362: 629–39.
40. De Saint-Martin A, Terzie J, Chistman D, et al. Superior sagittal sinus thrombosis and nephrotic syndrome: favourable outcome with low-molelular weight heparin. Arch Pediatr 1997;4:849–52.
41. Divekar AA, Ali US, Ronghe MD, et al. Superior sagittal sinus thrombosis in a child wih nephrotic syndrome. Pediatr Nephrol 1996;10:206–7.
42. Arnout MA. Cystic kidney diseases. In: Goldman L, Ausiello D, editors. Cecil textbook of medicine. 22nd edition. Saunders; 2004. p. 767–72.
43. Merlino G, Piani A, Dolso P, et al. Sleep disorders in patients with end-stage renal disease undergoing dialysis therapy. Nephrol Dial Transplant 2006;21:184–90.

44. Bastos JPC, Sousa RB, Nepomuceno LAM, et al. Sleep disturbances in patients on maintence hemodialysis: role of dialysis shift. Rev Assoc Med Bras 2007; 53(6):492–6.
45. Kryger MH. Management of obstructive sleep apnea-hypopnea syndrome: overview. In: Kryger MH, Roth T, Dement WC, editors. Principles and practice of sleep medicine. 3rd edition. Chapter 79. WB Saunders Company; 2000. p. 940–54.
46. Bolton CF. Peripheral neuropathies associated with chronic renal failure. Can J Neurol Sci 1980;7:89.
47. Asbury AK. Uremic neuropathy. In: Dyck PJ, Thomas PK, Lambert EH, editors. Peripheral neuropathy. 1st edition. Chapter 48. WB Saunders Company; 1975. p. 982–92.
48. Krishnan AV, Kiernan MC. Uremic neuropathy: clinical features and new pathological insights. Muscle Nerve 2007;35:273–90.
49. Van Ravenswaaij-Arts CMA, Kollée LAA, Hofman JCW, et al. Heart rate variability. Ann Intern Med 1993;118(6):436–47.
50. Kiernan M, Walters R, Andersen K, et al. Nerve excitability changes in chronic renal failure indicate membrane depolarization due to hyperkalemia. Brain 2002;125:1366–75.
51. Krishnan AV, Phoon RKS, Pussell BA, et al. Altered motor nerve excitability in end-stage kidney disease. Brain 2005;128:2164–74.
52. Kurata C, Uehara A, Ishikawa A. Improvement of cardiac sympathetic innervation by renal transplantation. J Nucl Med 2004;45:1114–20.
53. Keswani SC, Buldanlioglu U, Fischer A, et al. A novel endogenous erythropoietin mediated pathway prevents axonal degeneration. Ann Neurol 2004;56:815–26.
54. Locatelli F, Marcelli D, Conte F, et al. Comparison of mortality in ESRD patients on convective and diffusive extracorporeal treatments [The Registro Lombardo Dialisi E Trapianto]. Kidney Int. 1999;55(1):286–93.
55. Preston DC. Distal median neuropathies. In: Logigian EL, editor. Entrapment and other focal neuropathies. Neurologic Clinics 1999;17(3):407–24.
56. Kothari MJ. Ulnar neuropathy at the wrist. In Logigian EL, editor. Entrapment and other focal neuropathies. Neurologic Clinics 1999;17(3):463–76.
57. Campistol JM. Uremic myopathy. Kidney Int 2002;62(5):1901–13.
58. Feinfeld DA, Kurian B, Cheng JT, et al. Effect of oral l-carnitine on serum myoglobin in hemodialysis patients. Ren Fail 1996;18(1):91–6.
59. Alves FR, de A Quintanilha Ribeiro F. Revision about hearing loss in the Alport's syndrome, analysing the clinical, genetic and biomolecular aspects. Braz J Otorhinolaryngol 2005;71(6):813–9.
60. Kharrat M, Makni K, Kammoun K, et al. Autosomal dominant Alport's syndrome: study of a large Tunisian family. Saudi J Kidney Dis Transpl 2006;17(3):320–5.
61. Mandióroz M, Fernándes-Cadenas I, Montaner J. Neurological manifestations of Fabry disease. Rev Neurol 2006;43:739–45.
62. Tedeschi G, Bonavita S, Banerjek TK, et al. Diffuse central neural involvement in Fabry disease: a proton MRS imaging study. Neurology 1999;52:1663–7.
63. Schiffmann R, Askari H, Timmons M, et al. Weakly enzyme replacement therapy may slow decline of renal function in patients with Fabry disease who are on long-term biweekly dosing. J Am Soc Nephrol 2007;18(5):1368–70.
64. Chesney RW. Specific renal tubular disorders. In: Goldman L, Ausiello D, editors. Cecil textbook of medicine. 22nd edition. Saunders; 2004. p. 745–50 chapter. 122.
65. Chu CC, Huang CC, Chu NS. Recurrent hypokalemic muscle weakness as an initial manifestation of Wilson's disease. Nephron 1996;73(3):477–9.

66. Kalra V, Khurana D, Mittal R. Wilson's disease—early onset and lessons from a pediatric cohort in India. Indian Pediatr 2000;37(6):595–601.

67. Loi M. Lowe syndrome. Orphanet J Rare Dis 2006;18(1):16.

68. Charnas L, Bernar J, Pezeshkpour GH, et al. MRI findings and peripheral neuropathy in Lowe's syndrome. Neuropediatrics 1988;19(7):7–9.

69. Kraut JA, Sachs G. Hartnup disorder: unraveling the mystery. Trends Pharmacol Sci 2005;26(2):53–5.

70. Bröer S, Caranaugh JA, Resko JE. Neutral amino acid transport in epithelial cells and its malfunction in Hartnup disorder. Biochem Soc Trans 2005;33(Pt 1):233–6.

71. Rodríguez-Soriano J. Bartter and related syndromes: the puzzle is almost solved. Pediatr Nephrol 1998;12(4):315–27.

72. Cruz DN, Shaer AJ, Bia MJ, et al. Gitelman's syndrome revisited. An evaluation of symptoms and health-related quality of life. Kidney Int 2001;59:710–7.

73. Akinci B, Celik A, Saygili F, et al. A case of Gitelman's syndrome presenting with extreme hypokalemia and paralysis. Exp Clin Endocrinol Diabetes 2009;117(2):69–71.

74. Karet FE. Inherited distal renal tubular acidosis. J Am Soc Nephrol 2002;13:2178–84.

75. Comer DM, Droogan AG, Young IS, et al. Hypokalemic paralysis precipitated by distal renal tubular acidosis secondary to Sjögren's syndrome. Case report. Ann Clin Biochem 2008;45:221–5.

76. Fonte KF, Mont'Alverne FJA, Ribeiro EML, et al. Giant aneurysm of the intracavernous internal carotid artery associated with autosomal dominant polycystic kidney disease: case report. Arq Neuropsiquiatr 2006;64(3-D):881–4.

77. Burn DJ, Bates D. Neurology and the kidney. J Neurol Neurosurg Psychiatr 1998;65:810–21.

78. Gerschkovitch R, Sachs D, Clibovsky A, et al. Dentistry, neurology and nephrology: what is the connection? Nephrol Dial Transplant 2006;21:539–40.

79. Ito S, Nezu A, Matsumoto C, et al. Acute disseminated encephalomyelitis and post-streptococcal acute glomerulonephritis. Brain Dev 2002;24:88–90.

80. Bataller L, Graus F, Saiz A, et al. Spanish Opsoclonus-Myoclonus study group. Clinical outcome in adult onset idiopathic or paraneoplastic opsoclonus-myoclonus. Brain 2001;124(Pt 2):437–43.

81. Vigliani MC, Palmucci L, Polo P, et al. Paraneoplastic opsoclonus-myoclonus associated with renal cell carcinoma and responsive to tumor ablation. J Neurol Neurosurg Psychiatr 2001;70(6):814–5.

82. Evans B, Fagan C, Arnold T, et al. Paraneoplastic motor neuron disease and renal cell carcinoma: improvement after nephrectomy. Neurology 1990;40(6):960–2.

83. Cánovas D, Martínez JM, Viguera M, et al. Association of renal carcinoma with neuromyotonia and involvement of inferior motor neuron. Neurologia 2007;22(6):399–400.

84. Ammar H, Brown SH, Malani A, et al. A case of paraneoplasic cerebellar ataxia secondary to renal cell carcinoma. Southampt Med J 2008;101(5):556–7.

85. Bell BB, Tognoni PG, Bihrle R. Limbic encephalitis as a paraneoplastic manifestation of renal cell carcinoma. J Urol 1998;160(3 Pt1):828.

86. Kujawa KA, Niemi VR, Tomasi MA, et al. Ballistic-choreic movements as the presenting feature of renal cancer. Arch Neurol 2001;58:1133–5.

87. Roy MJ, May EF, Jabbari B. Life-threatening polyneuropathy heralding renal cell carcinoma. Mil Med 2002;167(12):986–9.

88. Solon AA, Gilbert CS, Meyer C. Myopathy as a paraneoplastic manifestation of renal cell carcinoma. Am J Med 1994;97(5):491–2.

89. Aragon Ching JB, Zujewski JA. CNS metastasis: an old problem in a new guise. Clin Cancer Res 2007;13:1644–5.
90. Pallud J, Nataf F, Roujeau T, et al. Intraventricular hemorrhage from a renal cell carcinoma pituitary metastasis. Acta Neurochir 2005;147(9):1003–4.
91. Sadamoto T, Yuki K, Migita K, et al. Solitary brain metastasis from renal cell carcinoma 15 years after nephrectomy: case report. Neurol Med Chir 2005; 45(8):423–7.
92. Such B, La Rochelle JC, Klatte T, et al. Brain metastasis from renal cell carcinoma: presentation, reccurrence and survival. Cancer 2008;113(7):1641–8.
93. Kuruvath S, Naidu S, Battacharyya M, et al. Spinal metastasis from renal cell carcinoma, 31 years following nephrectomy—case report. Clin Neuropathol 2007;26(4):176–9.
94. Alfieri A, Mazzoleni G, Schwartz A, et al. Renal cell carcinoma and intradural spinal metastasis with cauda equina infiltration: case report. Spine 2005; 30(1):161–3.
95. Varin S, Faure A, Bouc P, et al. Endoneurial metastasis of the sciatic nerve disclosing the relapse of a renal carcinoma, four years after its surgical treatment. Joint Bone Spine 2006;73(6):760–2.
96. Jhamb R, Gupta N, Garg S, et al. Diffuse lymphomatous infiltration of kidneys presenting as renal tubular acidosis and hypokalemic paralysis: case report. Croat Med J 2007;48:860–3.
97. Rosenbaum RB, Campbell SM, Rosenbaum JT. Clinical neurology of rheumatic disease. Butterworth-Heinemann; 1996. Chapter 8:135–162; Chapter 9:163–179; Chapter 11: 195–235.
98. Attur RP, Kandavar R, Kadavigere P, et al. Dialysis disequilibrium syndrome presenting as a focal neurological deficit. Hemodial Int 2008;12(3):313–5.
99. Hung SC, Hung SH, Tarng DC, et al. Thiamine deficiency and unexplained encephalopathy in hemodialysis and peritoneal dialysis patients. Am J Kidney Dis 2001;38:941–7.
100. Masafumi I, Toshiko I, Yanagihara C, et al. Wernicke's encephalopathy associated with hemodialysis: report of two cases and review of the literature. Clin Neurol Neurosurg 1999;101:118–21.
101. Zeir MG. The suddenly speechless florist on chronic dialysis: the unexpected threats of a flower shop? Nephrol Dial Tranplant 2006;21:223–5.
102. Descombes F, Dessibourg CA, Fellay G. Acute encephalopathy due to thiamine deficiency (Wernicke's encephalopathy) in a chronic hemodialysed patient: a case report. Clin Nephrol 1991;35:171–5.
103. Rob PM, Niederstadt C, Reusche E. Dementia in patients undergoing long-term dialysis: aetiology, differential diagnosis, epidemiology and management. CNS Drugs 2001;15(9):691–9.
104. Buono LM, Foroozan R, Savino PJ, et al. Posterior ischemic optic neuropathy after hemodialysis. Ophthalmology 2003;110:1216–8.
105. Servilla KS, Groggel GC. Anterior ischemic optic neuropathy as a complication of hemodialysis. Am J Kidney Dis 1986;8:61–3.
106. Basile C, Addabbo G, Montanaro A. Anterior ischemic optic neuropathy and dialysis: role of hypotension and anemia. J Nephrol 2001;14(5):420–3.
107. Kiss E, Keusch G, Zanetti M, et al. Dialysis-related amyloidosis revisited. Am J Roentgenol 2005;185(6):1460–7.
108. Gousheh J, Iranpour A. Association between carpal tunnel syndrome and arteriovenous fistula in hemodialysis patients. Plast Reconstr Surg 2005; 116(2):508–13.

109. Disse E, Thivolet C. Hypoglycemic coma in a diabetic patient on peritoneal dialysis due to interference of icodextrin metabolites with capillary blood glucose measurements. Diabetes Care 2004;27(9):2279.
110. Emder PJ, Howard NJ, Rosenberg AR. Non-ketotic hyperosmolar diabetic pre-coma due to pancreatitis in a boy on continuous ambulatory peritoneal dialysis. Nephron 1986;44(4):355–7.
111. Hinchey J, Chaves C, Appignani B, et al. A reversible posterior leukoencephal-opathy syndrome. N Engl J Med 1996;334(8):494–500.
112. Kaleyias J, Fauber E, Kothare SV. Tacrolimus induced subacute cerebellar ataxia. Europ J Paediatr Neurol 2006;10(2):86–9.
113. Yardimci N, Colak T, Sevmis S, et al. Neurologic complications after renal trans-plant. Exp Clin Transplant 2008;6(3):224–8.
114. Caillard S, Lachat V, Moulin B. Postransplant lymphoproliferative disorders in renal allograft recipients: report of 53 cases of a French multicenter study: PTLD French working group. Transpl Int 2000;13(Suppl 1):S388–93.
115. Tubman DE, Frick MB, Hanto DW. Lymphoma after organ transplantation: radiologic manifestations in the central nervous system, thorax and abdomen. Radiology 1983;149(3):625–31.
116. Jardim E, Takayanagui OM. Chagasic meningoencephalitis with detection of *Trypanosoma cruzi* in the cerebrospinal fluid of an immunodepressed patient. J Trop Med Hyg 1994;97(6):367–70.
117. Ferreira MS, Borges AS. Some aspects of protozoan infections in immunocom-promised patients—a review. Mem Inst Oswaldo Cruz 2002;97(4):443–57.
118. Crowder CD, Gyure KA, Drachenberg CB, et al. Successful outcome of progressive multifocal leukoencephalopathy in a renal transplant patient. Am J Transplant 2005;5(5):1151–8.

Neurologic Manifestations of Systemic Lupus Erythematosus in Children and Adults

Eyal Muscal, MD[a], Robin L. Brey, MD[b],*

KEYWORDS

- Collagen vascular disease • Systemic lupus erythematosus
- Neurologic disease • Autoantibodies • Cognitive dysfunction

Among the collagen vascular diseases neurologic manifestations have been most commonly recognized and well-studied in systemic lupus erythematosus (SLE, lupus). Neurologic manifestations are less prevalent in other systemic inflammatory and auto-immune disorders. Rheumatoid arthritis (RA) in adults, an erosive and potentially deforming inflammatory arthritis, has been associated with peripheral neuropathy, brain stem and spinal cord compression caused by a mass effect from pannus formation in the vertebral joints, and stroke caused by premature atherosclerotic vascular disease. Sjogren syndrome, characterized by dry eyes and dry mouth, has been associated with hemispheric and spinal cord lesions that can mimic the clinical and neuroradiographic features of multiple sclerosis. Scleroderma, characterized by skin hardening and fibrosis, may lead to peripheral neuropathy and trigeminal neuralgia in its systemic form (systemic sclerosis). This review focuses on the clinical presentation, pathophysiology, and treatment strategies of neuropsychiatric lupus (NPSLE) in children and adults.

SLE affects multiple organ systems in women 9 times more frequently than men. The prevalence is approximately 130/100,000 in the United States, with African Americans, Hispanics, and Asians more frequently affected than non-Hispanic whites.[1] The nervous system is commonly affected in children and adults with SLE,[2–7] is also

a Division of Pediatric Rheumatology, Texas Children's Hospital/Baylor College of Medicine, 6621 Fannin Street MC 3-2290, Houston, TX 77030, USA
b Department of Neurology, University of Texas Health Science Center at San Antonio, 7703 Floyd Curl Drive, Mail Code # 7883, San Antonio, TX 78229-3900, USA
* Corresponding author.
E-mail address: brey@uthscsa.edu (R.L. Brey).

Neurol Clin 28 (2010) 61–73
doi:10.1016/j.ncl.2009.09.004
0733-8619/09/$ – see front matter © 2010 Published by Elsevier Inc.

associated with a worse prognosis and more cumulative damage in children[4] and adults.[5,8] Neuropsychiatric lupus (NPSLE) manifestations can occur in the absence of either serologic activity or other systemic disease manifestations.[4] The American College of Rheumatology (ACR) established case definitions for 19 central and peripheral nervous system syndromes listed in **Box 1**.[9] Some of these are rarely seen in patients with SLE, and all occur in diseases other than SLE. Studies attempting to link NPSLE manifestations to underlying SLE-specific pathophysiologic processes are ongoing.

Box 1
Neuropsychiatric syndromes associated with SLE

NPSLE associated with the central nervous system
- Aseptic meningitis
- Cerebrovascular disease

  Stroke

  Transient ischemic attack

  Cerebral venous sinus thrombosis
- Cognitive disorders

  Delirium (acute confusional state)

  Dementia

  Mild cognitive impairment
- Demyelinating syndromes
- Headaches

  Tension headaches

  Migraine headaches
- Movement disorders (chorea)
- Psychiatric disorders

  Psychosis

  Mood disorders

  Anxiety disorder
- Seizure disorders
- Transverse myelopathy

NPSLE associated with peripheral nervous system
- Autonomic neuropathy
- Myasthenia gravis
- Peripheral neuropathy
- Sensorineural hearing loss

  Sudden onset

  Progressive

Cranial neuropathy

CLINICAL MANIFESTATIONS OF SLE
Prevalence of NPSLE Manifestations in Adults and Children

In adults, approximately 28% to 40% of NPSLE manifestations develop before or around the time of the diagnosis of SLE.[5] Estimates of the prevalence of NPSLE have ranged from 14% to more than 80% in adults[2,5,10–12] and 22% to 95% in children.[4,6,7,13,14] A retrospective study of NPSLE in 185 Chinese children in a 20-year period found that 11% had NPSLE manifestations at the time of diagnosis and an additional 16% developed them within 1 year. The mortality rate in this study was 45% in children with NPSLE and 17.4% in those without these manifestations.[7] A more recent prospective study of 256 pediatric SLE patients from Toronto followed for approximately 4 years confirmed the morbidity and cumulative organ damage associated with NPSLE manifestations; however, in this study only 6 patients (2.3%) died during the follow-up period.[14] The ethnic distribution of the children in this study was not given, and in adults, African American, Hispanic, and Asian SLE patients have a higher SLE-related disease morbidity, possibly contributing to the discrepant findings.

NPSLE in Adults

The ACR case definitions do not include the term "lupus cerebritis," which unfortunately continues to be misused for SLE patients with central nervous system (CNS) symptoms rather than more specific diagnostic terms.[9] Studies in adults using the ACR case definitions collectively have detected the presence of 14 to 17 of the 19 NPSLE syndromes and reported a fairly consistent prevalence of the following syndromes: total spectrum of headache (39%–61%), seizures (8%–18%), cerebrovascular disease (2%–8%), psychosis (3%–5%), cranial neuropathy (1.5%–2.1%), and movement disorder (1%). The range in the prevalence of mood disorders and cognitive dysfunction is much wider, with studies using systematic assessment of cognitive and psychiatric function finding a higher prevalence[2,5,10,15,16] than studies that only evaluated patients using sensitive instruments if "clinically indicated."[5] These studies testing cognitive function in every patient using sensitive psychiatric and neuropsychological instruments found the prevalence of the total spectrum of mood disorders to be between 69% and 74%, and the total range of cognitive disorders to be between 75% and 80%. In contrast, the study that did not do standardized psychiatric or cognitive assessments found that only 12.4% had mood disorder and 5.4% had evidence of cognitive dysfunction.[5] The number of patients reported with moderate to severe cognitive dysfunction in most studies is 25% to 40%, suggesting that the failure to test all patients in that study may have underestimated clinically important cognitive dysfunction.

The frequency of NPSLE in this large inception cohort study was 28% (158 of 572 patients), lower than other studies; the occurrence of neuropsychiatric events was associated with reduced quality of life and increased organ damage, irrespective of whether the particular event was judged to be SLE-related or not.[5] Whether or not this association strengthens or becomes more specific with time is currently being investigated, as more patients are being recruited and followed. Some additional information has been published recently by this group on short-term outcomes of NPSLE events on their inception cohort.[17] The maximum time of observation for determining short-term outcomes was 21 months (from up to 6 months before SLE diagnosis and up to 15 months after SLE diagnosis). Outcomes were determined using a physician-generated Likert score: death (1), much worse (2), worse (3), no change (4), improved (5), much improved (6), and resolved (7). Thus far, 271 (33.5%) of 890 patients had at least 1 NPSLE event and 90 had 2 or more events that included 15 different NPSLE syndromes (see **Box 1** for a complete list of the ACR NPSLE case definitions). The investigators found that 16.5% to 33.9% of the events (depending on which manifestation was being considered) were attributable directly to SLE and the remainder were caused by other concomitantly existing conditions. Short-term outcomes for patients with a neurologic event attributed to SLE were better than for those with an event not attributed to SLE. These data highlight an important clinical issue in caring for SLE patients with NPSLE manifestations; the ability to definitively attribute the neurologic manifestations appropriately is of paramount importance for diagnosis and treatment decisions.

A study from Hong Kong examined the direct and indirect costs of SLE in adults to determine the relationship between NPSLE and disease costs.[12] The overall prevalence of NPSLE in this cohort was 27%, with the most common manifestations being seizures and stroke. Patients with NPSLE in this study incurred twice the total disease-related costs than those without NPSLE manifestations, strengthening the need to find better treatment strategies to limit NPSLE-related disease activity and cumulative organ damage.

NPSLE in Children

There have been few comprehensive studies on NPSLE features and prevalence rates in children and adolescents. A reliance on adult data to understand NPSLE in childhood-onset lupus may ignore potential immunologic and brain structural differences between adults and children with the disease.[18] Neurologic involvement seems to be more severe in children who may accrue permanent organ damage at higher rates than adults.[19–21] In an older prospective study of NPSLE in children, nervous system manifestations were more common in a 6-year study period than glomerulonephritis (95% vs 55%, $P \leq .0001$).[6] The most prevalent NPSLE syndromes in this longitudinal study included headaches in 72% of children, mood disorder in 57%, cognitive dysfunction in 55%, seizure disorder in 51%, acute confusional disorder in 35%, peripheral nervous system impairment in 15%, psychosis in 12%, and stroke in 12%. The more recent prospective study of 256 children with SLE already mentioned confirmed the contribution of glomerulonephritis and nervous system manifestations in SLE-related morbidity over time.[14] A literature review of NPSLE in pediatric patients, with some contribution from the author's own clinical experience, concluded that long-term outcomes for pediatric patients with NPSLE was excellent, and confirmed Hiraki and colleagues'[14] finding of high overall survival (97%). However, in this study, patients who presented with seizures or stroke and had a high cumulative disease activity rate or frequent CNS flares were at higher risk for long-term nervous system damage. A study from Belgium comparing pediatric and adult SLE patients found that pediatric patients had more frequent renal disease and encephalopathy than adults.[22]

A retrospective study of NPSLE in children in the San Francisco area also found that NPSLE manifestations were common, occurred early in the course of the disease, and were not necessarily associated with disease activity outside the nervous system.[4] This was the first study to systematically assess the link between aPL and NPSLE manifestations in children. Although the presence of antiphospholipid antibodies was seen in 70% of children in this study (compared with approximately 25%–30% in adult SLE patients), the association of these antibodies with NPSLE was weak with the exception of cerebrovascular disease. The investigators suggest that there may be a different underlying pathophysiologic mechanism for noncerebrovascular NPSLE manifestations in children compared with adults, however, cognitive dysfunction, a manifestation that has been strongly linked to aPL in adults, was not systematically studied in these pediatric patients. This may have led to an underestimation of the importance of aPL overall in relation to NPSLE manifestations in children.

There are sparse data on neurocognitive impairment in children with SLE. Unlike adults with lupus, there is no validated clinical or research neuropsychologic testing battery for children with the disease. The few studies that have assessed neurocognitive status in children with SLE did not investigate for concurrent structural brain abnormalities. The Mini-Mental Status Examination (MMSE), known for its low sensitivity outside of dementia, showed a 55% prevalence rate of neurocognitive deficits in a total of 75 children.[6] In a 1990 study, 21 pediatric lupus patients had lower complex problem-solving scores compared with 11 patients with juvenile arthritis.[23] A recent study reported neurocognitive impairment in 59% (16 of 27) of children without previously diagnosed NPSLE.[24] The true prevalence rate and impact of neurocognitive impairment on academic performance and health-related quality of life status of children with lupus is still unknown.

More work is certainly needed in pediatric and adult SLE populations to better understand the underlying pathophysiology of NPSLE manifestations, and the similarities and differences between children and adults that may be important in treatment considerations.

PATHOPHYSIOLOGY AND PATHOGENESIS

The pathogenic causes of NPSLE manifestations are likely to be multifactorial and may involve autoantibody production, microangiopathy, intrathecal production of proinflammatory cytokines, and premature atherosclerosis.[25] Cellular and parenchymal changes in lupus murine models include neuronal cytotoxicity and atrophy of dendritic spines.[26] Cerebral spinal fluid from lupus-prone mice and adult patients with NPSLE reduce the viability of proliferating neural cell lines.[27] Postmortem histopathologic studies reveal a wide range of brain abnormalities caused by multifocal microinfarcts, cortical atrophy, gross infarcts, hemorrhage, ischemic demyelination, and patchy multiple sclerosis–like demyelination in people with SLE.[28] A microvasculopathy which was formerly attributed to deposition of immune complexes but is now suspected to arise from activation of complement, seems to be the most common microscopic brain findings in SLE.[29] Consistent with these small vessel changes, single photon emission computer tomography (SPECT) and MR spectroscopy studies suggest that cerebral atrophy and cognitive dysfunction in SLE patients may be related to chronic diffuse cerebral ischemia. However, all of these are nonspecific findings as patients without overt NPSLE manifestations also show these changes[25] and the brain can be pathologically normal in a patient with NPSLE manifestations.[28] This neuropathologic information along with brain imaging data discussed later strongly suggest that SLE may lead to abnormal neurophysiologic changes that are not necessarily accompanied by neuroanatomic abnormalities.

It is becoming clearer that the integrity of the blood-brain barrier is important in SLE-related neuropathology.[30] Processes leading to brain dysfunction in SLE probably involve abnormal endothelial-white blood cell interactions that allow proteins or cells access to the CNS. This may be a mechanism whereby autoantibody-mediated CNS effects can occur (see later discussion). Vascular endothelial cells can be stimulated by proinflammatory cytokines or autoantibodies that up-regulate the expression of adhesion proteins on their surface facilitating lymphocyte entry into the CNS.[31] Soluble serum levels of ICAM-1 increase with systemic disease activity in patients with SLE, for example, and normalize with remission,[32] strengthening the hypothesis that activated endothelial cells and a lack of integrity of the blood-brain barrier might be important requisites for disease activity in the brain.[33] Damage to the blood-brain barrier has also been suggested to be a risk factor for corticosteroid-induced psychiatric disorders in SLE.[34]

Various autoantibodies have been implicated in NPSLE manifestations, but the evidence is not consistent in all studies. Antiphospholipid antibodies (aPL), 1 of the most frequently studied, are a heterogeneous group of autoantibodies linked to thrombosis, recurrent fetal loss, and various neurologic manifestations in patients with and without SLE. The European Working Party on SLE studied the morbidity and mortality in patients with SLE for a 10-year period in a cohort of 1000 patients.[35] This is the best study of the risk of thrombotic events and aPL antibodies in people with SLE. At the beginning of this study, there were 204 (20.4%) patients with aCL IgG, 108 (10.8%) patients with aCL IgM, and 94 (9.4%) patients with lupus anticoagulant (LA). Thromboses were the most common cause of death in the last 5 years of follow-up and were always associated with antiphospholipid syndrome. The most common thrombotic events in these patients were strokes (11.8%), followed by myocardial infarction (7.4%), and pulmonary embolism (5.9%). This suggests an important role for aPL and recurrent thrombosis in patients with SLE.

aPL increases have also been associated with several different patterns of cognitive dysfunction in patients with SLE, depending on the study. Verbal memory deficits, decreased psychomotor speed, and decreased cognitive efficiency or productivity have all been significantly correlated to increased aPL levels in adult patients.

Three longitudinal studies have evaluated the relationship between serially obtained aPL levels and cognitive dysfunction in SLE patients.[3,36,37] All studies demonstrated that cognitive dysfunction was significantly associated with persistently positive aPL. Menon and colleagues[37] reported that SLE patients with persistently increased IgG aCL levels over a period of 2 to 3 years performed significantly worse than SLE patients with occasionally increased or never increased titers on various neuropsychological tests. These results were not observed with anti-DNA antibody titers or C3 (complement) levels. Attention, concentration, and psychomotor speed were the domains most affected. Hanly and colleagues[36] followed 51 female SLE patients for a 5-year period and found that persistent aCL IgG increases were associated with decreased psychomotor speed, whereas persistent aCL IgA increases were correlated with problems with executive functioning and reasoning abilities. They also found no association between cognitive deficits and anti-DNA antibodies. No cross-sectional relationship between cognitive dysfunction and aPL was found in this same population. Our group prospectively studied the relationship between aCL and anti-β2-glycoprotein 1 antibodies in 123 SLE patients for 3 years.[3] Factors significantly associated with cognitive decline were persistently positive aPL levels, prednisone use, diabetes, higher depression scores, and less education.

Anti-glutamate receptor antibodies may also play a role in cognitive dysfunction and psychiatric disease in patients with SLE. Diamond and colleagues[38] first demonstrated that a subset of lupus anti-DNA antibodies cross-reacts with the NR2 glutamate receptor in patients with SLE. This group showed that the NR2 receptor is recognized by murine and human anti-DNA antibodies and that these antibodies mediate apoptotic cell death of neurons in vitro and in vivo. The relationship between anti-glutamate receptor antibodies and NPSLE manifestations in humans with SLE has been conflicting. Most studies report that these antibodies are seen in 25% to 30% of patients with SLE.[39–41] Some studies find no cross-sectional relationship between anti-glutamate receptor antibodies and any specific clinical manifestations or cognitive dysfunction.[41,42] Others have reported an association between anti-glutamate receptor antibodies and cognitive dysfunction and depression,[40] or depression but not cognitive dysfunction.[42] A study by Kowal and colleagues[43] in an animal model suggests that anti-glutamate receptor antibodies are associated with cognitive dysfunction and hippocampal apoptosis only in the presence of disruption of the blood-brain barrier. It is possible that the magnitude and degree of dysfunction of the blood-brain in concert with the type and level of autoantibodies in human patients with SLE may be the determining factor regarding their pathogenicity in the brain.

Associations between autoantibodies, integrity of the blood-brain barrier and childhood NPSLE are not well understood. Lupus-related immune and vascular mechanisms may have different effects on children and adolescents because of impairment of normal developmental milestones. Gray and white matter damage may have more serious effects on patients in whom myelination in frontal structures is still ongoing.[44–46]

LABORATORY EVALUATION

There is no single diagnostic test that is sensitive and specific for SLE-related neuropsychiatric manifestations. The assessment of individual patients is based on clinical neurologic and rheumatologic evaluation, immunoserologic testing, brain imaging, and psychiatric and neuropsychological assessment. These examinations are used to support or refute the clinical diagnostic impression, exclude alternative explanations, and form the basis for prospective monitoring of clinical evolution and response to treatment interventions. An important consideration in the diagnostic approach to a patient with possible NPSLE manifestations is whether the particular clinical syndrome is caused by SLE-mediated organ dysfunction, a secondary phenomenon related to infection, medication side effects, or metabolic abnormalities (eg, uremia), or is caused by an unrelated condition. Infection is a major cause of CNS syndromes in hospitalized SLE patients.[47] Thus, it is always important to suspect infection in patients with SLE and CNS manifestations.

BRAIN IMAGING

Appenzeller and colleagues[48] have demonstrated a reduction in cerebral and corpus callosum volumes in adult SLE patients that are associated with disease duration and cognitive impairment and other CNS manifestations, but not total corticosteroid dose or the presence of aPL. Focal neurologic and neuropsychologic symptoms of SLE-related stroke correlate with structural magnetic resonance imaging (MRI) abnormalities. Using structural MRI, the majority (40%–80%) of abnormalities in NPSLE are small focal lesions concentrated in periventricular and subcortical white matter.[49] Cortical atrophy, ventricular dilation, diffuse white matter, and gross infarctions are also common. MRI reveals multiple discrete white matter lesions in periventricular, cortical/subcortical junction, and frontal lobe more commonly in patients with past NPSLE manifestations than in SLE patients without a history of NPSLE.[49,50] Disease duration, total corticosteroid dose, and a greater number of CNS manifestations, including isolated cognitive impairment, have been associated with hippocampal atrophy in patients with SLE.[51] A progression of hippocampal atrophy was associated with total corticosteroid dose and the number of NPSLE events in this study. These results complement the results using passive anti-glutamate receptor antibody infusion in mice with a disrupted blood-brain barrier, in whom hippocampal apoptosis was seen.[43] Brain MRI abnormalities were recently reported by our group in a consecutive cohort of 97 adult SLE patients enrolled within 9 months of diagnosis.[52] Brain atrophy was seen in 18% and focal lesions in 8% of patients, which suggests that the brain may be affected early in the course of SLE, even before the diagnosis of SLE is made; although perhaps worsened by high cumulative corticosteroid dose and NPSLE events, the development of brain atrophy and focal lesions is not dependent on these factors.

Visually analyzed fluorodeoxyglucose (FDG)-positron emission tomography (PET) consistently reveals abnormalities in prefrontal, parietal (inferior and superior), parietooccipital, posterior temporal, and occipital gray and white matter regions in active and quiescent NPSLE. Prefrontal, anterior cingulated, and inferior parietal white matter abnormalities have been seen during acute NPSLE but not during quiescent NPSLE. The metabolic disturbances in parietooccipital (peritrigonal) white matter remain an intriguing finding. Approximately 60% to 80% of active NPSLE patients consistently show bilateral parietooccipital white matter FDG-PET hypometabolism in the context of normal conventional MRI and no other PET abnormalities.[48]

Magnetic resonance spectroscopy (MRS) has revealed neurometabolic abnormalities even in white and gray matter that appears normal on conventional MRI.[53] Such abnormalities are believed to reflect neuronal injury or loss and demyelination and have been found during active and quiescent periods of NPSLE manifestations.[54] Kazora and colleagues[53] found a correlation between changes in cerebral white matter by MRS and cognitive impairment in SLE patients, even in the absence of overt NPSLE symptoms. Small cross-sectional studies on adults revealed white matter changes on diffusion tensor imaging (DTI, an MRI tool that assesses white matter microstructure) in patients with NPSLE and normal conventional MRIs. Lupus patients had findings suggestive of abnormal white matter integrity in frontal tracts, corpus callosal areas, and thalamus in these studies.[55,56] Measures of cerebral atrophy also correlated with markers of axonal and myelin loss on MRS and magnetization transfer imaging (MTI) in adult patients.[57] Data from DTI, MTI, and quantitative volumetric studies suggest that some of these newer imaging techniques may have promise as surrogates for CNS damage, and could be used as biomarkers in treatment trials.

There have been few prospective neuroimaging studies in children with SLE. Small prospective pediatric studies show cerebral atrophy and white matter lesions on traditional MRI, as has been seen in adult patients. SPECT brain abnormalities have been seen in pediatric SLE patients. However, a correlation between NPSLE manifestations and SPECT findings were not clearly evident[58]; the number of children studied was low (N = 7) and the neurologic manifestations were multiple or diffuse, whereas the SPECT abnormalities demonstrated focal hypoperfusion defects. Another study examined 24 children with SLE and 20 controls using anatomic brain MRI and MRS.[59] Seventy-five percent of the SLE patients had clinically evident NPSLE manifestations and 46% had abnormal anatomic brain MRI scans (3 in children without NPSLE manifestations). Four children had N-acetylaspartate/creatine (NAA/Cr) ratios that were significantly lower than the controls. Three children with relapses showed a correlation between the disease course and abnormal NAA/Cr ratios. Thus, MRS may be useful in monitoring the disease course and efficacy of pharmacologic treatment in children.

TREATMENT

The management of patients with NPSLE includes symptomatic and immunosuppressive therapies, but evidence for the efficacy of the treatment modalities commonly used is largely limited to uncontrolled clinical trials and anecdotal experience.[60] The key to treatment is to first establish the correct diagnosis by carefully following the guidelines for the diagnosis of NPSLE syndromes in the ACR 1999 case definitions.[9] For many NPSLE syndromes, symptomatic treatment may also be needed in addition to immunomodulatory therapy. Currently in the United States as many as 90% of SLE patients are treated with corticosteroids. Although this is the only FDA-approved drug for the treatment of SLE, evidence suggests that in addition to the well-known side effects of hyperlipidemia, diabetes, hypertensionm and osteopenia, corticosteroids also contribute to long-term morbidity in patients with SLE. Hydroxychloroquine is also commonly used to treat mild disease and seems to be safe to continue during pregnancy. Psychotropic medications (ie, antidepressants and atypical antipsychotics) may have an important adjunctive role in SLE patients with affective or psychotic disorder manifestations. Nonpharmacologic approaches are also important in SLE patients with psychiatric disorders and cognitive dysfunction. Haupt and colleagues[61] demonstrated the ability to improve coping using a novel psychological group intervention. Patients receiving this intervention showed a significant and sustained improvement in several symptoms, such as depression, anxiety, and overall mental burden. The control group, consisting of individuals placed on a waiting list, showed no such improvement.

Cyclophosphamide given as monthly intravenous (500–1000 mg/m^2) doses for a 6-month induction period followed by quarterly maintenance doses for a period of 2 years is a cytotoxic immunosuppressive treatment option with documented therapeutic benefits in the management of severe NPSLE manifestations unresponsive to other treatment modalities (nephritis and CNS manifestations).[62] A small, randomized, controlled clinical trial comparing long-term use of cyclophosphamide and methylprednisolone reported better overall therapeutic control of SLE-related neurologic manifestations (refractory seizures, peripheral and cranial neuropathy, and optic neuritis) with monthly intravenous cyclophosphamide,[63] with a similar incidence of new infections.

High-dose cyclophosphamide (200 mg/m^2), with or without autologous hematopoietic stem-cell transplantation has shown remarkable therapeutic benefits in cases of severe, life-threatening SLE with neuropsychiatric manifestations (and other organ involvement) that had been unresponsive to other treatment. The high-dose cyclophosphamide destroys lymphocytes but not bone marrow stem cells, thus allowing the immune system to be reconstituted with naive cellular elements. All studies of therapeutic modality have been open label and a controlled trial is currently being planned. In the 14 patients studied without stem-cell rescue, about 40% of patients have had a durable remission.[62] Burt and colleagues[64] have recently reported an open-label study of 50 treatment-refractory SLE patients treated with high-dose cyclophosphamide and stem-cell rescue. Intention-to-treat mortality was 2%. With a mean follow-up of 29 months, overall 5-year survival was 84% and the probability of a 5-year disease-free survival was 50%. Secondary analysis demonstrated stabilization of renal function and significant improvement in the SLE disease activity score, antinuclear antibody (ANA), anti-ds DNA, complement, and carbon monoxide lung diffusion capacity adjusted for hemoglobin. Although this represents significant benefit for SLE patients with severe and otherwise refractory disease, it is clearly not a cure for SLE. Fortunately, other drugs, currently in clinical trials, show great promise with potentially fewer side effects. Mycophenolate mofetil has been demonstrated to have a significantly higher complete response rate than intravenous cyclophosphamide in renal lupus and 2 open-label trials of rituximab also suggest benefit.[62]

There have been no published NPSLE treatment trials in pediatric populations. It is unclear whether children may warrant earlier and more aggressive therapies to preclude long-term neurologic sequelae.

SUMMARY

NPSLE manifestations are common in children and adults and a significant source of morbidity and mortality. The adoption of the NPSLE case definitions by the ACR has led to major advances in our ability to study nervous system manifestation of SLE and to identify homogeneous groups of patients from multiple studies for comparison purposes. The integrity of the blood-brain barrier seems to be important in preventing some brain pathology associated with SLE. It is possible that some of the autoantibodies that have been associated with NPSLE manifestations actually require a disrupted blood-brain barrier to exert their effect. Gaining a better understanding of this process should be a concerted focus of future research. Brain imaging is a powerful tool that can be used to better understand structural and functional changes in patients with SLE. It is possible that some of the newer brain imaging modalities will prove useful as biomarkers for SLE-related nervous system damage and for following treatment response.

REFERENCES

1. Danchenko N, Satia JA, Anthony MS. Epidemiology of systemic lupus erythematosus: a comparison of worldwide disease burden. Lupus 2006;15:308–18.
2. Brey RL, Holliday SL, Saklad AR, et al. Neuropsychiatric syndromes in lupus: prevalence using standardized definitions. Neurology 2002;58:1214–20.
3. McLaurin EY, Holliday SL, Williams P, et al. Predictors of cognitive dysfunction in patients with systemic lupus erythematosus. Neurology 2005;64:297–303.
4. Harel L, Sandborg C, Lee T, et al. Neuropsychiatric manifestations in pediatric systemic lupus erythematosus and association with antiphospholipid antibodies. J Rheumatol 2006;33:1873–7.
5. Hanly JG, Urowitz MB, Sanchez-Guerrero J, et al. Neuropsychiatric events at the time of diagnosis of systemic lupus erythematosus: an international inception cohort study. Arthritis Rheum 2007;56:265–73.
6. Sibbitt WL Jr, Brandt JR, Johnson CR, et al. The incidence and prevalence of neuropsychiatric syndromes in pediatric onset systemic lupus erythematosus. J Rheumatol 2002;29:1536–42.
7. Yu HH, Lee JH, Wang LC, et al. Neuropsychiatric manifestations in pediatric systemic lupus erythematosus: a 20-year study. Lupus 2006;15:651–7.
8. Bernatsky S, Clarke A, Gladman DD, et al. Mortality related to cerebrovascular disease in systemic lupus erythematosus. Lupus 2006;15:835–9.
9. The American College of Rheumatology nomenclature and case definitions for neuropsychiatric lupus syndromes. Arthritis Rheum 1999;42:599–608.
10. Ainiala H, Loukkola J, Peltola J, et al. The prevalence of neuropsychiatric syndromes in systemic lupus erythematosus. Neurology 2001;57:496–500.
11. Mikdashi J, Handwerger B. Predictors of neuropsychiatric damage in systemic lupus erythematosus: data from the Maryland lupus cohort. Rheumatology 2004;43:1555–60.
12. Zhu TY, Tam AS, Lee VWY, et al. Systemic lupus erythematosis with neuropsychiatric manifestations incurs high disease costs: a cost-of-illness study in Hong Kong. Rheumatology 2009;48:564–8.
13. Benseler SM, Silverman ED. Neuropsychiatric involvement in pediatric systemic lupus erythematosus. Lupus 2007;16:564–71.
14. Hiraki LT, Benseler SM, Tyrrell PN, et al. Clinical and laboratory characteristics and long-term outcomes of pediatric systemic lupus erythematosus: a longitudinal study. J Pediatr 2008;152:550–6.

15. Petri M, Naqibuddin M, Carson KA, et al. Cognitive function in a systemic lupus erythematosus inception cohort. J Rheumatol 2008;35(9):1776–81.
16. Costallat L, Bertolo M, Appenzeller S. The American College of Rheumatology nomenclature and case definitions for neuropsychiatric lupus syndromes: analysis of 527 patients. Lupus 2001;10:S32.
17. Hanly JG, Urowitz MB, Sanchez-Guerrero J, et al. Short-term outcome of neuropsychiatric events in systemic lupus erythematosus upon enrollment into an international inception cohort study. Arthritis Rheum 2008;59:721–9.
18. Carreno L, Lopez-Longo FJ, Monteagudo I, et al. Immunological and clinical differences between juvenile and adult onset of systemic lupus erythematosus. Lupus 1999;8(4):287–92.
19. Brunner HI, Silverman ED, To T, et al. Risk factors for damage in childhood-onset systemic lupus erythematosus: cumulative disease activity and medication use predict disease damage. Arthritis Rheum 2002;46(2):436–44.
20. Brunner HI, Gladman DD, Ibanez D, et al. Difference in disease features between childhood-onset and adult-onset systemic lupus erythematosus. Arthritis Rheum 2008;58(2):556–62.
21. Tucker LB, Uribe AG, Fernandez M, et al. Adolescent onset of lupus results in more aggressive disease and worse outcomes: results of a nested matched case-control study within LUMINA, a multiethnic US cohort (LUMINA LVII). Lupus 2008;17(4):314–22.
22. Hoffman IEA, Lauwerys BR, DeKeyser F, et al. Juvenile-onset systemic lupus erythemotosis: different clinical and serological pattern than adult-onset systemic lupus erythematosus. Ann Rheum Dis 2009;68:412–5.
23. Papero PH, Bluestein HG, White P, et al. Neuropsychologic deficits and anti-neuronal antibodies in pediatric systemic lupus erythematosus. Clin Exp Rheumatol 1990;8(4):417–24.
24. Brunner HI, Ruth NM, German A, et al. Initial validation of the Pediatric Automated Neuropsychological Assessment Metrics for childhood-onset systemic lupus erythematosus. Arthritis Rheum 2007;57(7):1174–82.
25. Hanly JG. Neuropsychiatric lupus. Curr Rheumatol Rep 2001;3:205–12.
26. Sakic B, Kolb B, Whishaw IQ, et al. Immunosuppression prevents neuronal atrophy in lupus-prone mice: evidence for brain damage induced by autoimmune disease? J Neuroimmunol 2000;111(1–2):93–101.
27. Sakic B, Kirkham DL, Ballok DA, et al. Proliferating brain cells are a target of neurotoxic CSF in systemic autoimmune disease. J Neuroimmunol 2005;169(1–2):68–85.
28. Hanly JG, Walsh NM, Sangalang V. Brain pathology in systemic lupus erythematosus. J Rheumatol 1992;19:732–41.
29. Belmont HM, Abramson SB, Lie JT. Pathology and pathogenesis of vascular injury in systemic lupus erythematosus. Interactions of inflammatory cells and activated endothelium. Arthritis Rheum 1996;39:9–22.
30. Abbott NJ, Mendonca LL, Dolman DE. The blood-brain barrier in systemic lupus erythematosus. Lupus 2003;12:908–15.
31. Zaccagni H, Fried J, Cornell J, et al. Soluble adhesion molecule levels, neuropsychiatric lupus and lupus-related damage. Front Biosci 2004;9:1654–9.
32. Spronk PE, Bootsma H, Huitema MG, et al. Levels of soluble VCAM-1, soluble ICAM-1, and soluble E-selectin during disease exacerbations in patients with systemic lupus erythematosus (SLE); a long term prospective study. Clin Exp Immunol 1994;97:439–44.
33. Ainiala H, Hietaharju A, Dastidar P, et al. Increased serum metalloproteinase 9 levels in systemic lupus erythematosus patients with neuropsychiatric

manifestations and brain magnetic resonance imaging abnormalities. Arthritis Rheum 2004;50:858–65.

34. Nishimura K, Harigai M, Omori M, et al. Blood-brain barrier damage as a risk factor for corticosteroid-induced psychiatric disorders in systemic lupus erythematosus. Psychoneuroendocrinology 2008;33:395–403.

35. Cervera R, Khamashta MA, Font J, et al. Morbidity and mortality in systemic lupus erythematosus during a 10-year period: a comparison of early and late manifestations in a cohort of 1,000 patients. Medicine 2003;82:299–308.

36. Hanly JG, Hong C, Smith S, et al. A prospective analysis of cognitive function and anticardiolipin antibodies in systemic lupus erythematosus. Arthritis Rheum 1999; 42(4):728–34.

37. Menon S, Jameson-Shortall E, Newman Hall-Craggs SP, et al. A longitudinal study of anticardiolipin antibody levels and cognitive functioning in systemic lupus erythematosus. Arthritis Rheum 1999;42(4):735–41.

38. DeGiorgio LA, Konstantinov KN, Lee SC, et al. A subset of lupus anti-DNA antibodies cross-reacts with the NR2 glutamate receptor in systemic lupus erythematosus [comment]. Nat Med 2001;7:1189–93.

39. Husebye ES, Sthoeger ZM, Dayan M, et al. Autoantibodies to a NR2A peptide of the glutamate/NMDA receptor in sera of patients with systemic lupus erythematosus. Ann Rheum Dis 2005;64:1210–3.

40. Omdal R, Brokstad K, Waterloo K, et al. Neuropsychiatric disturbances in SLE are associated with antibodies against NMDA receptors. Eur J Neurol 2005;12: 392–8.

41. Harrison M, Ravdin L, Volpe B, et al. Anti-NR2 antibody does not identify cognitive impairment in a general SLE population. Arthritis Rheum 2004;50: S596.

42. Lapteva L, Nowak M, Yarboro CH, et al. Anti-N-methyl-D-aspartate receptor antibodies, cognitive dysfunction, and depression in systemic lupus erythematosus. Arthritis Rheum 2006;54:2505–14.

43. Kowal C, Degiorgio LA, Lee JY, et al. Human lupus autoantibodies against NMDA receptors mediate cognitive impairment. Proc Natl Acad Sci U S A 2006;103: 19854–9.

44. Klingberg T, Vaidya CJ, Gabrieli JD, et al. Myelination and organization of the frontal white matter in children: a diffusion tensor MRI study. Neuroreport 1999;10(13): 2817–21.

45. Nagy Z, Westerberg H, Klingberg T. Maturation of white matter is associated with the development of cognitive functions during childhood. J Cogn Neurosci 2004; 16(7):1227–33.

46. Filley CM. The behavioral neurology of cerebral white matter. Neurology 1998; 50(6):1535–40.

47. Futrell N, Schultz LR, Millikan C. Central nervous system disease in patients with systemic lupus erythematosus. Neurology 1992;42:1649–57.

48. Appenzeller S, Rondina JM, Li LM, et al. Cerebral and corpus callosum atrophy in systemic lupus erythematosus. Arthritis Rheum 2005;52(9):2783–9.

49. Sibbitt WL Jr, Sibbitt RR, Brooks WM. Neuroimaging in neuropsychiatric systemic lupus erythematosus. Arthritis Rheum 1999;42:2026–38.

50. Abreu MR, Jakosky A, Folgerini M, et al. Neuropsychiatric systemic lupus erythematosus: correlation of brain MR imaging, CT, and SPECT. Clin Imaging 2005; 29:215–21.

51. Appenzeller S, Carnevalle AD, Li LM, et al. Hippocampal atrophy in systemic lupus erythematosus. Ann Rheum Dis 2006;65:1585–9.

52. Petri M, Naqibuddin M, Carson KA, et al. Brain magnetic resonance imaging in newly diagnosed systemic lupus erythematosus. J Rheumatol 2008;35(12): 2348–54.
53. Kozora E, Arciniegas DB, Filley CM, et al. Cognition, MRS neurometabolites, and MRI volumetrics in non-neuropsychiatric systemic lupus erythematosus: preliminary data. Cogn Behav Neurol 2005;18(3):159–62.
54. Chinn RJ, Wilkinson ID, Hall-Craggs MA, et al. Magnetic resonance imaging of the brain and cerebral proton spectroscopy in patients with systemic lupus erythematosus. Arthritis Rheum 1997;40:36–46.
55. Zhang L, Harrison M, Heier LA, et al. Diffusion changes in patients with systemic lupus erythematosus. Magn Reson Imaging 2007;25(3):399–405.
56. Hughes M, Sundgren PC, Fan X, et al. Diffusion tensor imaging in patients with acute onset of neuropsychiatric systemic lupus erythematosus: a prospective study of apparent diffusion coefficient, fractional anisotropy values, and eigenvalues in different regions of the brain. Acta Radiol 2007;48(2):213–22.
57. Bosma GP, Steens SC, Petropoulos H, et al. Multisequence magnetic resonance imaging study of neuropsychiatric systemic lupus erythematosus. Arthritis Rheum 2004;50(10):3195–202.
58. Falcini F, De Cristofaro MT, Ermini M, et al. Regional cerebral blood flow in juvenile systemic lupus erythematosus: a prospective SPECT study. Single photon emission computed tomography. J Rheumatol 1998;25(3):583–8.
59. Mortilla M, Ermini M, Nistri M, et al. Brain study using magnetic resonance imaging and proton MR spectroscopy in pediatric onset systemic lupus erythematosus. Clin Exp Rheumatol 2003;21(1):129–35.
60. O'Neill SG, Schrieber L. Immunotherapy of systemic lupus erythematosus. Autoimmun Rev 2005;4:395–402.
61. Haupt M, Millen S, Janner M, et al. Improvement of coping abilities in patients with systemic lupus erythematosus: a prospective study. Ann Rheum Dis 2005; 64:1618–23.
62. Petri M, Brodsky R. High-dose cyclophosphamide and stem cell transplantation for refractory systemic lupus erythematosus. JAMA 2006;295:559–60.
63. Barile-Fabris L, Ariza-Andraca R, Olguin-Ortega L, et al. Controlled clinical trial of IV cyclophosphamide versus IV methylprednisolone in severe neurological manifestations in systemic lupus erythematosus. Ann Rheum Dis 2005;64(4):620–5.
64. Burt RK, Traynor A, Statkute L, et al. Nonmyeloablative hematopoietic stem cell transplantation for systemic lupus erythematosus. JAMA 2006;295:527–35.

Neurologic Presentations of Gastrointestinal Disease

Ronald F. Pfeiffer, MD

KEYWORDS

- Gastrointestinal • Achalasia • Celiac disease
- Inflammatory bowel disease • Gastric surgery

In recent years, there has been increasing recognition of the presence of gastrointestinal (GI) dysfunction in the setting of neurologic diseases. Parkinson's disease is a particularly well-known example, but GI dysfunction also may occur in multiple sclerosis, stroke, and in various myopathic and peripheral neuropathic processes. There is much less awareness, however, that primary GI diseases may also display neurologic dysfunction as part of their clinical picture. This discourse focuses on some of those disease processes. Illnesses primarily targeting the GI tract are addressed and examples of primary esophageal, gastric, and intestinal disease processes are described. Hepatic dysfunction is addressed elsewhere in this issue, as are nutritional disturbances in which neurologic dysfunction may secondarily occur as a consequence of malabsorption.

ACHALASIA

Achalasia is a rare condition, with an annual incidence rate of approximately 0.5 per 100,000 and prevalence of approximately 8 per 100,000.[1] It is characterized by failure of the lower esophageal sphincter to relax after swallowing and by impaired esophageal peristalsis. The net result of these changes is a functional obstruction of food and liquid at the gastroesophageal junction. Individuals with achalasia experience dysphagia, often with regurgitation of swallowed food. They note a sensation of food being stuck in the throat, which may be accompanied by chest pain. Progressive weight loss frequently occurs. In a significant proportion of individuals with achalasia, dysphagia is actually not the initial clinical symptom.[2] Instead, individuals may initially experience regurgitation or may simply begin to eat more slowly. They may also develop unusual movements or postures, such as arching the neck or raising the arms, to aid in swallowing.

Department of Neurology, University of Tennessee Health Science Center, 855 Monroe Avenue, Memphis, TN 38163, USA
E-mail address: rpfeiffer@utmem.edu

Neurol Clin 28 (2010) 75–87
doi:10.1016/j.ncl.2009.09.007
0733-8619/09/$ – see front matter © 2010 Elsevier Inc. All rights reserved.

The primary pathophysiologic basis for achalasia seems to be loss of inhibitory neurons within the esophageal myenteric plexus that use nitric oxide and vasoactive intestinal polypeptide as neurotransmitters,[3,4] but the cause of the progressive ganglion cell loss is unknown. Viral and immunologic mechanisms have been proposed and a possible autoimmune basis has received the most attention.[5] Some investigators have suggested, however, that a primary neurodegenerative process might also be responsible for the development of achalasia, at least in a portion of patients. Lewy bodies have been documented within the esophageal myenteric plexus of individuals with achalasia and in persons with Parkinson's disease, where they are found primarily in inhibitory vasoactive intestinal polypeptide neurons.[6,7] Neuronal loss within the dorsal motor nucleus of the vagus has also been described in the setting of achalasia.[8] These pathologic abnormalities are also characteristic of Parkinson's disease. Reports of individuals suffering from achalasia and Parkinson's disease have been published.[9,10] Thus, it might be concluded that Parkinson's disease can be a cause of secondary achalasia or that in at least some patients, achalasia and Parkinson's disease share a common etiologic basis.

GASTRIC SURGERY

In the past, gastric surgery was primarily performed as a treatment for ulcer disease. With improved prevention and medical treatment of ulcers, gastric resection surgery is now rarely necessary. Instead, bariatric surgery, performed after failed dietary or medical management of obesity, has become the predominant form of gastric surgery in which neurologic complications may develop. If dietary and medical measures fail, bariatric surgery is considered in individuals with a body mass index of 35 or greater with an obesity-related comorbidity or with a body mass index of 40 or greater without an obesity-related comorbidity.[11]

A variety of surgical procedures have been developed in an effort to induce weight loss. Gastric restriction procedures (gastric stapling and laparoscopic banding) and gastric bypass procedures (Roux-en-Y gastric bypass) are performed most frequently. Neurologic complications may occur after both types.

The frequency with which neurologic complications occur is not entirely clear. Abarbanel and colleagues[12] studied 500 patients who had undergone gastric restriction surgery and noted the development of neurologic complications in 4.6% after 20 months of observation. In another retrospective study, however, 16% of 435 individuals undergoing bariatric surgery developed peripheral neuropathic complications compared with only 3% of 126 patients undergoing cholecystectomy.[13]

A variety of types of neuropathic involvement have been documented after bariatric surgery, including peripheral polyneuropathy, mononeuropathy, and radicular or plexus involvement (**Box 1**).[13] Peripheral polyneuropathy is typically chronic in character, although acute inflammatory demyelinating neuropathy has also been reported.[14] Carpal tunnel syndrome is the most frequently occurring mononeuropathy after bariatric surgery, comprising 79% of the reported cases in the series of Thaisetthawatkul and colleagues.[13] Ulnar, peroneal, radial, and sciatic nerve involvement were much less common. In this and other series, lateral femoral cutaneous neuropathy (meralgia paresthetica) has been described in 0.5% to 1.4% of individuals undergoing gastric bypass surgery.[12,13,15]

The etiology of peripheral neuropathic processes after bariatric surgery is probably multifactorial. Nutritional deficiency due to malabsorption is certainly responsible for some, but immunologic mechanisms have also been proposed,[13] and compression during or after surgery is likely responsible for most of the mononeuropathic injuries.

```
┌─────────────────────────────────────────────────────────────────────────┐
│ Box 1                                                                     │
│ Neurologic complications of obesity surgery                               │
├─────────────────────────────────────────────────────────────────────────┤
│ Neuropathy                                                                │
│     Polyneuropathy                                                        │
│     Mononeuropathy                                                        │
│         Carpal tunnel syndrome                                            │
│         Meralgia paresthetica                                             │
│         Others                                                            │
│     Radiculopathy                                                         │
│     Plexopathy                                                            │
│ Myopathy                                                                  │
│ Myelopathy                                                                │
│ Encephalopathy                                                            │
└─────────────────────────────────────────────────────────────────────────┘
```

Myopathic dysfunction has also been reported after bariatric surgery. Koffman and colleagues[14] noted muscle weakness in 7% of the 96 patients they studied. An acquired myotonic syndrome has been reported.[12] Postoperative rhabdomyolysis may also occur. In one report, it was noted in 1.4% of 353 patients undergoing bariatric surgery and attributed to the development of critical surface and deep tissue pressures during surgery.[16]

Myelopathy and encephalopathy have also been reported after bariatric surgery. In one report, myelopathy was actually the most frequent and disabling neurologic complication observed, with the myelopathy typically developing years after surgery.[17] Potentially treatable causes of myelopathy after gastric surgery include deficiency of vitamin B_{12}, folate, or pyridoxine; copper deficiency is yet another possible source.[11,14,17] Cortical dysfunction, bearing the characteristics of Wernicke's encephalopathy, complicated bariatric surgery in 25% of patients in one study.[14] It was noted much less frequently, however, in a larger prospective study.[12]

Deficiencies of multiple nutrients, including vitamin B_{12}, folate, pyridoxine, thiamine, vitamin D, and vitamin E, have been documented after bariatric surgery.[11] It is not clear, however, what role these deficiencies may play in the development of neurologic dysfunction in these patients, for even when deficiencies are corrected, improvement in neurologic function often does not follow.[17]

CELIAC DISEASE

The Greek physician, Aretaeus of Cappadocia, first described celiac disease (CD), also known as nontropical sprue or gluten-sensitive or gluten-induced enteropathy, in the first or second century CE.[18] The prevalence of CD, at least in American and European populations, has generally been estimated to be approximately 1%,[19] but recent studies suggest that the number of undiagnosed patients may be considerable and the prevalence much higher than previously proposed.[20] The classic clinical characterization of CD is that of diarrhea, malabsorption, weight loss, and gassy distension that develop as a consequence of damage to the mucosa of the small intestine, triggered by an immune-mediated response to gluten, the protein fraction of wheat (**Box 2**). Gluten contains two distinct proteins—glutenin and gliadin—and the pathophysiologic mechanism seems to be the production of IgA antibodies to gliadin.[21] Thus, individuals with classic CD display the presence antigliadin antibodies, IgG and IgA. They also display the presence of additional gliadin-related antibodies, such as antiendomysial and antitransglutaminase antibodies.

In recent years, however, it has become clear that the pathology of CD is not limited to the GI tract and that involvement of other systems within the body may occur. This has led some investigators to propose that the term, gluten sensitivity, be applied to individuals displaying more widespread involvement, reserving the label, CD, for those with evidence of enteropathy on small bowel biopsy.[18]

Neurologic dysfunction has been reported to develop in 6% to 12% of individuals with CD.[22–24] A variety of neurologic manifestations of gluten sensitivity are described, including peripheral neuropathy,[25] myopathy,[26] encephalopathy,[27] and myelopathy (**Box 3**).[18]

The entity that has received the most attention, however, has been labeled gluten ataxia. Progressive ataxia in patients with previously diagnosed CD was first described in 1966.[28] It was not until 30 years later, however, that Hadjivassiliou and colleagues[29–32] published the first of a series of reports in which they described the presence of antigliadin antibodies in individuals with sporadic, adult-onset ataxia of unknown etiology and ultimately coined the term, gluten ataxia, for individuals with this clinical presentation. In their reports, they documented the presence of antigliadin antibodies (IgG or IgA) in 41% (54/132) of individuals with sporadic idiopathic ataxia, compared with only 15% (5/33) of persons with clinically probable multiple system atrophy, 14% (8/59) of patients with familial ataxia, and 12% (149/1200) of normal controls.[32] In a second group of patients with sporadic idiopathic ataxia, assembled from another clinic, antigliadin antibodies were present in 32% (14/44). Other investigators have also reported elevations of antigliadin antibodies in patients with sporadic idiopathic ataxia but with lower frequencies, ranging from 11% to 27%.[22,33–35] This finding has not been universal, however, and some investigators have not encountered this elevation in their study populations.[36,37]

Whether or not gluten ataxia genuinely exists as a distinct entity remains a subject of debate.[36,38] The nonspecificity of antigliadin antibodies, reflected in the fact that antigliadin antibodies are present in significant numbers of normal controls, is one point of contention. Moreover, antigliadin antibodies have been noted to be present in 44% of a group of 52 patients with Huntington's disease, prompting speculation that antigliadin antibodies might simply be an epiphenomenon in certain neurodegenerative diseases.[39] The absence of any clearly defined pathophysiologic mechanism that might account for the cerebellar dysfunction in affected individuals has been another criticism of the concept of gluten ataxia as a distinct clinical entity. A chronic, immune-mediated inflammatory process, however, has been proposed as responsible for the

---

Box 2
Gastrointestinal features of celiac disease

Diarrhea

Malabsorption

Weight loss

Gassy distension

Box 3
Neurologic complications of celiac disease
Ataxia
Peripheral neuropathy
Myopathy
Myelopathy
Encephalopathy

cerebellar damage[40] and autopsy examination in several affected individuals has demonstrated Purkinje cell loss and lymphocytic infiltration within the cerebellum and posterior columns of the spinal cord.[30] More recently, Hadjivassiliou and colleagues[41] have reported that individuals with gluten ataxia, independent of intestinal involvement, demonstrate antitransglutaminase 6 IgG and IgA antibodies, whereas antitransglutaminase 2 IgA antibodies are present in persons with GI disease. They also report that postmortem examination has demonstrated cerebellar IgA deposits that contain transglutaminase 6.

The potential importance of recognizing the presence of gluten ataxia is that the disorder may respond to a gluten-free diet,[18,42] although this remains controversial. Intravenous immunoglobulin therapy has been reported as effective in ameliorating cerebellar ataxia in individuals with antigliadin antibodies.[43]

INFLAMMATORY BOWEL DISEASE

Inflammatory bowel disease (IBD) encompasses several disease entities characterized by inflammation within the intestine. Ulcerative colitis (UC) and Crohn's disease (CrD), the latter also known as regional enteritis or granulomatous colitis, are the two most common and well-recognized members of this group. UC was first described by Wilks in 1859[44] whereas CrD was not delineated until 1932.[45] These two conditions share many clinical and even pathologic features but also display distinct differences (**Table 1**).

In Europe and North America, which are relatively high-incidence areas, the incidence of UC is in the range of 3 to 15 per 100,000.[46] CrD shows an even more pronounced geographic variation than UC and in Europe and North America displays a distinct north-south gradient, with a higher incidence rate in northern latitudes. In Europe and North America, incidence rates of 6 to 10 per 100,000 have been reported. In other parts of the world, such as Asia, the previously low incidence of CrD seems to be growing.[47,48]

Table 1		
Gastrointestinal features of inflammatory bowel disease		
Feature	Crohn's Disease	Ulcerative Colitis
Abdominal pain	Frequent	Unusual
Diarrhea	Frequent	Frequent
Rectal bleeding	Occasional	Frequent
Weight loss	Frequent	Unusual
Fistula and stricture	Frequent	Rare

The etiology of UC and CrD is uncertain. Genetic factors seem to be operative in both but especially in CrD.[49,50] Environmental factors also seem important and some investigators have even suggested a link between CrD and *Mycobacterium avium* subspecies *paratuberculosis* infection.[47,51] Other environmental factors, such as stress and the use of some pharmacologic agents (antibiotics and nonsteroidal anti-inflammatory drugs), have also been implicated, perhaps functioning to alter mucosal barrier integrity, stimulate immune responses, or change the bacterial microenvironment within the gut.[52]

Within the GI tract, CrD is characterized by focal inflammation that may develop at any level, including the mouth,[53] but is most prone to involve the distal small intestine and proximal colon. A cobblestone appearance to the intestinal mucosa, the consequence of enlarging and coalescing ulcers, is characteristic and noncaseating granulomas may also develop. Transmural spread of the inflammation can lead to fistula formation, and fibrosis with stricture formation is common. In contrast, UC is confined to the colon and is characterized by diffuse inflammation of the colonic mucosa and submucosa.

Neurologic involvement in IBD is uncommon but occurs. Estimates of the presence of neurologic involvement in IBD range from 0.2% to 35.7%.[54] Peripheral and central nervous system involvement occurs (**Table 2**). Although nutritional deficiency, infection, and other processes may secondarily involve the nervous system, primary neurologic involvement can be precipitated by autoimmune factors.

Peripheral neuropathy is probably the most frequent neurologic complication of CrD and UC.[55,56] In a detailed review of neurologic complications of IBD, peripheral neuropathy accounted for 31.5% of patients with neurologic involvement.[55] Focal (mononeuropathy, cranial neuropathy, brachial plexopathy), multifocal (mononeuritis multiplex, multifocal motor neuropathy), and generalized (acute or chronic inflammatory demyelinating neuropathy, small or large fiber axonal sensorimotor neuropathy) neuropathic processes have all been identified in patients with IBD.[54,55,57–60] In the experience of one group of investigators, in patients with generalized peripheral neuropathy, axonal involvement is present in approximately 70%, a demyelinating pattern in 30%.[60] Although in some instances, peripheral nerve involvement in IBD is secondary to extrinsic insults, such as nutritional deficiency and medication-induced neuropathy, primary involvement, presumably on an autoimmune basis, also occurs.

Specific patterns of cranial nerve involvement have been described in IBD. Auditory nerve involvement, in the form of acute sensorineural hearing loss or chronic subclinical hearing impairment, may occur in the setting of UC.[61–65] In contrast, Melkersson-Rosenthal syndrome, characterized by recurrent facial nerve palsy along with intermittent orofacial swelling and fissuring of the tongue, has been reported in patients with CrD and even proposed as part of the pathologic spectrum of CD because both conditions are characterized by the formation of noncaseating granulomas.[66,67]

If joint and muscle involvement are included, musculoskeletal involvement is the most frequent extraintestinal manifestation of IBD.[68,69] Muscle involvement alone, however, is less common. In a report by Lossos and colleagues,[55] it accounted for 16% of IBD cases with neurologic involvement. Myopathic involvement occurs more frequently in CrD than UC but has been described in both. A variety of inflammatory myopathic processes are described in patients with IBD, including dermatomyositis, polymyositis, granulomatous myositis, and rimmed vacuole myopathy.[55,70–72] Myositic symptoms usually coincide with GI disease activity but may occasionally precede the development of GI symptoms.[71,73]

Table 2
Neurologic complications of inflammatory bowel disease

Peripheral neuropathy
  Generalized
    Demyelinating
      Acute inflammatory demyelinating polyneuropathy
      Chronic inflammatory demyelinating polyneuropathy
    Axonal
      Large fiber axonal sensorimotor polyneuropathy
      Small fiber axonal polyneuropathy
  Focal
    Mononeuropathy
    Cranial neuropathy
      Sensorineural hearing loss (UC)
      Melkersson-Rosenthal syndrome (CrD)
    Brachial plexopathy
  Multifocal
    Mononeuritis multiplex
    Multifocal motor neuropathy
Myopathy
  Inflammatory myopathy
  Focal myositis
Myelopathy
Cerebrovascular events
  Large vessel stroke
  Small vessel stroke
  Vasculitis
  Venous sinus thrombosis

Focal involvement of muscle may also occur, primarily in CrD. Focal myositis involving the gastrocnemius[74] and other muscles[75] has been reported. Abscess formation in the psoas or other muscles is also a potential complication of CrD. Psoas muscle abscess is characterized by flank, pelvic, or abdominal pain, usually associated with fever and leukocytosis, and diagnosis is confirmed by ultrasound or CT.

Slowly progressive myelopathy may also develop in the setting of IBD and accounted for 26% of patients with neurologic involvement in the experience of Lossos and colleagues.[55] Although it has been reported in UC,[76] it occurs more often in individuals with CrD, where vitamin B_{12} deficiency as a consequence of surgical resection of the terminal ileum is sometimes responsible.[77,78] In patients with CrD, a more acute myelopathy or cauda equina syndrome may develop secondary to extension of fistulas to the epidural or subdural space, with consequent empyema.[79-82]

An association between IBD, especially UC, and multiple sclerosis has been reported by many investigators.[83-86] In a recent study, the odds ratio for multiple sclerosis between patients with IBD and normal controls was 1.5 using one large database and 1.6 using another.[87] Although in some instances, the onset of demyelinating disease has correlated with the use of infliximab for treatment of IBD,[88,89] the fact that IBD also confers a higher risk for the development of other autoimmune diseases suggests that a dysfunctional immune system is more likely responsible in most instances.[87]

Cerebrovascular events are rare, yet important, neurologic complications of IBD. They have been reported more frequently in CrD than UC but may occur in both.[90] A wide variety of cerebrovascular processes are reported in IBD. Large vessel and small vessel disease may result in stroke.[91,92] Cerebral vasculitis, presumably on an autoimmune basis, may also occur.[93–96] Venous involvement, with venous sinus thrombosis, may occur in UC and CrD, but more frequently in UC.[97–99] The etiology of cerebrovascular events in IBD is likely multifactorial. Reports of hypercoagulability due to elevations of factors V and VIII and fibrinogen, decreased antithrombin III, or the presence of anticardiolipin or lupus anticoagulant antibodies have all been published, as have suggestions that hyperhomocysteinemia, vitamin B_{12}, and pyridoxine deficiency may play a role in some individuals.[91,100–105]

SUMMARY

It is becoming increasingly clear that many disease processes once believed mono-symptomatic actually affect multiple systems within the body. The examples discussed in this article comprise only a fraction of the conditions in which neurologic dysfunction may appear in the setting of GI disease. Perhaps this should not be surprising, given the similarities between the two systems, particularly with regard to the enteric nervous system and the central nervous system. It is thus important for neurologists and gastroenterologists to remember that neurogastroenterology is a bidirectional concept and that neurologists be aware of potential GI dysfunction in their patients, just as gastroenterologists must be familiar with the possibility of neurologic dysfunction in the patients they are treating.

REFERENCES

1. Mayberry JF. Epidemiology and demographics of achalasia. Gastrointest Endosc Clin N Am 2001;11(2):235–8.
2. Trugman AM, Quinn CC, Shaffer HA. Esophageal disorders and surgery. In: Biller J, editor. The interface of neurology and internal medicine. Philadelphia: Lippincott Williams & Wilkins; 2008. p. 217–21.
3. Goyal RK, Hirano I. The enteric nervous system. N Engl J Med 1996;334(17): 1106–15.
4. Mearin F, Mourelle M, Guarner F, et al. Patients with achalasia lack nitric oxide synthase in the gastro-oesophageal junction. Eur J Clin Invest 1993;23(11): 724–8.
5. Walzer N, Hirano I. Achalasia. Gastroenterol Clin North Am 2008;37(4):807–25.
6. Qualman SJ, Haupt HM, Yang P, et al. Esophageal Lewy bodies associated with ganglion cell loss in achalasia. Similarity to Parkinson's disease. Gastroenterology 1984;87(4):848–56.
7. Wakabayashi K, Takahashi H, Takeda S, et al. Parkinson's disease: the presence of Lewy bodies in Auerbach's and Meissner's plexuses. Acta Neuropathol 1988; 76(3):217–21.
8. Johnston BT, Colcher A, Li Q, et al. Repetitive proximal esophageal contractions: a new manometric finding and a possible further link between Parkinson's disease and achalasia. Dysphagia 2001;16(3):186–9.
9. Yoshimura N, Shoji M, Matsui T. An autopsy case of Parkinson's disease manifesting hyperphagia and dysphagia followed by severe achalasia (disorder of motility) of the esophagus. No To Shinkei 1982;34(8):741–6 [in Japanese].

10. Mitani M, Kawamoto K, Funakawa I, et al. A case of esophageal achalasia followed by Parkinson's disease. Rinsho Shinkeigaku 2005;45(8):607–9 [In Japanese].
11. Koffman BM, Daboul I. Bariatric surgery. In: Biller J, editor. The interface of neurology and internal medicine. Philadelphia: Lippincott Williams & Wilkins; 2008. p. 250–5.
12. Abarbanel JM, Berginer VM, Osimani A, et al. Neurologic complications after gastric restriction surgery for morbid obesity. Neurology 1987;37(2):196–200.
13. Thaisetthawatkul P, Collazo-Clavell ML, Sarr MG, et al. A controlled study of peripheral neuropathy after bariatric surgery. Neurology 2004;63(8):1462–70.
14. Koffman BM, Greenfield LJ, Ali II, et al. Neurologic complications after surgery for obesity. Muscle Nerve 2006;33(2):166–76.
15. Macgregor AM, Thoburn EK. Meralgia paresthetica following bariatric surgery. Obes Surg 1999;9(4):364–8.
16. Khurana RN, Baudendistel TE, Morgan EF, et al. Postoperative rhabdomyolysis following laparoscopic gastric bypass in the morbidly obese. Arch Surg 2004; 139(1):73–6.
17. Juhasz-Pocsine K, Rudnicki SA, Archer RL, et al. Neurologic complications of gastric bypass surgery for morbid obesity. Neurology 2007;68(21):1843–50.
18. Hadjivassiliou M, Sanders DS. Neurologic manifestations of gluten sensitivity. In: Biller J, editor. The interface of neurology and internal medicine. Philadelphia: Lippincott Williams & Wilkins; 2008. p. 233–7.
19. Green PHR, Cellier C. Celiac disease. N Engl J Med 2007;357(17):1731–43.
20. Vilppula A, Collin P, Mäki M, et al. Undetected celiac disease in the elderly: a biopsy-proven population-based study. Dig Liver Dis 2008;40(10):809–13.
21. Lycke N, Kilander A, Nilsson LA, et al. Production of antibodies to gliadin in intestinal mucosa of patients with coeliac disease: a study at the single cell level. Gut 1989;30(1):72–7.
22. Pellecchia MT, Scala R, Filla A, et al. Idiopathic cerebellar ataxia associated with celiac disease: lack of distinctive neurological features. J Neurol Neurosurg Psychiatr 1999;66(1):32–5.
23. Lagerqvist C, Ivarsson A, Juto P, et al. Screening for adult coeliac disease— which serological marker(s) to use? J Intern Med 2001;250(3):241–8.
24. Vaknin A, Eliakim R, Ackerman Z, et al. Neurological abnormalities associated with celiac disease. J Neurol 2004;251(11):1393–7.
25. Hadjivassiliou M, Grünewald RA, Kandler RH, et al. Neuropathy associated with gluten sensitivity. J Neurol Neurosurg Psychiatr 2006;77(11):1262–6.
26. Hadjivassiliou M, Chattopadhyay AK, Grünewald RA, et al. Myopathy associated with gluten sensitivity. Muscle Nerve 2007;35(4):443–50.
27. Hadjivassiliou M, Grünewald RA, Lawden M, et al. Headache and CNS white matter abnormalities associated with gluten sensitivity. Neurology 2001;56(3):385–8.
28. Cooke WT, Smith WT. Neurological disorders associated with adult coeliac disease. Brain 1966;89(4):683–722.
29. Hadjivassiliou M, Boscolo S, Davies-Jones GA, et al. The humoral response in the pathogenesis of gluten ataxia. Neurology 2002;58(8):1221–6.
30. Hadjivassiliou M, Grünewald RA, Chattopadhyay AK, et al. Clinical, radiological, neurophysiological, and neuropathological characteristics of gluten ataxia. Lancet 1998;352(9140):1582–5.
31. Hadjivassiliou M, Gibson A, Davies-Jones GA, et al. Does cryptic gluten sensitivity play a part in neurological illness? Lancet 1996;347(8998):369–71.

32. Hadjivassiliou M, Grünewald R, Sharrack B, et al. Gluten ataxia in perspective: epidemiology, genetic susceptibility and clinical characteristics. Brain 2003; 126(Pt 3):685–91.
33. Bürk K, Bösch S, Müller CA, et al. Sporadic cerebellar ataxia associated with gluten sensitivity. Brain 2001;124(Pt 5):1013–9.
34. Bushara KO, Goebel SU, Shill H, et al. Gluten sensitivity in sporadic and hereditary cerebellar ataxia. Ann Neurol 2001;49(4):540–3.
35. Luostarinen LK, Collin PO, Peräaho MJ, et al. Coeliac disease in patients with cerebellar ataxia of unknown origin. Annu Mediaev 2001;33(6):445–9.
36. Abele M, Schöls L, Schwartz S, et al. Prevalence of antigliadin antibodies in ataxia patients. Neurology 2003;60(10):1674–5.
37. Combarros O, Infante J, López-Hoyos M, et al. Celiac disease and idiopathic cerebellar ataxia. Neurology 2000;54(12):2346.
38. Wills AJ, Unsworth DJ. The neurology of gluten sensitivity: separating the wheat from the chaff. Curr Opin Neurol 2002;15(5):519–23.
39. Bushara KO, Nance M, Gomez CM. Antigliadin antibodies in Huntington's disease. Neurology 2004;62(1):132–3.
40. Zelnik N, Pacht A, Obeid R, et al. Range of neurologic disorders in patients with celiac disease. Pediatrics 2004;113(6):1672–6.
41. Hadjivassiliou M, Aeschlimann P, Strigun A, et al. Autoantibodies in gluten ataxia recognize a novel neuronal transglutaminase. Ann Neurol 2008;64(3):332–43.
42. Hadjivassiliou M, Davies-Jones GA, Sanders DS, et al. Dietary treatment of gluten ataxia. J Neurol Neurosurg Psychiatr 2003;74(9):1221–4.
43. Nanri K, Okita M, Takeguchi M, et al. Intravenous immunoglobulin therapy for autoantibody-positive cerebellar ataxia. Intern Med 2009;48(10):783–90.
44. Wilks S. Lectures on pathological anatomy. London: Longmans; 1859.
45. Crohn BB, Ginzburg K, Oppenheimer GD. Regional ileitis: a pathological and clinical entity. JAMA 1932;99:1323–8.
46. Pfeiffer RF, Shanahan F. Inflammatory bowel disease. In: Biller J, editor. The interface of neurology and internal medicine. Philadelphia: Lippincott Williams & Wilkins; 2008. p. 228–32.
47. Hermon-Taylor J. *Mycobacterium avium* subspecies *paratuberculosis*, Crohn's disease and the Doomsday Scenario. Gut Pathog 2009;1(1):15.
48. Goh KL, Xiao S-D. Inflammatory bowel disease: a survey of the epidemiology in Asia. J Dig Dis 2009;10(1):1–6.
49. Philpott DJ, Viala J. Towards an understanding of the role of NOD2/CARD15 in the pathogenesis of Crohn's disease. Best Pract Res Clin Gastroenterol 2004; 18(3):555–68.
50. Mathew CG, Lewis CM. Genetics of inflammatory bowel disease: progress and prospects. Hum Mol Genet 2004;13 Spec No 1:R161–8.
51. Sartor RB. Does *Mycobacterium avium* subspecies *paratuberculosis* cause Crohn's disease? Gut 2005;54(7):896–8.
52. Sartor RB. Mechanisms of disease: pathogenesis of Crohn's disease and ulcerative colitis. Nat Clin Pract Gastroenterol Hepatol 2006;3(7):390–407.
53. William T, Marsch W-C, Schmidt F, et al. Early oral presentation of Crohn's disease. J Dtsch Dermatol Ges 2007;5(8):678–9.
54. Oliveira GR, Teles BC, Brasil EF, et al. Peripheral neuropathy and neurological disorders in an unselected Brazilian population-based cohort of IBD patients. Inflamm Bowel Dis 2008;14(3):389–95.
55. Lossos A, River Y, Eliakim A, et al. Neurologic aspects of inflammatory bowel disease. Neurology 1995;45(3 Pt 1):416–21.

56. Elsehety A, Bertorini TE. Neurologic and neuropsychiatric complications of Crohn's disease. Southampt Med J 1997;90(6):606–10.
57. Coert JH, Dellon AL. Neuropathy related to Crohn's disease treated by peripheral nerve decompression. Scand J Plast Recontr Surg Hand Surg 2003; 37(4):243–4.
58. Demarquay JF, Caroli-Bosc FX, Buckley M, et al. Right-sided sciatalgia complicating Crohn's disease. Am J Gastroenterol 1998;93(11):2296–8.
59. Greco F, Pavone P, Falsaperla R, et al. Peripheral neuropathy as first sign of ulcerative colitis in a child. J Clin Gastroenterol 2004;38(2):115–7.
60. Gondim FA, Brannagan TH III, Sander HW, et al. Peripheral neuropathy in patients with inflammatory bowel disease. Brain 2005;128(Pt 4):867–79.
61. Summers RW, Harker L. Ulcerative colitis and sensorineural hearing loss: is there a relationship? J Clin Gastroenterol 1982;4(3):251–2.
62. Kumar BN, Walsh RM, Wilson PS, et al. Sensorineural hearing loss and ulcerative colitis. J Laryngol Otol 1997;111(3):277–8.
63. Weber RS, Jenkins HA, Coker NJ. Sensorineural hearing loss associated with ulcerative colitis. A case report. Arch Otolaryngol 1984;110(12):810–2.
64. Hollanders D. Sensorineural deafness—a new complication of ulcerative colitis? Postgrad Med J 1986;62(730):753–5.
65. Kumar BN, Smith MS, Walsh RM, et al. Sensorineural hearing loss in ulcerative colitis. Clin Otolaryngol Allied Sci 2000;25(2):143–5.
66. Lloyd DA, Payton KB, Guenther L, et al. Melkersson-Rosenthal syndrome and Crohn's disease: one disease or two? Report of a case and discussion of the literature. J Clin Gastroenterol 1994;18(3):213–7.
67. Ratzinger G, Sepp N, Vogetseder W, et al. Cheilitis granulomatosa and Melkersson-Rosenthal syndrome: evaluation of gastrointestinal involvement and therapeutic regimens in a series of 14 patients. J Eur Acad Dermatol Venereol 2007;21(8):1065–70.
68. Bourikas LA, Papadakis KA. Musculoskeletal manifestations of inflammatory bowel disease. Inflamm Bowel Dis 2009 [Epub ahead of print].
69. Fornaciari G, Salvarani C, Beltrami M, et al. Musculoskeletal manifestations in inflammatory bowel disease. Can J Gastroenterol 2001;15(6):399–403.
70. Chugh S, Dilawari JB, Sawhney IM, et al. Polymyositis associated with ulcerative colitis. Gut 1993;34(4):567–9.
71. Leibowitz G, Eliakim R, Amir G, et al. Dermatomyositis associated with Crohn's disease. J Clin Gastroenterol 1994;18(1):48–52.
72. Ménard DB, Haddad H, Blain JG, et al. Granulomatous myositis and myopathy associated with Crohn's disease. N Engl J Med 1976;295(15):818–9.
73. Al-Kawas FH. Myositis associated with Crohn's colitis. Am J Gastroenterol 1986; 81(7):583–5.
74. Christopoulos C, Savva S, Pylarinou S, et al. Localised gastrocnemius myositis in Crohn's disease. Clin Rheumatol 2003;22(2):143–5.
75. Berger P, Wolf R, Flierman A, et al. Myositis as the first manifestation of an exacerbation of Crohn's disease. Ned Tijdschr Geneeskd 2007;151(23):1295–8 [in Dutch].
76. Ray DW, Bridger J, Hawnaur J, et al. Transverse myelitis as the presentation of Jo-1 antibody syndrome (myositis and fibrosing alveolitis) in long-standing ulcerative colitis. Br J Rheumatol 1993;32(12):1105–8.
77. Best CN. Subacute combined degeneration of spinal cord after extensive resection of ileum in Crohn's disease: report of a case. Br J Med 1959; 2(5156):862–4.

78. Baker SM, Bogoch A. Subacute combined degeneration of the spinal cord after ileal resection and folic acid administration in Crohn's disease. Neurology 1973; 23(1):40–1.

79. Hershkowitz S, Link R, Ravden M, et al. Spinal empyema in Crohn's disease. J Clin Gastroenterol 1990;12(1):67–9.

80. Sacher M, Göpfrich H, Hochberger O. Crohn's disease penetrating into the spinal canal. Acta Paediatr Scand 1989;78(4):647–9.

81. Gelfenbeyn M, Goodkin R, Kliot M. Sterile recurrent spinal epidural abscess in a patient with Crohn's disease: a case report. Surg Neurol 2006;65(2):178–84.

82. Frank B, Dörr F, Penkert G, et al. An epidural spinal abscess with caudal symptoms as a complication of Crohn's disease. Dtsch Med Wochenschr 1991; 116(35):1313–6 [in German].

83. Gupta G, Gelfand JM, Lewis JD. Increased risk for demyelinating diseases in patients with inflammatory bowel disease. Gastroenterology 2005;129(3): 819–26.

84. Kimura K, Hunter SF, Thollander MS, et al. Concurrence of inflammatory bowel disease and multiple sclerosis. Mayo Clin Proc 2000;75(8):802–6.

85. Rang EH, Brooke BN, Hermon-Taylor J. Association of ulcerative colitis with multiple sclerosis. Lancet 1982;2(8297):555.

86. Bernstein CN, Wajda A, Blanchard JF. The clustering of other inflammatory diseases in inflammatory bowel disease: a population-based study. Gastroenterology 2005;129:827–36.

87. Cohen R, Robinson D, Paramore C, et al. Autoimmune disease concomitance among inflammatory bowel disease patients in the United States, 2001–2002. Inflamm Bowel Dis 2008;14(6):738–43.

88. Freeman HJ, Flak B. Demyelination-like syndrome in Crohn's disease after infliximab therapy. Can J Gastroenterol 2005;19(5):313–6.

89. Thomas CW Jr, Weinshenker BG, Sandborn WJ. Demyelination during anti-tumor necrosis factor alpha therapy with infliximab for Crohn's disease. Inflamm Bowel Dis 2004;10(1):28–31.

90. Talbot RW, Heppell J, Dozois RR, et al. Vascular complications of inflammatory bowel disease. Mayo Clin Proc 1986;61(2):140–5.

91. Younes-Mhenni S, Derex L, Berruyer M, et al. Large-artery stroke in a young patient with Crohn's disease. Role of vitamin B_6 deficiency-induced hyperhomocysteinemia. J Neurol Sci 2004;221(1–2):113–5.

92. Fukuhara T, Tsuchida S, Kinugasa K, et al. A case of pontine lacunar infarction with ulcerative colitis. Clin Neurol Neurosurg 1993;95(2):159–62.

93. Gobbelé R, Reith W, Block F. Cerebral vasculitis as a concomitant neurological illness in Crohn's disease. Nervenarzt 2000;71(4):299–304 [in German].

94. Pandian JD, Henderson RD, O'Sullivan JD, et al. Cerebral vasculitis in ulcerative colitis. Arch Neurol 2006;63(5):780.

95. Liu YS, Fang YH, Ruan LX, et al. Takayasu's arteritis associated with Crohn's disease. J Zhejiang Univ Sci B 2009;10(8):631–4.

96. Holzer K, Esposito L, Stimmer H, et al. Cerebral vasculitis mimicking migraine with aura in a patient with Crohn's disease. Acta Neurol Belg 2009;109(1):44–8.

97. Johns DR. Cerebrovascular complications of inflammatory bowel disease. Am J Gastroenterol 1991;86(3):367–70.

98. Garcia-Moncó JC, Gómez Beldarrain M. Superior sagittal sinus thrombosis complicating Crohn's disease. Neurology 1991;41(8):1324–5.

99. Samal SC, Patra S, Reddy DC, et al. Cerebral venous sinus thrombosis as a presenting feature of Crohn's disease. Indian J Gastroenterol 2004;23(4):148–9.

100. Musio F, Older SA, Jenkins T, et al. Case report: cerebral venous thrombosis as a manifestation of acute ulcerative colitis. Am J Med Sci 1993;305(1):28–35.
101. Danese S, Papa A, Saibeni S, et al. Inflammation and coagulation in inflammatory bowel disease: the clot thickens. Am J Gastroenterol 2007;102(1):174–86.
102. Mevorach D, Goldberg Y, Gomori JM, et al. Antiphospholipid syndrome manifested by ischemic stroke in a patient with Crohn's disease. J Clin Gastroenterol 1996;22(2):141–3.
103. Mahmood A, Needham J, Prosser J, et al. Prevalence of hyperhomocysteinaemia, activated protein C resistance and prothrombin gene mutation in inflammatory bowel disease. Eur J Gastroenterol Hepatol 2005;17(7):739–44.
104. Oldenburg B, Van Tuyl BA, van der Griend R, et al. Risk factors for thromboembolic complications in inflammatory bowel disease: the role of hyperhomocysteinaemia. Dig Dis Sci 2005;50(2):235–40.
105. Penix LP. Ischemic strokes secondary to vitamin B_{12} deficiency-induced hyperhomocysteinemia. Neurology 1998;51(2):622–4.

Neurologic Presentations of Hepatic Disease

Meghan K. Harris, MD, Debra Elliott, MD,
Robert N. Schwendimann, MD, Alireza Minagar, MD, FAAN*,
Stephen L. Jaffe, MD

KEYWORDS

- Hepatic encephalopathy • [1]H-MR spectroscopy
- Hepatic cirrhosis • Hyperammonemia

Hepatic encephalopathy (HE) is a neuropsychiatric syndrome that develops in the context of portosystemic venous shunting, in the presence or absence of intrinsic hepatic disease.[1] HE is clinically characterized by altered sensorium and a spectrum of neuropsychiatric abnormalities. Several hypotheses have been proposed to explain the underlying pathogenic mechanisms of altered brain function associated with advanced hepatic disease and portosystemic shunting. HE may lead to coma and death; however, in many cases it is reversible. This article discusses the most recent developments in understanding the pathophysiology of HE and its diagnosis and management.

EPIDEMIOLOGY AND CLINICAL FEATURES

Amodio and colleagues[2] reported a 20% prevalence of cognitive abnormalities diagnosed by neuropsychological evaluation in patients with hepatic cirrhosis. Two other studies from the United Kingdom[3] and Japan[4] on the rate of development of HE in patients who underwent transjugular intrahepatic portosystemic shunts reported rates of 29.9% and 52%, respectively. HE is a frequent complication of advanced cirrhotic hepatic disease, and its development is often regarded as an indication for hepatic transplantation. Apart from neuropsychiatric abnormalities, other clinical manifestations of advanced hepatic disease that usually co-occur with HE include ascites, jaundice, and gastrointestinal (GI) variceal hemorrhage. Clinically, and based on the underlying hepatic pathology, HE is categorized into 3 major groups[5]: type A, encephalopathy from acute liver failure (ALF); type B, in which encephalopathy is caused by portosystemic shunting in the absence of intrinsic hepatic disease; and type C, in

Department of Neurology, Louisiana State University Health Sciences Center, 1501 Kings Highway, Shreveport, LA 71130, USA
* Corresponding author.
E-mail address: aminag@lsuhsc.edu (A. Minagar).

Neurol Clin 28 (2010) 89–105
doi:10.1016/j.ncl.2009.09.016
0733-8619/09/$ – see front matter © 2010 Published by Elsevier Inc.

neurologic.theclinics.com

which HE occurs with hepatic cirrhosis and portal hypertension with portosystemic shunting. A list of potential precipitating factors of HE is given in **Box 1**.

Patients with HE present with a wide range of clinical manifestations ranging from subtle changes in mentation with memory dysfunction to confusion with somnolence and disorientation and, finally, to stupor and coma. Often patients may have minimal hepatic encephalopathy (MHE), which is characterized by normal neurologic findings except for mild cognitive difficulties usually associated with attention deficits detected only by neuropsychological testing.[1] Those with overt HE typically have symptoms that begin with mental confusion and decreased motor activity. Often within a few days, patients may progress to a comatose state. Patients with HE may demonstrate flapping tremor or asterixis, and the smell of fetor hepaticus may be detected in their exhaled breath. Extrapyramidal symptoms may develop, such as tremor and various movement disorders. Occasionally seizures and increased intracranial pressure (ICP), with corticospinal tract involvement, occur. In some patients, rigidity may be observed

---

Box 1
List of precipitating factors for development of HE

Elevated nitrogen load due to
  GI bleeding
  Uremia
  Excessive dietary protein intake
Electrolyte abnormalities
  Hypokalemia
  Acidosis
  Hyponatremia
Infective processes
  Urinary tract, skin, or respiratory infections
  Spontaneous bacterial peritonitis
  Helicobacter pylori infection
Superimposed hepatic injury
  Drug-induced liver disease
  Viral hepatitis
Drugs
  Acetaminophen
  Valproic acid
  Benzodiazepines
  Narcotics
  Diuretics
  Anesthetic agents (eg, halothane)
  High-dose acetylsalicylic acid
  Alcohol abuse
Terminal hepatic disease and hepatocellular carcinoma

during passive extension or flexion of muscle groups, and some comatose patients may develop decerebrate posturing. The West Haven Classification System is generally used to grade HE (**Box 2**).[5,6]

PATHOPHYSIOLOGY

The pathophysiology of HE results from interactions among various neurotoxic compounds within the central nervous system (CNS). Development of HE in the context of hepatic cirrhosis is a clinical reflection of functional disturbances of cells involved in neurotransmission. Low-grade cerebral edema, when imaged by ^{1}H magnetic resonance ([1]H-MR) spectroscopy in patients with cirrhosis, shows increases in the metabolites glutamine/glutamate and decreases in myoinositol, providing evidence of glial edema.[7,8] Elevated serum concentrations of ammonia, hyponatremia, benzodiazepines, and proinflammatory cytokines are relevant to the development of astrocyte swelling and oxidative stress. At a molecular level, this low-grade cerebral edema is associated with an increased production of reactive oxygen and nitrogen oxide species, ultimately leading to changes in protein expression and RNA modifications, which in turn disrupts brain function.[9]

Potential neurotoxins that, as a result of alteration in their levels, may act synergistically and result in development of HE include ammonia, manganese, proinflammatory cytokines (tumor necrosis factor [TNF]-α, interleukin [IL]-1β, IL-6), mercaptans, phenols, and octanoic acid.[10] Selective alterations in blood-brain barrier (BBB) permeability and enhanced γ-aminobutyric acid (GABA)-mediated (GABAergic) transmission involving endogenous benzodiazepines are also believed to contribute to the pathogenesis of HE.[10]

Box 2
West Haven criteria for semiquantitative grading of HE

Grade	Criteria
1	Trivial lack of awareness
	Euphoria or anxiety
	Shortened attention span
	Impaired performance of addition
2	Lethargy or apathy
	Minimal disorientation for time or place
	Subtle personality change
	Inappropriate behavior
	Impaired performance of subtraction
3	Somnolence to semistupor, but responsive to verbal stimuli
	Confusion
	Gross disorientation
4	Coma (unresponsive to verbal or noxious stimuli)

From Ference P, Lockwood A, Mullen K, et al. Hepatic encephalopathy definition, nomenclature, diagnosis, and qualification: final report of the working party at the 11th World Congress of Gastroenterology, Vienna, 1998. Hepatology 2002;35(3):718.

ROLE OF AMMONIA IN PATHOGENESIS OF HE

Various clinical and laboratory observations have supported the role of ammonia in the pathophysiology of HE.[11,12] Ammonia is produced in the GI tract by bacterial degradation of amino acids, urea, and amines. Enterocytes, via the enzyme glutaminase, also convert glutamine to glutamate and ammonia.[13] In normal circumstances, the liver converts ammonia to urea by the Krebs-Henseleit cycle, and ammonia is consumed in other organs when glutamate is converted to glutamine via glutamine synthetase (GS). In patients with cirrhosis, a decrease in the number of hepatocytes reduces the process of ammonia detoxification, and portosystemic shunting detours ammonia-containing blood away from the liver into the systemic circulation, leading to hyperammonemia.

In the brain, astrocytes are the cells that contain the enzyme GS. One key function of the astrocyte is to protect the brain from excessive neuroexcitation. The astrocytes accomplish this by uptake of excess ammonia and glutamate, converting these compounds to glutamine by glutamate synthetase.[14] Glutamine accumulation within the astrocytes acutely leads to cell swelling and chronically results in formation of Alzheimer type II astrocytosis in the cerebral cortex. As previously noted, [1]H-MR spectroscopic studies in HE patients confirm the glial edema transformation.[7,8] Swelling of the astrocytes seems to be a consequence of the osmolytic action, which in turn results from intracellular build up of glutamine, the "osmotic glutamine hypothesis." It was previously believed that glutamine was not a toxic substance and that glutamate synthesis within the astrocyte was effective in protecting neurons from elevated circulating ammonia.[15] However, there is now evidence to suggest that glutamine is much more harmful than previously believed. Researchers who proposed that glutamine played a toxic role in HE development tested their theory by administering methionine sulfoximine (MSO), an inhibitor of GS, to rats.[16,17] They observed that MSO decreased the death rate in rats after acute ammonia intoxication. Moreover, it has been demonstrated that a reduction in cerebral glutamine accumulation by using MSO reversed several pathophysiologic and metabolic manifestations of experimentally induced HE. Decrease in overall cerebral edema,[18,19] reduced astrocyte swelling in vivo[20] and in cell culture,[21,22] prevention of the increase of ICP,[20] decrease in cerebral blood flow,[23] enhanced extracellular potassium activity,[24] decrease in ammonia-induced reactive oxygen species (ROS) production,[25,26] and decrease in the mitochondrial permeability transition (MPT) were all observed.[27,28]

Glutamine may affect neurons adversely by decreasing the extracellular fluid volume of the brain, which in turn may decrease diffusion of molecules and may increase accumulation of excitotoxic neurotransmitters and other neurotoxic compounds.[29,30] Brain MR imaging findings in cirrhotic patients and in those with MHE demonstrate that cerebral edema becomes more pronounced as the underlying pathology worsens.[8,31–34] These [1]H-MR spectroscopic abnormalities improve after hepatic transplantation[35] or after routine treatment of HE. Using quantitative cerebral mapping by MR imaging, Shah and colleagues[32] measured localized water content in a cohort of 38 subjects with HE. These investigators detected a significant general increase in cerebral water content in white matter, whereas water content of gray matter was generally unchanged. Based on the results of this study, the severity of HE correlated with the degree of elevated water content in frontal and occipital white matter, globus pallidus, anterior limb of internal capsule, and putamen. Such correlation between water content and severity of HE was not detected for the occipital and frontal cortices, the thalamus, and posterior limb of the internal capsule.

Apart from hyperammonemia, which is a major player in the pathogenesis of HE, elevated levels of benzodiazepines, hyponatremia, and proinflammatory cytokines can exacerbate astrocyte swelling. These neurotoxic factors may exert a synergistic effect, which may explain precipitation of HE after exposure to certain insults such as hemorrhage, infection, use of sedative-hypnotics, dehydration following use of diuretics, or electrolyte abnormalities.[10] Why cirrhotic patients are so sensitive to these metabolic and infectious insults and develop HE remains largely unknown. However, it is hypothesized that under hyperammonemic conditions, certain organic osmolytes, such as myoinositol and taurine, are significantly depleted from astrocytes (as a compensatory mechanism to glutamine-induced osmotic insult) and this pathologic metabolic state sensitizes astrocytes to further swelling from other pathologic mechanisms involved in the pathogenesis of HE.[35]

ROLE OF OXIDATIVE AND NITROSATIVE STRESS IN DEVELOPMENT OF HE

The potential role of oxidative and nitrosative stress in the pathogenesis of HE has been explored in various human, animal, and cell culture studies.[36–39] Based on the evidence obtained, elevated ammonia, changes in inflammatory cytokines, benzodiazepines, and hyponatremia evoke generation of reactive oxygen and nitrogen species, including nitric oxide (NO), through the N-methyl-D-aspartate (NMDA) receptor and Ca^{2+}-dependent mechanisms.[26,40–43] Activation of NMDA receptors occurs under these circumstances as a result of a depolarization-induced removal of Mg^{2+} blockade and autocrine amplification due to astroglial glutamate release.[9] The role of NMDA receptors in the pathogenesis of HE may differ between ALF and chronic hyperammonemia. Acute hyperammonemia in the context of ALF leads to excessive NMDA receptor activation and neuronal degeneration. However, in chronic liver failure, the activity of the glutamate-NO-cGMP pathway is impaired, and such abnormality may contribute to the cognitive decline observed in patients with HE.[44] A recent study on rats with ALF by Cauli and colleagues[45] demonstrated that blocking of brain NMDA receptors by continuous administration of MK-801 or memantine through miniosmotic pumps can delay or prevent animal death.

Available data suggest that astrocyte swelling and elevated ammonia trigger P47 (Phox)-dependent reduced nicotinamide adenine dinucleotide phosphate (NADPH) oxidase–catalyzed ROS generation, whereas Ca^{2+}/calmodulin-dependent isoforms of NO synthase are involved in astrocyte swelling–induced NO synthesis and protein tyrosine nitration.[42]

According to the "Trojan Horse" concept proposed by Albrecht and Norenberg,[15] glutamine acts as a carrier for ammonia whereby it induces negative effects in the cell. These investigators hypothesized that mitochondria within the astrocytes actively accumulate glutamine, followed by cleavage of glutamine by phosphate-activated glutaminase, causing an intramitochondrial elevation of ammonia-generating ROS via induction of the MPT.[15] The MPT is a Ca^{2+}-dependent process associated with the collapse of the inner mitochondrial membrane potential due to the opening of the permeability transition pore. This collapse leads to mitochondrial dysfunction, energy failure, and further generation of free radicals.[46–48] Other research suggests that it is ammonia itself, along with hypo-osmotic astrocyte swelling, that initially produces oxidative stress without the participation of mitochondria; thus, MPT may be induced as a consequence of oxidative stress rather than being its cause.[9] The astrocyte swelling during HE leading to formation of ROS and reactive nitrogen oxide species (RNOS) can affect the respiratory chain of neighboring neurons and contribute to the impaired brain energy metabolism and neuronal transmission. Oxidative stress, along with NMDA receptor activation, causes astrocyte swelling, which in turn generates further oxidative stress,[49,50] causing a vicious damaging cycle.[9]

Astrocyte swelling–induced formation of ROS/RNOS may cause tyrosine nitration of proteins. Tyrosine nitration of astrocytic proteins occurs in vitro in response to astrocytic swelling,[42] ammonia,[40] benzodiazepines,[41] or proinflammatory cytokines.[51] Elevated levels of nitrotyrosine have been detected in astrocytes near the BBB. It has been suggested that protein tyrosine nitration may affect transastrocytic substrate transport, thereby causing selective alterations in BBB permeability.[9] Further investigation is required to determine the complete role of protein tyrosine nitration in the pathogenesis of HE.

RNA OXIDATION

RNA oxidation plays a part in the pathogenesis of HE. RNA oxidation leads to its impaired translation with generation of dysfunctional proteins or decreased synthesis. Through a recent in vitro and in vivo study of cultured rat astrocytes, vital mouse brain slices, and rat brain in vivo, Görg and colleagues[51] demonstrated that elevated ammonia levels, TNF-α, benzodiazepines, and hypo-osmotic swelling induce RNA oxidation in these cells. The RNA oxidation is a highly sensitive marker for oxidative stress. The RNA molecule is more vulnerable to damage than DNA because of its single-stranded structure. In these rat studies,[52] ROS hydroxylated guanosine to 8-oxy-7,8-dihydro-29-guanosine (8OHG), which is detected in the astrocytes and neuronal cytosol of ammonia-intoxicated rats. This product was also found in granular dendritic structures and in postsynaptic dendritic regions associated with an RNA-binding splicing protein. These findings suggest that oxidative stress in HE modifies the RNA species involved in granular RNA transport along dendrites.[52] These researchers concluded that RNA oxidation might alter gene expression and local protein synthesis, thus providing another link between the formation of ROS/RNOS and ammonia toxicity in HE.

MANGANESE

Under normal circumstances, manganese is eliminated via the hepatobiliary system. In cirrhotic patients, serum and brain manganese levels are elevated; the bilateral hyperintense signal usually seen in the globus pallidus observed on T1-weighted MR images is attributed to manganese deposition.[53] Plasma-binding proteins, including albumin, modify the quantity of manganese transported across the BBB.[54] Hypoalbuminemia is a frequent finding in chronic liver disease; therefore, decreased protein binding could result in increased BBB transport of manganese in this condition.[55]

ROLE OF GABAERGIC TONE IN HE

The hypothesis concerning the role of "GABAergic tone" in HE was developed using animal models of ALF and implies that neuronal activity in hepatic coma is similar to that induced by GABAergic neural mechanisms.[56] Several mechanisms have been proposed to explain increased GABAergic tone: increased brain GABA, increased number of GABA-A receptors, increased concentration in brain of endogenous benzodiazepine-like compounds that would increase activation of GABA-A receptors, increased concentration in brain of neurosteroids that would increase activation of GABA-A receptors, and enhanced activation of GABA receptors by ammonia.[44] Although few studies have found evidence contradicting any of these mechanisms,[57,58] some support the concept that hyperammonemia is responsible for the apparent increase in GABAergic tone in HE by enhancing activation of GABA-A receptors through a direct effect or via increase in neurosteroids that positively modulate these receptors.[44,59–62]

Zinc, which is a negative modulator of GABA-A receptor mediated currents, may also play a role in the pathogenesis of HE, although its mechanism is not completely understood.[63] What is known is that ammonia, TNF-α, benzodiazepines, and osmotic astrocyte swelling activate an NO-dependent mobilization of zinc that may augment GABAergic neurotransmission.[9] A consequence of this action is a translocation of stimulatory protein 1 (SP1), which participates in the expression of the peripheral benzodiazepine receptor (PBR).[64,65] The PBR is upregulated in HE[66,67] and plays a role in MPT involving the oxidative stress response toward benzodiazepines and is involved in the production of neurosteroids[56] that have a positive GABA-A receptor modulatory activity. This process could also account for the increased GABAergic tone seen in patients with HE.[68] Another study also suggests that ammonia-induced astrocyte swelling, and the subsequent increase in MPT, could involve PBR.[69]

DIAGNOSTIC ASSESSMENT

Obtaining a thorough history, with emphasis on identification of predisposing factors for HE, and a detailed medical examination, with particular attention to manifestations of HE such as asterixis, are essential steps in the diagnosis of HE. Laboratory evaluation for HE consists of routine biochemical tests, including liver function tests and serum ammonia levels, examination of ascitic fluid for identification of a polymorphonuclear count higher than $250/mL^3$, ascitic fluid culture, and a coagulation profile. Neuropsychological assessment with cognitive testing may assist the clinician in identifying patients in the early stages of HE while they still seem to be clinically normal. Electroencephalography (EEG) in HE may reveal, in addition to nonspecific diffuse slowing of cortical activity, the more specific abnormalities of bilateral synchronous delta waves and triphasic waves observed mainly in frontal brain areas. Although EEG may facilitate diagnosis, there is no definite correlation between the severity of EEG abnormalities and the stages of HE.

Neuroimaging may or may not contribute toward the diagnosis of HE. Computed tomography of the brain may be normal or may reveal cerebral edema in acute stages and cerebral atrophy in chronic cases. Brain MR imaging is more sensitive for demonstrating cerebral edema and its response to treatment. MR imaging can exclude other neurologic pathology, and, in cirrhotic patients, MR imaging reveals typical bilateral pallidal hyperintensity on T1-weighted images, probably reflecting manganese deposition (**Fig. 1**).[70,71] However, pallidal hyperintense signal does not correlate with the clinical stage of HE. The fast, fluid-attenuated inversion recovery (FLAIR) T2-weighted sequence is a novel MR technique that, in patients with HE, shows hyperintense signals along the hemispheric white matter in or around the corticospinal tract (**Fig. 2**). [1]H-MR spectroscopy reveals abnormalities of cerebral osmolytes, including myoinositol, glutamate/glutamine, and choline (**Fig. 3**). A pattern of decreased myoinositol and elevated glutamate/glutamine is associated with HE.[71,72]

DIFFERENTIAL DIAGNOSIS

Several medical disorders are differentially diagnosed as HE. Other metabolic encephalopathies, such as those caused by uremia, sepsis, hypoxia, hypoglycemia, diabetic ketoacidosis, hypercapnia, and hypothyroidism, may mimic the clinical picture of HE. Other disorders to be considered include transient ischemic attack, subdural

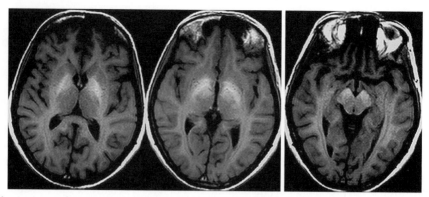

Fig. 1. Transverse T1-weighted MR images of a patient with chronic liver failure and parkinsonism. Note the bilateral and symmetric hyperintense signals involving globus pallidus and anterior brainstem. (*From* Rovira A, Alonso J, Cordoba J. MR imaging findings in hepatic encephalopathy. AJNR Am J Neuroradiol 2008;29(9):1614; with permission.)

hematoma, intracranial hemorrhage, ischemic stroke, CNS abscess, encephalitis, meningitis, CNS neoplasms, alcoholism, and epilepsy.

MANAGEMENT OF HE

HE is the result of several synergistic factors in the context of hepatic failure, and, therefore, a variety of treatments have been proposed. In ALF, the only procedure with a favorable outcome is hepatic transplantation. Patients may have to wait long periods until a "match liver" becomes available; therefore, the ensuing

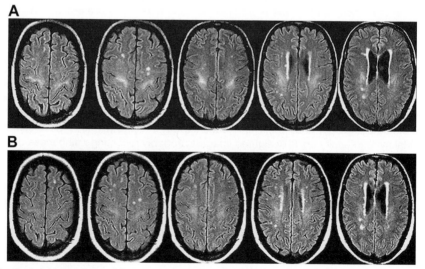

Fig. 2. Axial T2-weighted fast FLAIR images of a patient with hepatic cirrhosis during an episode of HE. Note the symmetric hyperintense signals along the corticospinal tracts in both cerebral hemispheres (*A*). The abnormal hyperintense signals resolved almost completely during a follow-up study obtained few months later, when the patient showed no overt HE (*B*). (*From* Rovira A, Alonso J, Cordoba J. MR imaging findings in hepatic encephalopathy. AJNR Am J Neuroradiol 2008;29(9):1617; with permission.)

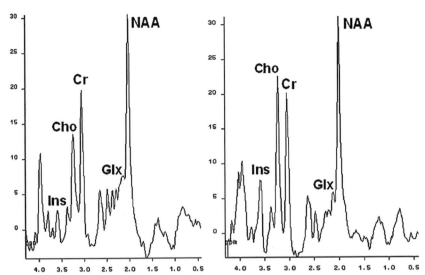

Fig. 3. [1]H-MR spectroscopy water-suppressed proton spectra of an 8-mL voxel located in the parietal region including predominantly normal-appearing white matter in a patient with cirrhosis before (*left*) and after (*right*) liver transplantation, recorded with a stimulated echo acquisition mode pulse sequence (TR/TE, 1600/20 ms; acquisitions, 256). The main resonances correspond to *N*-acetylaspartate (NAA, 2.0 ppm), glutamine/glutamate (Glx, 2.1–2.5 ppm), creatine/phosphocreatine (Cr, 3.02 ppm), choline-containing compounds (Cho, 3.2 ppm), and myoinositol (Ins, 3.55 ppm). The initial spectrum shows an increase in the glutamate/glutamine region and a decrease in the myoinositol and choline resonances. These abnormalities normalized after liver transplantation. Normal NAA indices are seen in both examinations. (*From* Rovira A, Alonso J, Cordoba J. MR imaging findings in hepatic encephalopathy. AJNR Am J Neuroradiol 2008;29(9):1615; with permission.)

encephalopathy must be attenuated in the meantime for the patient to survive until the time of operation. Chronic liver failure and cirrhosis are also accompanied by degrees of cognitive dysfunction progressing to severe encephalopathy, particularly when associated with "acute on chronic" liver disease. Preventive and acute therapies are crucial in minimizing morbidity and mortality in these cases.

The first steps toward successful management consist of early recognition of the HE with prevention of the development of neurologic symptoms. To that end, all cirrhotic patients, or those with portosystemic shunting, should be considered at high risk for MHE. Between 60% and 84% of cirrhotic patients may have MHE on careful neuro-psychological testing or use of the portosystemic encephalopathy (PSE) syndrome test.[5,73,74] Because MHE is associated with numerous neuropsychological problems, including impaired driving ability,[75] treatment at this stage should result in improvement in test performance and may improve quality of life.[76] Treatment options for MHE and HE include lowering the levels of ammonia and other toxins with medications or cautious dietary restriction. It is also important to identify and eradicate confounding influences, such as *Helicobacter pylori* infection, bacterial peritonitis, GI bleeding, and electrolyte imbalance, particularly hyponatremia. Because fluid restriction in hyponatremia is often unsatisfactory, vasopressin antagonism at the renal tubule by vaptans can now be used in short-term and long-term management, but it requires careful monitoring to make sure the patient's fluid intake is adequate (see **Box 1**).[77] Care should also be taken to eliminate medications, such as sedatives, that may also contribute to impaired cognition, and abstinence from alcohol must be enforced.[78]

Overzealous protein restriction may worsen the patient's health because of the resultant catabolic state and protein energy malnutrition.[79] A daily protein intake of 0.8 to 1.2 g/kg body weight is therefore recommended, decreasing to 20 g/d only during acute attacks of HE. Vegetable proteins are better tolerated than fish, meat, or dairy protein, and will improve nitrogen balance without worsening HE. Branched-chain amino acids can be administered orally up to 0.25 g/kg in patients intolerant of dietary protein.[78] A mainstay of treatment is the use of nonabsorbable disaccharides, such as lactulose, which decrease ammonia absorption. Lactulose, given orally at doses of 30 to 60 g/d (titrated to 2–3 semisoft stools per day), can be administered long-term with no serious side effects, but compliance may be an issue in two-thirds of patients.[80] There are alternatives that have been shown to be just as effective, such as probiotics and antibiotics. Treatment with probiotics, which modify the microflora of the gut, has been advocated for patients with MHE and has been shown to improve neuropsychiatric scores compared with placebo.[81] Probiotics have been shown to be as effective as lactulose treatment.[82] Delivering the probiotic in yogurt offers patients an inexpensive, palatable, and easily acceptable form of treatment.[80] Yogurt is derived from the fermentation of lactic acid in milk and contains natural bacteria, including the beneficial *Lactobacillus bulgaricus*. Yogurt ingestion is associated with a decrease in pathogenic urease-producing bacteria, such as *Escherichia coli*, *Fusobacterium*, and staphylococci.

Intercurrent *H pylori* infection has been associated with high serum ammonia levels and worsening of HE. Eradication with clarithromycin and tinidazole plus omeprazole was associated with a lower incidence of HE and lower ammonia and plasma endo-toxin (lipopolysaccharide) levels.[83,84] Certain antibiotics have shown efficacy in HE treatment regardless of *H pylori* status, the most popular being rifaximin. This antibi-otic is poorly absorbed from the GI tract and has effects similar to probiotics in the reduction of ammonia and other gut toxins (ie, mercaptans and benzodiazepines). It is used to prevent and treat traveler's diarrhea due to *E coli* and gastritis from *H pylori*.[85] Although there is a demand for better designed placebo-controlled studies, 2 recent reviews have demonstrated that rifaximin has superior efficacy, with more rapid improvement of HE symptoms, compared with lactulose, and that treatment with rifaximin results in fewer and shorter hospitalizations and, thus, lower hospital costs.[86,87] Another meta-analysis found rifaximin lacking in superiority regarding the presence of symptoms of acute or chronic encephalopathy and diarrhea, but slightly superior with respect to abdominal pain compared with nonabsorbable disaccha-rides.[88] Rifaximin was associated with better tolerability than comparative drugs, including paromomycin, neomycin, and lactulose, in all reviews. Once ammonia has been absorbed into the blood, measures to improve detoxification by the liver and other organs can be undertaken to blunt its harmful effects. Ornithine and aspartate are significant substrates for the conversion of ammonia to urea and glutamine. To this end, exogenous administration of L-ornithine-L-aspartate (LOLA) has been studied. A review of publications concerning the effectiveness and safety of LOLA treatment found that it significantly improved overt HE compared with placebo but was not effective in MHE.[89]

Concerning the CNS, other therapies have been directed toward the correction of impaired neurotransmitter function in HE. Patients who succumb to hepatic coma have been found to have increased acetylcholinesterase (AChE) activity in the pres-ence of normal choline acetyltransferase. Animal models have suggested that this increase is independent of ammonia levels and, therefore, separate treatment may

be warranted. Preliminary studies in rats suggest that the AChE inhibitor rivastigmine improved memory deficits and resulted in a 25% inhibition of AChE activity.[90] No studies in humans have been published at this time. Neurosteroid inhibitors may also, theoretically, be used to lower levels of neurosteroids, such as pregnenolone, allopregnanolone, and tetrahydrodesoxycorticosterone (THDOC), and thus improve the altered neurotransmission found in HE, which results in increased GABA tone. Indomethacin is an inhibitor of the 3α-hydroxysteroid dehydrogenase enzyme involved in neurosteroid synthesis in the brain. Animal studies have shown that intraperitoneal indomethacin can ameliorate locomotor dysfunction in rats with encephalopathic behavioral changes 4 weeks after portocaval anastomosis, with associated normalization of brain levels of allopregnanolone and THDOC.[91] However, another study reveals that hepatic failure in rats, induced by intraperitoneal injection of thioacetamide, worsened when given indomethacin as compared with normal saline injections 3 days after disease induction. The investigators determined that higher mortality and morbidity was likely caused by the inhibition of prostacyclin, which aggravated hepatic damage.[92] This might suggest that protection of prostacyclin during indomethacin treatment would further enhance its benefit. In humans with ALF, parenteral indomethacin has been found to significantly lower increased ICP and improve compromised cerebral perfusion pressure (CPP), which are prominent causes of death in this condition.[93]

Other therapies used to reduce intracranial hypertension in acutely ill patients while awaiting recovery of the liver or liver transplant include the use of hypothermia, hyperventilation, hypertonic saline, mannitol, and sedation with propofol or thiopental.[94,95] Not all have been studied in controlled randomized trials. Although early fluid resuscitation is important, these patients cannot metabolize lactate normally. Therefore, Hartmann solution, lactated Ringer solution, normal saline, and colloid solutions with high chloride content, which may result in hyperchloremic metabolic acidosis, are discouraged.[96,97] Some suggest that invasive ICP and hemodynamic monitoring are necessary despite the presence of profound coagulopathy and that noninvasive monitoring via various neuroimaging procedures is inadequate and impractical.[97] Others point out that a possible risk/benefit ratio has not been proven in terms of a better neurologic outcome, given that the risk of bleeding complications is 10%.[98,99] Coagulopathy may be temporarily ameliorated by infusion of platelets, fresh frozen plasma, and cryoprecipitate to cover procedures and decrease the risk of intracerebral hemorrhage. A target CPP of more than 55 mm Hg will maintain adequate cerebral oxygenation; placing the patient in a 20° head-up position will assist in reducing ICP without compromising the mean arterial pressure and CPP.[97] Hyperventilation is best saved for emergency treatment of impending herniation because of its short-term effectiveness. Mild hypothermia, to a temperature of 35 to 36°C, may reduce ICP without the side effects of more aggressive cooling, such as worsening coagulopathy, immune suppression, and insulin resistance.[97] Trials are now being developed to study hypothermia in ALF in a randomized controlled fashion.[100]

Treatment of the underlying hepatic failure with liver or hepatocyte transplantation is the most lasting and successful treatment of ALF-induced cerebral edema. Until successful treatment can be accomplished, patients with "acute on chronic" liver failure (AoCLF) can be placed on artificial liver devices for short periods of time to maintain life. Three major extracorporeal systems are currently used: single-pass albumin dialysis (SPAD), the molecular adsorbent recycling system (MARS), and Prometheus, which entails fractionated plasma separation and adsorption.[99] The latter 2 systems have been proved retrospectively to improve encephalopathy and decrease bilirubinemia and, in some cases, have caused hemodynamic improvement;

however, they do not lower cytokine levels.[101] Seventy percent of patients with AoCLF treated with such ex vivo techniques became medically stable enough to survive liver transplantation within a 2- to 3-week period. However, those with severe liver failure (Mayo End-Stage Liver Disease [MELD] scores >35) and those who did not undergo transplantation had a 3-month survival rate of less than 20%, and those with primary liver dysfunction after transplant did not survive.[101] Controversy exists concerning the true benefits of these intensive and expensive therapies and the problems associated with them. There have been reports of MARS treatment worsening coagulopathy and bleeding, causing hypoglycemia due to the use of glucose-poor dialysate, and altering the pharmacokinetics of antibiotics and antifungals. Prometheus does not improve blood pressure and the hyperdynamic state as well as MARS, and clotting may be problematic. These treatments should only be performed by institutions that have liver transplantation available.[102] SPAD may be a less expensive and more convenient approach and more successful than MARS in eliminating ammonia and bilirubin, but it has not been as extensively studied.[102,103]

Development of a bioartificial liver using hepatocytes is underway. Porcine hepatocytes are more available than human cells, so most studies use the porcine system in which plasma or ultrafiltrate is perfused through the hepatocytes to metabolize toxins. Early reports suggest an improved survival rate over controls provided with routine medical treatment. Because of cross-species incompatibility complications, the use of cryopreserved mature human hepatocytes from discarded livers, fetal human hepatocytes, and stem cells is being investigated. Immortalized C3A human hepatocytes from a hepatoblastoma are used in an extracorporeal liver assist device, which has been shown to improve bilirubin and ammonia levels and encephalopathy but not mortality, when liver transplantation is not available. So far, safety has been demonstrated, but there is concern about risks of malignancy from the C3A hepatocytes.[102]

REFERENCES

1. Munoz SJ. Hepatic encephalopathy. Med Clin North Am 2008;92(4):795–812.
2. Amodio P, Del Picollo F, Marchetti P, et al. Clinical features and survival of cirrhotic patients with subclinical cognitive alterations detected by the number connection test and computerized psychometrictests. Hepatology 1999;29(6): 1662–7.
3. Tripathi D, Helmy A, Macbeth K, et al. Ten years' follow-up of 472 patients following transjugular intrahepatic portosystemic stent–shunt insertion at a single centre. Eur J Gastroenterol Hepatol 2004;16(1):9–18.
4. Mamiya Y, Kanazawa H, Kimura Y, et al. Hepatic encephalopathy after transjugular intrahepatic portosystemic shunt. Hepatol Res 2004;30(3):162–8.
5. Ferenci P, Lockwood A, Mullen K, et al. Hepatic encephalopathy—definition, nomenclature, diagnosis, and qualification: final report of the working party at the 11th World Congress of Gastroenterology, Vienna, 1998. Hepatology 2002; 35(3):716–21.
6. Atterbury CE, Maddrey WC, Conn HO. Neomycin-sorbitol and lactulose in the treatment of acute portal-systemic encephalopathy: a controlled, double-blind clinical trial. Am J Dig Dis 1978;23(5):398–405.
7. Häussinger D. Low grade cerebral edema and the pathogenesis of hepatic encephalopathy in cirrhosis. Hepatology 2006;43(6):1187–90.
8. Häussinger D, Laubenberger J, vom Dahl S, et al. Proton magnetic resonance spectroscopy studies on human brain myoinositol in hypo-osmolarity and hepatic encephalopathy. Gastroenterology 1994;107(5):1475–80.

9. Häussinger D, Schliess F. Pathogenetic mechanisms of hepatic encephalopathy. Gut 2008;57(8):1156–65.

10. Butterworth RF. Pathophysiology of hepatic encephalopathy: the concept of synergism. Hepatol Res 2008;38:S116–21.

11. Norenberg MD. Astrocytic–ammonia interactions in hepatic encephalopathy. Semin Liver Dis 1996;16(3):245–53.

12. Ong JP, Aggarwal A, Krieger D, et al. Correlation between ammonia levels and the severity of hepatic encephalopathy. Am J Med 2003;114(3):188–93.

13. Chatauret N, Butterworth RF. Effects of liver failure on inter-organ trafficking of ammonia: implications for the treatment of hepatic encephalopathy. J Gastroenterol Hepatol 2004;19:S219–23.

14. Norenberg MD, Martinez-Hernandez A. Fine structural localization of glutamine synthetase in astrocytes of rat brain. Brain Res 1979;161(2):303–10.

15. Albrecht J, Norenberg MD. Glutamine: a Trojan horse in ammonia neurotoxicity. Hepatology 2006;44(4):788–94.

16. Warren KS, Schenker S. Effect of an inhibitor of glutamine synthesis (methionine sulfoximine) on ammonia toxicity and metabolism. J Lab Clin Med 1964;64: 442–9.

17. Lamar C Jr, Sellinger OZ. The inhibition in vivo of cerebral glutamine synthetase and glutamine transferase by the convulsant methionine sulfoximine. Biochem Pharmacol 1965;14:489–506.

18. Takahashi H, Koehler RC, Brusilow SW, et al. Inhibition of brain glutamine accumulation prevents cerebral edema in hyperammonemic rats. Am J Physiol 1991;261:H825–9.

19. Blei AT, Olafsson S, Therrien G, et al. Ammonia-induced brain edema and intracranial hypertension in rats after portacaval anastomosis. Hepatology 1994;19(6):1437–44.

20. Willard-Mack CL, Koehler RC, Hirata T, et al. Inhibition of glutamine synthetase reduces ammonia-induced astrocyte swelling in rat. Neuroscience 1996;71(2): 589–99.

21. Isaacks RE, Bender AS, Kim CY, et al. Effect of ammonia and methionine sulfoximine on myo-inositol transport in cultured astrocytes. Neurochem Res 1999; 24(1):51–9.

22. Zwingmann C, Flogel U, Pfeuffer J, et al. Effects of ammonia exposition on glioma cells: changes in cell volume and organic osmolytes studied by diffusion-weighted and high-resolution NMR spectroscopy. Dev Neurosci 2000;22(5–6):463–71.

23. Master S, Gottstein J, Blei AT. Cerebral blood flow and the development of ammonia-induced brain edema in rats after portacaval anastomosis. Hepatology 1999;30(4):876–80.

24. Sugimoto H, Koehler RC, Wilson DA, et al. Methionine sulfoximine, a glutamine synthetase inhibitor, attenuates increased extracellular potassium activity during acute hyperammonemia. J Cereb Blood Flow Metab 1997;17(1):44–9.

25. Norenberg MD, Jayakumar AR, Rama Rao KV. Oxidative stress in the pathogenesis of hepatic encephalopathy. Metab Brain Dis 2004;19(3–4):313–29.

26. Murthy CR, Rama Rao KV, Bai G, et al. Ammonia-induced production of free radicals in primary cultures of rat astrocytes. J Neurosci Res 2001;66(2): 282–8.

27. Bai G, Rama Rao KV, Murthy CR, et al. Ammonia induces the mitochondrial permeability transition in primary cultures of rat astrocytes. J Neurosci Res 2001;66(5):981–91.

28. Rama Rao KV, Jayakumar AR, Norenberg MD. Ammonia neurotoxicity: role of the mitochondrial permeability transition. Metab Brain Dis 2003;18:113–27.
29. Sykova E. Glia and volume transmission during physiological and pathological states. J Neural Transm 2005;112:137–47.
30. Simard M, Nedergaard M. The neurobiology of glia in the context of water and ion homeostasis. Neuroscience 2004;129(4):877–96.
31. Shah NJ, Neeb H, Kircheis G, et al. Quantitative T1 and water content mapping in hepatic encephalopathy. In: Häussinger D, Kircheis G, Schliess F, editors. Hepatic encephalopathy and nitrogen metabolism. Dordrecht (The Netherlands): Springer; 2006. p. 273–83.
32. Shah NJ, Neeb H, Kircheis G, et al. Quantitative cerebral water content mapping in hepatic encephalopathy. Neuroimage 2008;41(3):706–17.
33. Laubenberger J, Häussinger D, Bayer S, et al. Proton magnetic resonance spectroscopy of the brain in symptomatic and asymptomatic patients with liver cirrhosis. Gastroenterology 1997;112(5):1610–6.
34. Cordoba J, Alonso J, Rovira A, et al. The development of low grade cerebral edema in cirrhosis is supported by the evolution of (1)H-magnetic resonance abnormalities after liver transplantation. J Hepatol 2001;35(5):598–604.
35. Shawcross DL, Balata S, Olde-Damink SW, et al. Low myoinositol and high glutamine levels in brain are associated with neuropsychological deterioration after induced hyperammonemia. Am J Physiol 2004;287:G503–9.
36. Negru T, Ghiea V, Pasarica D. Oxidative injury and other metabolic disorders in hepatic encephalopathy. Rom J Physiol 1999;36(1–2):29–36.
37. Harrison PM, Wendon JA, Gimson AE, et al. Improvement by acetylcysteine of hemodynamics and oxygen transport in fulminant hepatic failure. N Engl J Med 1991;324(26):1852–7.
38. Sushma S, Dasarathy S, Tandon RK, et al. Sodium benzoate in the treatment of acute hepatic encephalopathy: a double-blind randomized trial. Hepatology 1992;16(1):138–44.
39. Wendon JA, Harrison PM, Keays R, et al. Cerebral blood flow and metabolism in fulminant liver failure. Hepatology 1994;19(6):1407–13.
40. Schliess F, Görg B, Fischer R, et al. Ammonia induces MK-801-sensitive nitration and phosphorylation of protein tyrosine residues in rat astrocytes. FASEB J 2002;16(7):739–41.
41. Görg B, Foster N, Reinehr RM, et al. Benzodiazepine-induced protein tyrosine nitration in rat astrocytes. Hepatology 2003;37(2):334–42.
42. Schliess F, Foster N, Görg B, et al. Astrocyte swelling increases protein tyrosine nitration in cultured rat astrocytes. Glia 2004;47(1):21–9.
43. Reinehr R, Görg B, Becker S, et al. Hypoosmotic swelling and ammonia increase oxidative stress by NADPH oxidase in cultured astrocytes and vital brain slices. Glia 2007;55(7):758–71.
44. Llansola M, Rodrigo R, Monfort P, et al. NMDA receptors in hyperammonemia and hepatic encephalopathy. Metab Brain Dis 2007;22(3–4):321–5.
45. Cauli O, Rodrigo R, Llansola M, et al. Glutamatergic and gabaergic neurotransmission and neuronal circuits in hepatic encephalopathy. Metab Brain Dis 2009; 24(1):69–80.
46. Zoratti M, Szabo I. The mitochondrial permeability transition. Biochim Biophys Acta 1995;1241(2):139–76.
47. Bernardi P, Colonna R, Costantini P, et al. The mitochondrial permeability transition. Biofactors 1998;8(3–4):273–81.

48. Zoratti M, Szabo I, De Marchi U. Mitochondrial permeability transitions: how many doors to the house? Biochim Biophys Acta 2005;1706(1–2):40–52.
49. Schliess F, Görg B, Häussinger D. Pathogenetic interplay between osmotic and oxidative stress: the hepatic encephalopathy paradigm. Biol Chem 2006; 387(10–11):1363–70.
50. Schliess F, Görg B, Reinehr RM, et al. Osmotic and oxidative stress in hepatic encephalopathy. In: Häussinger D, Kircheis G, Schliess F, editors. Hepatic encephalopathy and nitrogen metabolism. Dordrecht, The Netherlands: Springer; 2006. p. 20–42.
51. Görg B, Bidmon HJ, Keitel V, et al. Inflammatory cytokines induce protein tyrosine nitration in rat astrocytes. Arch Biochem Biophys 2006;449(1–2): 104–14.
52. Görg B, Qvartskhava N, Keitel V, et al. Ammonia increases RNA oxidation in cultured astrocytes and brain in vivo. Hepatology 2008;48(2):567–79.
53. Pomier-Layrargues G, Spahr L, Butterworth RF. Increased manganese concentrations in pallidum of cirrhotic patients. Lancet 1995;345(8951):735.
54. Rabin O, Hegedus L, Bourre JM, et al. Rapid brain uptake of manganese(II) across the blood-brain barrier. J Neurochem 1993;61(2):509–17.
55. Butterworth RF, Spahr L, Fontaine S, et al. Manganese toxicity, dopaminergic dysfunction and hepatic encephalopathy. Metab Brain Dis 1995;10(4):259–67.
56. Schafer DF, Jones EA. Hepatic encephalopathy and the gamma-aminobutyric acid neurotransmitter system. Lancet 1982;1(8262):18–20.
57. Ahboucha S, Pomier-Layrargues G, Butterworth RF. Increased brain concentrations of endogenous (non-benzodiazepine) GABA-A receptor ligands in human HE. Metab Brain Dis 2004;19(3–4):241–51.
58. Ahboucha S, Araqi F, Layrargues GP, et al. Differential effects of ammonia on the benzodiazepine modulatory site on the GABA-A receptor of human brain. Neurochem Int 2005;47(1–2):58–63.
59. Itzhak Y, Roig-Cantisano A, Dombro RS, et al. Acute liver failure and hyperammonemia increase peripheral-type benzodiazepine receptor binding and pregnenolone synthesis in mouse brain. Brain Res 1995;705(1–2):345–8.
60. Norenberg MD, Itzhak Y, Bender AS. The peripheral benzodiazepine receptor and neurosteroids in HE. Adv Exp Med Biol 1997;420:95–111.
61. Takahashi K, Kameda H, Kataoka M, et al. Ammonia potentiates GABAA response in dissociated rat cortical neurons. Neurosci Lett 1993;151(1):51–4.
62. Ha JH, Basile AS. Modulation of ligand binding to components of the GABAA receptor complex by ammonia: implications for the pathogenesis of hyperammonemic syndromes. Brain Res 1996;720(1–2):35–44.
63. Celentano JJ, Gyenes M, Gibbs TT, et al. Negative modulation of the gamma-aminobutyric acid response by extracellular zinc. Mol Pharmacol 1991;40(5): 766–73.
64. Kruczek C, Görg B, Keitel V, et al. Hypoosmolarity and ammonia affect zinc homeostasis in cultured rat astrocytes. Glia 2009;57(1):79–92.
65. Giatzakis C, Papadopoulos V. Differential utilization of the promoter of peripheral-type benzodiazepine receptor by steroidogenic versus nonsteroidogenic cell lines and the role of Sp1 and Sp3 in the regulation of basal activity. Endocrinology 2004;145(3):1113–23.
66. Giguere JF, Hamel E, Butterworth RF. Increased densities of binding sites for the 'peripheral-type' benzodiazepine receptor ligand [3H]PK 11195 in rat brain following portacaval anastomosis. Brain Res 1992;585(1–2):295–8.

67. Lavoie J, Layrargues GP, Butterworth RF. Increased densities of peripheral-type benzodiazepine receptors in brain autopsy samples from cirrhotic patients with hepatic encephalopathy. Hepatology 1990;11(5):874–8.

68. Butterworth RF. The astrocytic (peripheral-type) benzodiazepine receptor: role in the pathogenesis of portal-systemic encephalopathy. Neurochem Int 2000; 36(4–5):411–6.

69. Panickar KS, Jayakumar AR, Rama Rao KV, et al. Downregulation of the 18-kDa translocator protein: effects on the ammonia-induced mitochondrial permeability transition and cell swelling in cultured astrocytes. Glia 2007;55(16):1720–7.

70. Kulisevski J, Pujol J, Balanzo J, et al. Pallidal hyperintensity on magnetic reso-nance imaging in cirrhotic patients: clinical correlations. Hepatology 1992; 16(6):1382–8.

71. Rovira A, Alonso J, Cordoba J. MR imaging findings in hepatic encephalopathy. AJNR Am J Neuroradiol 2008;29(9):1612–21.

72. Kreis R, Ross BD, Farrow NA, et al. Metabolic disorders of the brain in chronic hepatic encephalopathy detected with H-1 MR spectroscopy. Radiology 1992; 182(1):19–27.

73. Dhiman RK, Chawla YK. Minimal hepatic encephalopathy: time to recognize and treat. Trop Gastroenterol 2008;29(1):6–12.

74. Weissenborn K, Ennen JC, Schomerus H, et al. Neuropsychological character-ization of hepatic encephalopathy. J Hepatol 2001;34(5):768–73.

75. Bajaj JS. Management options for minimal hepatic encephalopathy. Expert Rev Gastroenterol Hepatol 2008;2(6):785–90.

76. Zhou YQ, Chen SY, Jiang LD, et al. Development and evaluation of the quality of life instrument in chronic liver disease patients with minimal hepatic encephalop-athy. J Gastroenterol Hepatol 2009;24(3):408–15.

77. Ginès P, Guevera M. Hyponatremia in cirrhosis: pathogenesis, clinical signifi-cance, and management. Hepatology 2008;48(3):1002–10.

78. Gerber T, Schomerus H. Hepatic encephalopathy in liver cirrhosis. Drugs 2000; 60(6):1353–70.

79. Merli M, Riggio O. Dietary and nutritional indications in hepatic encephalopathy. Metab Brain Dis 2009;24(1):211–21.

80. Leevy CB, Phillips JA. Hospitalizations during the use of rifaximin versus lactulose for the treatment of hepatic encephalopathy. Dig Dis Sci 2007;52(3): 737–41.

81. Bajaj JS, Saeian K, Christensen KM, et al. Probiotic yogurt for the treatment of hepatic encephalopathy. Am J Gastroenterol 2008;103(7):1707–15.

82. Sharma P, Sharma BC, Puri V, et al. An open-label randomized controlled trial of lactulose and probiotics in the treatment of minimal hepatic encephalopathy. Eur J Gastroenterol Hepatol 2008;20(6):506–11.

83. Chen SJ, Wang LJ, Zhu Q, et al. Effect of *H. pylori* infection and its eradication on hyperammonemia and hepatic encephalopathy in cirrhotic patients. World J Gastroenterol 2008;14(12):1914–8.

84. Abdel-Hady H, Zaki A, Badra G, et al. *Helicobacter pylori* infection in hepatic encephalopathy: relationship to plasma endotoxins and blood ammonia. Hepatol Res 2007;37(12):1026–33.

85. Gerard L, Garey KW, DuPont HL. Rifaximin: a nonabsorbably refamycin antibi-otic for use in nonsystemic gastrointestinal infections. Expert Rev Anti Infect Ther 2005;3(2):201–11.

86. Maclayton DO, Eaton-Maxwell A. Rifaximin for treatment of hepatic encephalop-athy. Ann Pharmacother 2009;43(1):77–84.

87. Lawrence KR, Klee JA. Rifaximin for the treatment of hepatic encephalopathy. Pharmacotherapy 2008;28(8):1019–32.
88. Jiang Q, Jiang XH, Zheng MH, et al. Rifaximin versus nonabsorbable disaccharides in the management of hepatic encephalopathy: a meta-analysis. Eur J Gastroenterol Hepatol 2008;20(11):1064–70.
89. Jiang Q, Jiang XH, Zheng MH, et al. L-Ornithine-L-aspartate in the management of hepatic encephalopathy: a meta-analysis. J Gastroenterol Hepatol 2009; 24(1):9–14.
90. García-Ayllón MS, Cauli O, Silveyra MX, et al. Brain cholinergic impairment in liver failure. Brain 2008;131(Pt 11):2946–56.
91. Ahboucha S, Jiang W, Chatauret N, et al. Indomethacin improves locomotor deficit and reduces brain concentrations of neuroinhibitory steroids in rats following portacaval anastomosis. Neurogastroenterol Motil 2008;20:949–57.
92. Chu CJ, Hsiao CC, Wang TF, et al. Prostacyclin inhibition by indomethacin aggravates hepatic damage and encephalopathy in rats with thioacetamide-induced fulminant hepatic failure. World J Gastroenterol 2005;11(2):232–6.
93. Tofteng F, Larsen FS. The effect of indomethacin on intracranial pressure, cerebral perfusion and extracellular lactate and glutamate concentrations in patients with fulminant hepatic failure. J Cereb Blood Flow Metab 2004;24: 798–804.
94. Raghavan M, Marik PE. Therapy of intracranial hypertension in patients with fulminant hepatic failure. Neurocrit Care 2006;4(2):179–89.
95. Detry O, DeRoover A, Honoré P, et al. Brain edema and intracranial hypertension in fulminant hepatic failure: pathophysiology and management. World J Gastroenterol 2006;12(46):7405–12.
96. Rehm M, Orth V, Scheingraber S, et al. Acid-base changes caused by 5% albumin versus 6% hydroxyethyl starch solution in patients undergoing actue normovolemic hemodilution: a randomized prospective study. Anesthesiology 2000;93:1174–83.
97. Auzinger G, Wendon J. Intensive care management of acute liver failure. Curr Opin Crit Care 2008;14(2):179–88.
98. Vaquero J, Fontana RJ, Larson AM, et al. Complications and use of intracranial pressure monitoring in patients with acute liver failure and severe encephalopathy. Liver Transpl 2005;11:1581.
99. Bacher A, Zimpfer M. Hot topics in liver intensive care. Transplant Proc 2008; 40(4):1179–82.
100. Stravitz RT, Lee WM, Kramer AH, et al. Therapeutic hypothermia for acute liver failure: toward a randomized, controlled trial in patients with advanced hepatic encephalopathy. Neurocrit Care 2008;9(1):90–6.
101. Faenza S, Baraldi O, Bernardi M, et al. Mars and Prometheus: our clinical experience in acute chronic liver failure. Transplant Proc 2008;40:1169–71.
102. Phua J, Lee KH. Liver support devices. Curr Opin Crit Care 2008;14(2):208–15.
103. Sauer IM, Goetz M, Steffen I, et al. In vitro comparison of the molecular adsorbent recirculation system (MARS) and single-pas albumin dialysis (SPAD). Hepatology 2008;39:1408–14.

Neurologic Presentations of Nutritional Deficiencies

Neeraj Kumar, MD

KEYWORDS

- Nutritional deficiency • Neurologic complications

Optimal functioning of the central and peripheral nervous system is dependent on a constant supply of appropriate nutrients. Neurologic signs occur late in malnutrition. Deficiency diseases such as kwashiorkor and marasmus are endemic in underdeveloped countries. Individuals at risk in developed countries include the poor and homeless, the elderly, patients on prolonged or inadequate parenteral nutrition, individuals with food fads or eating disorders such as anorexia nervosa and bulimia, those suffering from malnutrition secondary to chronic alcoholism, and patients with pernicious anemia or disorders that result in malabsorption such as sprue, celiac disease, and inflammatory bowel disease. Of particular concern in the developed world is the epidemic of obesity. The increasing rates of bariatric surgery have been accompanied by neurologic complications related to nutrient deficiencies. The preventable and potentially treatable nature of these disorders makes this an important subject. Prognosis depends on prompt recognition and institution of appropriate therapy.

Particularly important for optimal functioning of the nervous system are the B-group vitamins (vitamin B_{12}, thiamine, niacin, and pyridoxine), vitamin E, copper, and folic acid. Not infrequently multiple nutritional deficiencies coexist. The first section of this review discusses neurologic manifestations related to deficiency of key nutrients such as vitamin B_{12}, folate, copper, vitamin E, thiamine, and others. **Table 1** summarizes the salient aspects covered in this section. The second section addresses neurologic complications related to bariatric surgery. The third sections includes neurologic presentations caused by nutrient deficiencies in the setting of alcoholism. The concluding section addresses neurologic deficiency diseases that have a geographic predilection. Many of these latter conditions are seen in tropical or developing countries, and are often caused by multiple coexisting deficiencies.

The interested reader is directed to some recent review articles and book chapters for additional references.[1–10]

Department of Neurology, Mayo Clinic College of Medicine, Mayo Clinic, 200 First Street, SW, Rochester, MN 55905, USA
E-mail address: kumar.neeraj@mayo.edu

Neurol Clin 28 (2010) 107–170
doi:10.1016/j.ncl.2009.09.006
0733-8619/09/$ – see front matter © 2010 Elsevier Inc. All rights reserved.

neurologic.theclinics.com

Table 1
Summary of sources, causes of deficiency, neurologic significance, laboratory tests, and treatment of deficiency states related to Cbl, folate, copper, vitamin E, thiamine, niacin, and pyridoxine

Nutrient	Sources	Major Causes of Deficiency	Neurologic Significance Associated with Deficiency	Laboratory Tests	Treatment	Additional Comments
Cobalamin	Meats, egg, milk, fortified cereals, legumes	Pernicious anemia, elderly (caused by atrophic gastritis and food-Cbl malabsorption), gastric surgery, acid reduction therapy, gastrointestinal disease, parasitic infestation by fish tapeworm, hereditary enzyme defects, N_2O toxicity, rarely strict vegetarianism, often unknown	Myelopathy or myeloneuropathy, peripheral neuropathy, neuropsychiatric manifestations, optic neuropathy, autonomic dysfunction	Serum Cbl, serum MMA, plasma total Hcy, hematologic tests (anemia, macrocytosis, neutrophil hypersegmentation), Schilling test, serum gastrin, intrinsic factor and parietal cell antibodies	IM B_{12} 1000 µg twice weekly for 2 weeks (or 100 µg twice weekly for 2 weeks), followed by weekly for 2 months and monthly thereafter or IM B_{12} 1000 µg daily for the first week, followed by weekly for the first month, then monthly thereafter; CyanoCbl is the form commonly used in United States, hydroxoCbl is the form preferred in parts of Europe; it requires less frequent injections and may be more allergenic	Even in the presence of severe malabsorption, 2–5 years may pass before cobalamin deficiency develops Disturbance in cobalamin metabolism in AIDS-associated myelopathy

Folate	In virtually all foods (spinach, yeast, peanuts, liver, beans such as kidney beans and lima beans, broccoli are particularly rich sources) (grains and cereals are fortified with folic acid)	Alcoholism, gastrointestinal disease, folate antagonists (eg, methotrexate, trimethoprim), errors of folate metabolism. Folate deficiency generally coexists with other nutrient deficiencies	Neurologic manifestations are rare and indistinguishable from those caused by Cbl deficiency	Serum folate, RBC folate (more reliable indicator of tissue stores than serum folate), plasma total Hcy	Oral folate 1 mg 3 times a day followed by a maintenance dose of 1 mg a day; for acutely ill patients 1–5 mg/d (parenteral); supplementation with 0.4 mg/d in women in child bearing as for prophylaxis against neural tube defects	Clinically significant depletion of body folate stores may be seen in weeks-months. Higher requirements in pregnancy, lactation, methotrexate toxicity. Folate in foods have a bioavailability of less than 50%, folic acid supplements are in the monoglutamate form and have a bioavailability approaching 100%. The reduced folates in food are labile and readily lost under certain cooking conditions such as boiling

(continued on next page)

Table 1 *(continued)*

Nutrient	Sources	Major Causes of Deficiency	Neurologic Significance Associated with Deficiency	Laboratory Tests	Treatment	Additional Comments
Copper	Organ meats, seafood, nuts, mushroom, cocoa, chocolate, beans, whole grain products	Gastric surgery, zinc toxicity, gastrointestinal disease, total parenteral nutrition and enteral feeding, rarely acquired dietary deficiency, often unknown	Myelopathy or myeloneuropathy	Serum and urinary copper, serum ceruloplasmin, serum and urinary zinc, hematologic parameters (anemia, neutropenia, vacuolated myeloid precursors, ringed sideroblasts, iron-containing plasma cells)	Oral elemental copper: 8 mg/d for a week, 6 mg/d for the second week, 4 mg/d for the third week and 2 mg/d thereafter	Hyperzincemia of indeterminate cause may be present even in the absence of excess zinc ingestion Speculative if copper deficiency may have been responsible for subacute myelo-optic neuropathy (secondary to clioquinol)
Vitamin E	Vegetable oils (sunflower and olive), leafy vegetables, fruits, meats, nuts, cereals	Chronic cholestasis (particularly in children), pancreatic insufficiency, gastrointestinal disease, AVED, homozygous hypobetalipo-proteinemia, abetalipo-proteinemia, chylomicron retention disease	Spinocerebellar syndrome with peripheral neuropathy, ophthalmoplegia, pigmentary retinopathy	Serum vitamin E Ratio of serum α-tocopherol to sum of serum cholesterol and triglycerides	Vitamin E ranging from 200 mg/d to 200 mg/kg/d (oral, intramuscular); supplementation of bile slats in some patients	Vitamin E deficiency is virtually never the consequence of a dietary inadequacy Neurologic findings are rare in vitamin E-deficient adults with chronic cholestasis Vitamin E bioavailability is dependent on food fat

	Sources	Risk factors	Neurologic presentation	Diagnostic test	Treatment	Comments
Thiamin	Enriched, fortified, or whole grain products, organ meats	Recurrent vomiting, gastric surgery, alcoholism, dieting, increased demand with marginal nutritional status	Beriberi (dry, wet, infantile), WE, KS	Urinary thiamin, serum thiamin, erythrocyte transketolase activation assay, RBC thiamin diphosphate	50–300 mg/d of thiamine (intravenous, intramuscular, oral); higher doses may be required in WE; infantile beriberi: 5–20 mg of parenteral thiamine	At risk patients should receive parenteral thiamine before administration of glucose or parenteral nutrition
Niacin	Meat, fish, poultry, enriched bread, fortified cereals	Corn as primary carbohydrate source, alcoholism, malabsorption, carcinoid and Hartnup syndrome	Encephalopathy (peripheral neuropathy)	Urinary excretion of methylated niacin metabolites	25–50 mg of nicotinic acid (intramuscular, oral)	
Pyridoxine	Meat, fish, eggs, soybeans, nuts, dairy products	B_6 antagonists (INH, hydralazine, penicillamine), alcoholism, gastrointestinal disease	Infantile seizures, peripheral neuropathy (pure sensory neuropathy with toxicity)	Plasma pyridoxal phosphate	50–100 mg of pyridoxine daily (oral); pyridoxine supplementation in patients on isoniazid	

Abbreviations: AVED, ataxia with vitamin E deficiency; Cbl, cobalamin; Hcy, homocysteine; IM, intramuscular; INH, isoniazid; KS, Korsakoff syndrome; MMA, methylmalonic acid; RBC, red blood cell; WE, Wernicke encephalopathy.

From Kumar N. Nutritional neuropathies. Neurol Clin 2007; 25(1): 209-55

NEUROLOGIC MANIFESTATIONS RELATED TO DEFICIENCIES OF KEY NUTRIENTS
Vitamin B_{12}

Even though vitamin B_{12} (B_{12}) refers specifically to cyanocobalamin, the terms cobalamin (Cbl), B_{12}, and vitamin B_{12} are generally used interchangeably. Cbl is required as a cofactor in several enzymatic reactions. The 2 active forms of Cbl are methylCbl and adenosylCbl (**Fig. 1**).[11] **Fig. 1** shows the biochemical pathways involved in Cbl metabolism and **Fig. 2** shows the steps involved in the gastrointestinal processing and absorption of Cbl. Cbl is transferred across the intestinal mucosa into portal blood where it binds to transCbl II (TCII). The liver takes up approximately 50% of the Cbl and the rest is transported to other tissues. TCII-bound Cbl is taken up by cells through TCII receptor-mediated endocytosis. Cbl bound to transcobalamin II (holoTC) is the fraction of total vitamin B_{12} available for tissue uptake. Intracellular lysosomal degradation releases Cbl for conversion to methylCbl or adenosylCbl. Most of the Cbl secreted in the bile is reabsorbed. The estimated daily losses of Cbl are minute compared with body stores. Hence, even in the presence of severe malabsorption, 2 to 5 years may pass before Cbl deficiency develops.[12] Similarly, a clinical relapse in pernicious anemia after interrupting Cbl therapy takes approximately 5 years before it is recognized.

Causes of deficiency

Not infrequently the cause of Cbl deficiency is unknown. Most patients with clinically expressed Cbl deficiency have malabsorption related to intrinsic factor such as that seen in pernicious anemia. Cbl deficiency is particularly common in the elderly and is most likely caused by the high incidence of atrophic gastritis and achlorhydria-induced food-Cbl malabsorption.[13,14] Food-bound Cbl malabsorption is rarely associated with clinically significant deficiency. Cbl deficiency is commonly seen following gastric surgery. Partial gastrectomy and bariatric surgery cause food-bound Cbl malabsorption; partial gastrectomy may also be associated with loss of intrinsic factor.[15–18] Acid reduction therapy such as with H_2 blockers and prolonged use of drugs like metformin can also cause Cbl deficiency.[19,20] Other causes of Cbl deficiency include conditions associated with malabsorption such as ileal disease or resection, bacterial overgrowth, pancreatic disease, and tropical sprue. *Helicobacter pylori* infection of the stomach may be associated with mucosal atrophy, hypochlorhydria, and impaired splitting of bound Cbl from food proteins. Competition for Cbl secondary to parasitic infestation by the fish tapeworm *Diphyllobothrium latum* may cause Cbl deficiency. Certain hereditary enzymatic defects can also manifest as disorders of Cbl metabolism.[21] Increased prevalence of B_{12} deficiency has been recognized in patients infected with human immunodeficiency virus (HIV) with neurologic symptoms but the precise clinical significance of this is unclear.[22,23] In AIDS-associated myelopathy the Cbl- and folate-dependent transmethylation pathway is depressed and cerebrospinal fluid and serum levels of *S*-adenosyl methionine are reduced.[24] Despite low B_{12} levels in many patients with AIDS, serum homocysteine (Hcy) and methylmalonic acid (MMA) levels are normal and Cbl supplementation fails to improve clinical manifestations.

Nitrous oxide (N_2O, "laughing gas") is a commonly used inhalational anesthetic that has been abused because of its euphoriant properties. N_2O irreversibly oxidizes the cobalt core of Cbl and renders methylCbl inactive.[25] Clinical manifestations of Cbl deficiency appear relatively rapidly with N_2O toxicity because the metabolism is blocked at the cellular level, but they may be delayed up to 8 weeks.[26,27] Postoperative neurologic dysfunction can be seen with N_2O exposure during routine anesthesia

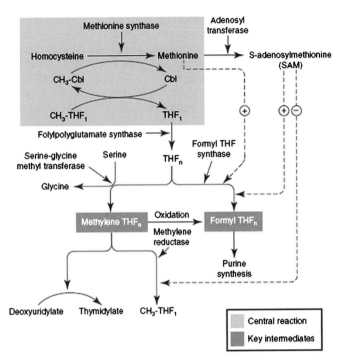

Cobalamin (Cbl); CH_3 = methyl group; THF_1 and THF_n =
monoglutamated and polyglutamated forms of tetrahydrofolate

Fig. 1. Biochemistry of cobalamin and folate deficiency. MethylCbl is a cofactor for a cytosolic enzyme, methionine synthase, in a methyl-transfer reaction that converts homocysteine (Hcy) to methionine. Methionine is adenosylated to SAM, a methyl group donor required for biologic methylation reactions involving proteins, neurotransmitters, and phospholipids. Decreased SAM production leads to reduced myelin basic protein methylation and white matter vacuolization in Cbl deficiency. Methionine also facilitates the formation of formyl-tetrahydrofolate (THF), which is involved in purine synthesis. During the process of methionine formation methylTHF donates the methyl group and is converted into THF, a precursor for purine and pyrimidine synthesis. Impaired DNA synthesis could interfere with oligodendrocyte growth and myelin production. AdenosylCbl is a cofactor for L-methylmalonyl CoA (CoA) mutase, which catalyzes the conversion of L-methylmalonyl CoA to succinyl CoA in an isomerization reaction. Accumulation of methylmalonate and propionate may provide abnormal substrates for fatty acid synthesis. The branched-chain and abnormal odd-number carbon fatty acids may be incorporated into the myelin sheath. The biologically active folates are in the THF form. MethylTHF is the predominant folate and is required for the Cbl-dependent remethylation of Hcy to methionine. Methylation of deoxyuridylate to thymidylate is mediated by methyleneTHF. Impairment of this reaction results in accumulation of uracil, which replaces the decreased thymine in nucleoprotein synthesis and initiates the process that leads to megaloblastic anemia. CH_3, methyl group; Cbl, cobalamin; THF_1 and THF_n, monoglutamated and polyglutamated forms of tetrahydrofolate. (*Adapted from* Tefferi A, Pruthi RK. The biochemical basis of cobalamin deficiency. Mayo Clin Proc 1994;69:185; with permission.)

if subclinical Cbl deficiency is present.[26,28] N_2O toxicity caused by inhalant abuse has been reported among dentists, other medical personnel, and university students.[29–31]

Vitamin B_{12} deficiency is only rarely the consequence of diminished dietary intake. Strict vegetarians may rarely develop mild Cbl deficiency after years. The low vitamin

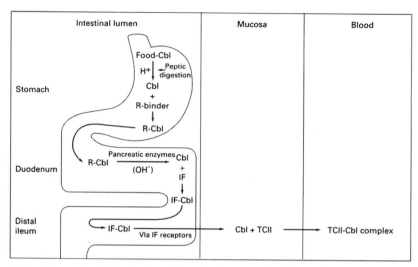

Fig. 2. Physiology of cobalamin absorption. In the stomach, Cbl bound to food is dissociated from proteins in the presence of acid and pepsin. The released Cbl binds to R proteins secreted by salivary glands and gastric mucosa. In the small intestine, pancreatic proteases partially degrade the R protein-Cbl complex at neutral pH and release Cbl, which then binds with IF. IF is a Cbl-binding protein secreted by gastric parietal cells. The IF-Cbl complex binds to specific receptors in the ileal mucosa and is internalized. In addition to the IF-mediated absorption of ingested Cbl, there is a nonspecific absorption of Cbl that occurs by passive diffusion at all mucosal sites. This is a relatively inefficient process by which 1–2% of the ingested amount is absorbed. Cbl, cobalamin; H^+, acidic, OH^-, alkaline; IF, intrinsic factor. (*Adapted from* Tefferi A, Pruthi RK. The biochemical basis of cobalamin deficiency. Mayo Clin Proc 1994;69:183; with permission.)

B_{12} level noted in vegetarians is often without clinical consequences. Clinical manifestations are more likely when poor intake begins in childhood wherein limited stores and growth requirements act as additional confounders.

Clinical significance

Neurologic manifestations may be the earliest and often the only manifestation of Cbl deficiency.[32–38] The severity of the hematologic and neurologic manifestations may be inversely related in a particular patient. Relapses are generally associated with the same neurologic phenotype. The commonly recognized neurologic manifestations may include a myelopathy with or without an associated neuropathy, cognitive impairment, optic neuropathy (impaired vision, optic atrophy, centrocecal scotomas), and paresthesias without abnormal signs.

The best characterized neurologic manifestation of Cbl deficiency is a myelopathy that has commonly been referred to as subacute combined degeneration. The neurologic features typically include a spastic paraparesis, extensor plantar response, and impaired perception of position and vibration. Accompanying optic nerve involvement may be present. The most severely involved regions are the cervical and upper thoracic posterior columns. Changes are also seen in the lateral columns. Involvement of the anterior columns is rare. Spongiform changes and foci of myelin and axon destruction are seen in the spinal cord white matter. There is myelin loss followed by axonal degeneration and gliosis. Neuropsychiatric manifestations include decreased memory, personality change, psychosis, and rarely delirium.[34,36] High total vitamin B_{12} intake or higher vitamin B_{12} concentrations and MMA levels have been associated with slower cognitive decline among the very elderly.[39,40] A recent study of Cbl status and rate of brain volume loss in community-dwelling elderly individuals noted that decrease in brain volume was greater among those with lower Cbl and holoTC levels and higher plasma total Hcy and MMA levels.[41]

Rarely reported neurologic manifestations related to Cbl deficiency include cerebellar ataxia, orthostatic tremors, ophthalmoplegia, vocal cord paralysis, a syringomyelia-like distribution of motor and sensory deficits, and autonomic dysfunction.[42–49]

Clinical, electrophysiologic, and pathologic involvement of the peripheral nervous system has been described with Cbl deficiency. In a recent study Cbl deficiency was detected in 27 of 324 patients with a polyneuropathy.[50] Clues to possible B_{12} deficiency in a patient with polyneuropathy included a relatively sudden onset of symptoms, findings suggestive of an associated myelopathy, onset of symptoms in the hands, macrocytic red blood cells, and the presence of a risk factor for Cbl deficiency.

Serum Cbl can be normal in some patients with Cbl deficiency and serum MMA and total Hcy levels are useful in diagnosing patients with Cbl deficiency.[12,51–55] The sensitivity of the available metabolic tests for Cbl deficiency has facilitated the development of the concept of subclinical Cbl deficiency.[56,57] This refers to biochemical evidence of Cbl deficiency in the absence of hematologic or neurologic manifestations. These biochemical findings should respond to Cbl therapy if Cbl deficiency is their true cause. The frequency of subclinical Cbl deficiency is estimated to be at least 10 times that of clinical Cbl deficiency and its incidence increases with age.[57–59] The cause of subclinical Cbl deficiency includes food-bound Cbl malabsorption but is frequently unknown; the course is often stationary.[60,61] Some of these individuals may have subtle neurologic and neurophysiologic abnormalities of uncertain significance that may respond to Cbl therapy.[62,63] The presence of a low Cbl level in association with neurologic manifestations does not imply cause and effect or indicate the presence of metabolic Cbl deficiency. The incidence of cryptogenic polyneuropathy, cognitive impairment, and Cbl deficiency increases with age and Cbl deficiency may be a chance occurrence rather than causative. Although Cbl levels are frequently low in the elderly, up to one-third are falsely low by clinical and metabolic criteria, and many of the remainder are clinically innocent.[13,58,64,65] The clinical impact of subclinical Cbl deficiency and its appropriate management are uncertain. If it is unclear whether an elevated MMA or Hcy level is caused by Cbl deficiency, the response to empirical parenteral B_{12} replacement can be assessed.

Investigations
Serum Cbl determination has been the mainstay for evaluating Cbl status.[12,65,66] The older microbiologic and radioisotopic assays have been replaced by immunologically based chemiluminescence assays. Although it is a widely used screening test, serum Cbl measurement has technical and interpretive problems and lacks sensitivity and specificity for the diagnosis of Cbl deficiency (**Table 2**).[12,52–54,57,58,66–71] Levels of serum MMA and plasma total Hcy are useful as ancillary diagnostic tests.[12,51–55] The specificity of MMA is superior to that of plasma Hcy. Although plasma total Hcy is a very sensitive indicator of Cbl deficiency, its major limitation is its poor specificity. **Table 2** indicates causes other than Cbl deficiency that can result in abnormal levels of Cbl, MMA, and Hcy. Hcy should be measured either fasting or after an oral methionine load. Immediate refrigeration of the blood sample is important because levels of Hcy increase if whole blood is left at room temperature for hours. Measuring MMA and Hcy is also useful in patients with N_2O toxicity and those with inherited metabolic disorders. In these conditions vitamin B_{12}-dependent pathways are impaired despite

Table 2
Common causes, other than Cbl deficiency, for abnormal Cbl, MMA, and Hcy levels[56,57,66]

Cbl	MMA	Hcy
Decrease (falsely low)	*Increase*	*Increase*
Pregnancy	Renal insufficiency	Renal insufficiency
Transcobalamin I deficiency	Volume contraction (possible)	Volume contraction
Folate deficiency	Bacterial contamination of gut (possible)	Folate deficiency
Other diseases: HIV infection, myeloma	MMCoA mutase deficiency	Vitamin B_6 deficiency
Drugs: anticonvulsants, oral contraceptives, radionuclide isotope studies	Other MMA-related enzyme defects	Other diseases: hypothyroidism, renal transplant, leukemia, psoriasis, alcohol abuse
Idiopathic	Infancy, pregnancy	Inappropriate sample collection and processing
Increase (falsely normal)	*Decrease*	Drugs: isoniazid, colestipol, niacin, L-DOPA
Renal failure	Antibiotic-related reductions in bowel flora	Enzyme defects: cystathionine β-synthase deficiency, MTHFR deficiency
Intestinal bacterial overgrowth		Age, males, increased muscle mass
Transcobalamin II deficiency Abnormal Cbl-binding protein		
Liver disease (increase haptocorrin concentration)		
Myeloproliferative disorders (polycythemia vera, chronic myelogenous leukemia) (increase haptocorrin concentration)		

Abbreviations: Cbl, cobalamin; Hcy, homocysteine; HIV, human immunodeficiency virus; MMA, methylmalonic acid; MMCoA, L-methylmalonyl coenzyme A; MTHFR, methylene tetrahydrofolate reductase.

normal vitamin B_{12} levels. Vitamin B_{12} bound to holoTC is the fraction of total vitamin B_{12} available for tissue uptake and therefore has been proposed by some as a potentially useful alternative indicator of vitamin B_{12} status.[72–80]

An increase in the mean corpuscular volume may precede development of anemia.[81] The presence of neutrophil hypersegmentation may be a sensitive marker for Cbl deficiency and may be seen in the absence of anemia or macrocytosis. Megaloblastic bone marrow changes may be seen.

To determine the cause of Cbl deficiency, tests directed at determining the cause of malabsorption are undertaken. Concerns regarding cost, accuracy, and radiation exposure have led to a significant decrease in the availability of the Schilling test.[82] Elevated serum gastrin and decreased pepsinogen I levels are seen in 80% to 90% of patients with pernicious anemia but the specificity of these tests is limited.[83] Elevated gastrin levels are a marker for hypochlorhydria or achlorhydria, which are invariably seen with pernicious anemia. Elevated gastrin levels may be seen in up to

30% of the elderly.[14] Elevated serum gastrin levels are approximately 70% specific and sensitive for pernicious anemia.[84] Anti-intrinsic factor antibodies are specific (>95%) but lack sensitivity and are found in approximately 50% to 70% of patients with pernicious anemia.[85–87] Studies suggest that antiparietal cell antibodies may not be seen as commonly as was earlier believed and therefore have limited usefulness.[87] False-positive results for the gastric parietal cell antibody are common. They may be seen in 10% of people more than 70 years old and are also present in other autoimmune endocrinopathies. A common approach is to combine the specific but insensitive intrinsic factor antibody test with the sensitive but nonspecific serum gastrin or pepsinogen level in patients with Cbl deficiency.[65]

Electrophysiologic abnormalities include nerve conduction studies suggestive of a sensorimotor axonopathy, and abnormalities on somatosensory evoked potentials, visual evoked potentials, and motor evoked potentials.[88,89]

Magnetic resonance imaging (MRI) abnormalities include a signal change in the subcortical white matter and posterior and lateral columns.[89–92] Similar spinal cord MRI findings are seen with nitrous oxide toxicity.[31] Brain T2-hyperintensities seen in Cbl deficiency may show significant improvement with vitamin B_{12} replacement[93] Contrast enhancement involving the dorsal or lateral columns may be present.[94,95] The dorsal column may show a decreased signal on T1-weighted images.[95] Other reported findings include cord atrophy and anterior column involvement.[96,97] Treatment may be accompanied by reversal of cord swelling, contrast enhancement, and signal change.[89,90,92,95,97] Increased T2 signals involving the cerebellum are also reported.[47,98] Rarely striking diffuse white matter abnormalities suggestive of a leukoencephalopathy may be seen.[47,99]

Management

The goals of treatment are to reverse the signs and symptoms of deficiency, replete body stores, ascertain the cause of deficiency, and monitor response to therapy. With normal Cbl absorption, oral administration of 3 to 5 μg of cyanoCbl may suffice. In patients with food-bound Cbl malabsorption caused by achlorhydria, 50 to 100 μg of cyanoCbl given orally is often adequate.[100] More recent studies have shown blunted metabolic responses in elderly persons with subclinical deficiency until oral doses reached 500 μg or more.[101–103] Patients with Cbl deficiency caused by achlorhydria-induced food-bound Cbl malabsorption show normal absorption of crystalline B_{12} but are unable to digest and absorb Cbl in food because of achlorhydria. The more common situation is one of impaired absorption where parenteral therapy is required. A short course of daily or weekly therapy is often followed by monthly maintenance therapy (see **Table 1**). If the oral dose is large enough, even patients with an absorption defect may respond to oral Cbl.[104] The response to oral therapy is less predictable and relapse occurs following cessation of oral therapy sooner than with parenteral regimens.[33,105]

Patients with pernicious anemia have a higher risk of gastric cancer and carcinoids, and therefore should undergo endoscopy.[106] Patients with pernicious anemia also have a higher frequency of thyroid disease and iron deficiency and should be screened for these conditions.[107,108]

Patients with B_{12} deficiency are prone to develop neurologic deterioration following N_2O anesthesia. This situation is preventable by prophylactic vitamin B_{12} given weeks before surgery in individuals with a borderline B_{12} level who are expected to receive N_2O anesthesia. Intramuscular B_{12} should be given to patients with acute N_2O poisoning. Methionine supplementation has also been proposed as a first-line therapy.[109] With chronic exposure, immediate cessation of exposure should be ensured. In AIDS-associated myelopathy, a possible benefit of administration of the S-adenosyl methionine precursor, L-methionine, was suggested by a pilot study but not confirmed in a subsequent double-blind study.[110,111]

Response to treatment may relate to the extent of involvement and delay in starting treatment.[36] Remission correlates inversely with the time lapsed between symptom onset and initiation of therapy. Response of the neurologic manifestations is variable, may be incomplete, often starts in the first week, and is complete in 6 months.[65] Response of the hematologic derangements is prompt and complete. Reticulocyte count begins to increase within 3 days and peaks around 7 days. Red blood cell count begins to increase by 7 days and is followed by a decline in mean corpuscular volume with normalization by 8 weeks. MMA and Hcy levels normalize by 10 to 14 days. Cbl and holoTC levels increase after injection regardless of the benefit. Hence, MMA and Hcy are more reliable for monitoring response to therapy. In patients with severe Cbl deficiency, replacement therapy may be accompanied by hypokalemia as a result of proliferation of bone marrow cells that use potassium. The clinical significance of this hypokalemia is unproven.[65,112]

HydroxoCbl is commonly used in parts of Europe. It is more allergenic but has superior retention and may permit injections every 2 to 3 months.[113] Compared with hydroxoCbl, cyanoCbl binds to serum proteins less well and is excreted more rapidly.[114] Intranasal administration of hydroxoCbl has been associated with fast absorption and normalization of Cbl levels.[115] Advantages of delivering Cbl by the nasal or sublingual route are unproven. Oral preparations of intrinsic factor are available but not reliable. Antibodies to intrinsic factor may nullify its effectiveness in the intestinal lumen.

Neurologically affected patients may have high folate levels.[38] Inappropriate folate therapy may delay recognition of the Cbl deficiency and cause neurologic deterioration. Anemia caused by Cbl deficiency often responds to folate therapy but the response is incomplete and transient. It is unclear if routine folate supplementation may compromise the early diagnosis of the hematologic manifestations or worsen the neurologic consequences.

Folic Acid

Folate functions as a coenzyme or cosubstrate by modifying, accepting, or transferring 1 carbon moiety in single-carbon reactions involved in the metabolism of nucleic and amino acids. The biologically active folates are in the tetrahydrofolate (THF) form. MethylTHF is the predominant folate and is required for the Cbl-dependent remethylation of Hcy to methionine (see **Fig. 1**). Methylation of deoxyuridylate to thymidylate is mediated by methyleneTHF (see **Fig. 1**). Impairment of this reaction results in accumulation of uracil, which replaces the decreased thymine in nucleoprotein synthesis and initiates the process that leads to megaloblastic anemia. Folate is absorbed by a saturable mechanism that occurs in the proximal small intestines and an unsaturable mechanism that predominates in the ileum. The saturable process is mediated by the reduced folate carrier located in the cellular brush border membranes.[116] In the enterocyte, folate is converted into methylTHF and a carrier-mediated mechanism exports it into the bloodstream. The absorbed folate is cleared from the bloodstream and enters various compartments. The reduced folate carrier is also involved in cellular uptake of reduced folates in tissues. Cellular folate uptake also occurs via passive diffusion. Once internalized, folate undergoes polyglutamation, which permits its attachment to enzymes. Polyglutamated folates have greater metabolic activity and are better retained by cells compared with monoglutamated folates.[117] Serum folate levels decrease within 3 weeks after reduced folate intake or absorption, red blood cell folate declines weeks later, and clinically significant depletion of folate stores may be seen within months.[118] Clinical features of folate deficiency occur more rapidly with low stores or coexisting alcoholism. The ratio of body stores to daily requirement is 100:1.[119] Daily folate losses may approximate 1% to 2% of body stores.

Causes of deficiency

Folate deficiency rarely exists in the pure state. It is often associated with conditions that affect other nutrients. Hence, attribution of neurologic manifestations to folate deficiency requires exclusion of other potential causes. Populations at increased risk of folate deficiency include alcoholics, premature infants, and adolescents. Increased folate requirements are seen in pregnancy, lactation, and chronic hemolytic anemia. Folate deficiency may also result from restricted diets such as those used to manage phenylketonuria. Folate deficiency may be seen with small bowel disorders associated with malabsorption such as tropical sprue, celiac disease, bacterial overgrowth syndrome, giardiasis, and inflammatory bowel disease. Folate absorption may be decreased in conditions associated with reduced gastric secretions such as gastric surgery, atrophic gastritis, acid-suppressive therapy, and acid neutralization by treatment of pancreatic insufficiency.[120–122] Drugs such as aminopterin, methotrexate, pyrimethamine, trimethoprim, and triamterene act as folate antagonists and produce folate deficiency by inhibiting dihydrofolate reductase.[123] The mechanism by which anticonvulsants, antituberculosis drugs, sulfasalazine, and oral contraceptives result in folate deficiency is uncertain. Methotrexate can causes leukoencephalopathy associated with marked increase in cerebrospinal fluid homocysteine.

Clinical significance

Theoretically folate deficiency could cause the same deficits as those seen with Cbl deficiency because of its importance in the production of methionine, S-adenosyl methionine (SAM), and THF. For reasons that are not clear, neurologic manifestations like those seen in Cbl deficiency are rare in folate deficiency.[124,125] The myeloneuropathy or neuropathy or megaloblastic anemia seen in association with folate deficiency is indistinguishable from Cbl deficiency.[126–130]

Folate deficiency has been associated with affective disorders.[131] A low folate level may be seen in elderly asymptomatic individuals, particularly in patients with psychiatric disease and Alzheimer dementia.[132] In recent years there has been some evidence to suggest that chronic folate deficiency may increase the risk of cardiovascular disease, cerebrovascular disease, peripheral vascular disease, venous thrombosis, and may cause cognitive impairment.[124,125] In one study, moderate reduction of Hcy levels with folate, Cbl, and vitamin B_6 had no effect on vascular outcomes in patients with stroke at 2 years follow-up.[133] Low folate levels may be a risk factor for cognitive decline in high-functioning older adults.[134] In another population-based study in the elderly, high folate intake was associated with cognitive decline.[39] The precise significance of these observations awaits further studies.

Folate deficiency causes increased frequency of neural tube defects in babies born to folate-deficient mothers.[125] Congenital errors of folate metabolism can be related either to defective transport of folate through various cells or to defective intracellular use of folate caused by some enzyme deficiencies. These are often associated with severe central neurologic dysfunction.[135] Hereditary deficiency of cystathionine β-synthase leads to hyperhomocysteinemia and hyperhomocysteinuria. The homozygous form lead to mental retardation, premature atherosclerosis, and seizures associated with markedly elevated Hcy levels and heretozygous individuals have milder elevation in Hcy levels with increased vascular risk. A more common condition is

C-to-T substitution at codon 677 in the gene coding for *N5*, *N10*-methylene tetrahydrofolate reductase (MTHFR). Homozygotes for this condition (C677T) mutation have mildly increased Hcy levels and increased vascular risk.

Investigations

Microbiologic assays for folate measurement have largely been replaced by radioisotopic assays. More recently automated immunologic methods using chemiluminescence or other nonisotopic detection are used. Folate results are dependent on the method used and laboratory where they were performed.[136] Plasma Hcy levels have been shown to be elevated in 86% of patients with clinically significant folate deficiency.[54] Metabolic folate deficiency, as suggested by elevated plasma total Hcy levels that improve with folate therapy, can be seen in asymptomatic individuals.[124] Generally a serum folate level of 2.5 µg/L has been taken as the cutoff for folate deficiency. It has been noted that plasma Hcy levels are slightly elevated and respond to folate supplementation in persons with folate levels as high as 5 µg/L.[137] This has led to the suggestion that serum folate levels between 2.5 and 5 µg/L may indicate a mildly compromised folate status. Serum folate fluctuates daily and does not correlate with tissue stores.[138] Red blood cell folate is more reliable than plasma folate because its levels are less affected by short-term fluctuations in intake.[139] However, red blood cell folate assay is subject to greater variation depending on the method and laboratory.[136] Reticulocytes have a higher folate content than mature red blood cells. Their presence can affect red blood cell folate levels as can blood transfusions.

Management

In women of childbearing age with epilepsy daily folate supplement of 0.4 mg is recommended for prophylaxis against neural tube defects. With documented folate deficiency an oral dose of 1 mg 3 times a day may be followed by a maintenance dose of 1 mg a day (see **Table 1**). Daily doses as high as 20 mg may be needed in patients with malabsorption. Acutely ill patients may need parenteral administration in a dose of 1 to 5 mg. Despite malabsorption patients respond to oral folic acid because it is readily absorbed by nonspecific mechanisms. Even in high doses, toxicity caused by folic acid is rare.[140] Coexisting Cbl deficiency should be ruled out before instituting folate therapy. Reduced folates such as folinic acid (N5-formylTHF) is required only when folate metabolism is impaired by drugs such as methotrexate or by an inborn error of metabolism. Plasma Hcy is likely the best biochemical tool for monitoring response to therapy; it decreases within a few days of instituting folate therapy but does not respond to inappropriate Cbl therapy.[141] Because folate deficiency is generally seen in association with a broader dietary inadequacy, the associated comorbidities need to be addressed.

Copper

Copper is a component of enzymes that have a critical role in maintaining the structure and function of the nervous system (**Table 3**). **Fig. 3** shows the pathways involved in copper absorption and excretion and the sites of defect in Menkes disease and Wilson disease.

Causes of deficiency

Because of the ubiquitous distribution of copper and a low daily requirement, acquired dietary copper deficiency is rare. Copper deficiency may occur in premature or low birth weight infants and in malnourished infants.[142] Copper deficiency may be a complication of total parenteral or enteral nutrition.[143,144] Other causes of copper

Table 3
Copper-dependent enzymes and their function

Enzyme	Function
Cytochrome c oxidase	Electron transport and oxidative phosphorylation
Copper/zinc superoxide dismutase	Antioxidant defense
Tyrosinase	Melanin synthesis
Dopamine β-hydroxylase	Catecholamine biosynthesis
Lysyl oxidase	Cross-linking of collagen and elastin
Peptidylglycine α-amidating monooxygenase	Neuropeptide and peptide hormone processing
Ceruloplasmin	Brain iron homeostasis
Hephaestin	Link between copper and iron metabolism

deficiency include nephrotic syndrome, glomerulonephritis, and enteropathies associated with malabsorption such as celiac disease, cystic fibrosis, Crohn disease, sprue, bacterial overgrowth, and others.[143,145–148] The commonest identified cause of copper deficiency in patients with a copper deficiency myelopathy has been reported to be a prior history of gastric surgery.[146,149–160] The duration between gastric surgery and onset of neurologic symptoms may range from less than a year to 24 years.[155,157] Excessive zinc ingestion is a well-recognized cause of copper deficiency.[146,156,161–166] Parenteral zinc overloading during chronic hemodialysis has also been associated with copper deficiency myelopathy.[167] In addition to the common use of zinc in the prevention or treatment of common colds and sinusitis, zinc therapy has been used for conditions such as acrodermatitis enteropathica, treatment of decubitus ulcers, sickle cell disease, celiac disease, memory impairment, and acne. Unusual sources of excess zinc have included patients who consumed excessive amounts of denture cream for long periods and patients swallowing zinc-containing coins.[163,165,166,168] An elevated serum zinc level in the absence of exogenous zinc ingestion may also be seen.[154,157,163,169–174] The significance of hyperzincemia seen in the absence of exogenous zinc ingestion is unclear.[171,175,176] Treatment with the copper-chelating agent tetrathiomolybdate has been reported to cause copper deficiency.[177] Clioquinol is an antibacterial drug that was used indiscriminately in Japan and other parts of the world before 1970. Clioquinol is also a copper chelator. The myelo-optic neuropathy seen with copper deficiency is similar to that reported with clioquinol; it has recently been speculated that copper deficiency may have been the mechanism of clioquinol toxicity.[178,179] Often the cause of copper deficiency is unclear. Emerging knowledge about copper transport may help clarify the cause of idiopathic hypocupremia.[180] The presence of multiple causes of copper deficiency can increase the chances of development of a clinically significant deficiency state.[146] Other nutrient deficiencies can coexist with copper deficiency.[146,147]

Clinical significance

Menkes disease is a copper deficiency-related disease in humans and is caused by congenital copper deficiency. Impaired biliary copper excretion underlies copper toxicity in Wilson disease. Copper deficiency-associated myelopathy has been described in ruminants and other animal species and has been called swayback or enzootic ataxia. The well-recognized hematologic manifestations of copper deficiency in humans include anemia and neutropenia.[160,163] Thrombocytopenia and resulting

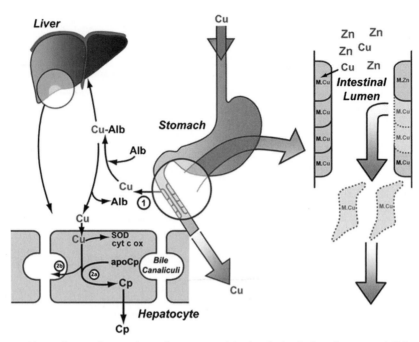

Fig. 3. Absorption and excretion of copper and basis of zinc-induced copper deficiency. Copper is probably absorbed from the stomach and proximal intestines. The Menkes P-type ATPase (*ATP7A*) is responsible for copper trafficking to the secretory pathway for efflux from enterocytes and other cells. Absorbed copper is bound to plasma albumin and amino acids in the portal blood and taken to the liver where it is incorporated into ceruloplasmin and released into the plasma. The Wilson P-type ATPase (*ATP7B*) is responsible for copper trafficking to the secretory pathway for ceruloplasmin biosynthesis and for endosome formation before biliary secretion. Copper distributes to the cornea, bone, brain, and kidneys. Bile is the major pathway for copper excretion. Excretion of copper into the gastrointestinal tract is the major pathway that regulates copper homeostasis and prevents deficiency or toxicity. Excessive zinc ingestion is a well-recognized cause of copper deficiency. The zinc-induced inhibition of copper absorption could be the result of competition for a common transporter or a consequence of induction of metallothionein in enterocytes. Metallothionein is an intracellular ligand and copper has a higher affinity for metallothionein than zinc. Zinc causes an upregulation of metallothionein production in the enterocytes. Copper displaces zinc from metallothionein, binds preferentially to the metallothionein, remains in the enterocytes, and is lost in the stools as the intestinal cells are sloughed off. Failure to mobilize absorbed copper from intestinal cells forms the basis of Menkes disease (1). In Wilson disease there is decreased incorporation of copper into ceruloplasmin (2a) and impaired biliary excretion of copper (2b). Cu, copper; Zn, zinc; Cp, ceruloplasmin; M, metallothionein; alb, albumin; SOD, superoxide dismutase; cyt c ox, cytochrome c oxidase. (*Adapted from* Kumar N. Copper deficiency myelopathy (human swayback). Mayo Clin Proc 2006;81:1378; with permission.)

pancytopenia is relatively rare. Typical bone marrow findings include a left shift in granulocytic and erythroid maturation with cytoplasmic vacuolization in erythroid and myeloid precursors.[150,160,163,181,182] Ringed sideroblasts and hemosiderin containing plasma cells may be present. Erythroid hyperplasia with decreased myeloid to erythroid ratio and dyserythropoiesis including megaloblastic changes may be seen. Patients may be given a diagnosis of sideroblastic anemia or myelodysplastic syndrome or aplastic anemia.

Only in recent years have the neurologic manifestations of acquired copper deficiency in humans been recognized.[145–167,169–172,174,182–188] The neurologic syndrome caused by acquired copper deficiency may be present without the hematologic manifestations. The most common manifestation is a myelopathy or myeloneuropathy that resembles the subacute combined degeneration seen with vitamin B_{12} deficiency.[145,146,149,151–155,157,158,161,162,164–167,171,172,174,182–187] It presents with a spastic gait and prominent sensory ataxia. The sensory ataxia is primarily caused by dorsal column dysfunction. Clinical or electrophysiologic evidence of an associated axonal peripheral neuropathy is common.[157,186,189] A wrist drop or foot drop may be present.[154,185,189] Peripheral neuropathy without myelopathy, central nervous system (CNS) demyelination, myopathy with myelopathy, optic neuropathy with myelopathy, optic neuritis with peripheral neuropathy, a sensory ganglionopathy, and cognitive impairment have also been described in association with copper deficiency but the significance of these reported associations needs further study.[145,146,150,158,165,169,170,188] Progressive, asymmetric weakness or electrodiagnostic evidence of denervation suggestive of lower motor neuron disease has also been reported.[156,165] One patient with myelo-optic neuropathy related to copper deficiency reported severe hyposmia and hypogeusia.[146] Copper and vitamin B_{12} deficiency may coexist.[154,158,163,174,190] Continued neurologic deterioration in patients with a history of B_{12}-related myelopathy who have a normal B_{12} level while on replacement therapy should be evaluated for copper deficiency.

Investigations

Laboratory indicators of copper deficiency include reduced serum copper or ceruloplasmin, and reduced urinary copper excretion. Urinary copper excretion may be normal. It declines only when dietary copper is very low. Changes in serum copper levels usually parallel the ceruloplasmin concentration. Ceruloplasmin is an acute-phase reactant and the increase in ceruloplasmin is probably responsible for the increase in serum copper levels seen in various conditions such as pregnancy, oral contraceptive use, liver disease, malignancy, hematologic disease, myocardial infections, smoking, diabetes, uremia, and various inflammatory and infections diseases. Copper deficiency could be masked under these conditions. It has been suggested that serum copper may be inadequate for assessing total body copper stores and activity of copper enzymes such as erythrocyte superoxide dismutase and platelet or leukocyte cytochrome c oxidase may be a better indicator of metabolically active copper stores.[191,192] A low serum copper or ceruloplasmin level can be seen in Wilson disease or the Wilson disease heterozygote state. Serum ceruloplasmin is absent in aceruloplasminemia. Hence, the laboratory detection of a low serum copper level does not imply copper deficiency.[193] Urinary zinc excretion is normal or elevated. Serum zinc elevation may be seen in the absence of exogenous zinc ingestion. The commonest abnormality on the spine MRI is increased T2 signal involving the dorsal column **(Fig. 4)**.[46,154,157,166,174,184,186] The cervical cord is most commonly involved and contrast enhancement is not present. Nonspecific areas of increased signal involving the subcortical white matter have been reported but are of uncertain significance.[154] A more confluent subcortical white matter signal or periventricular lesions are suggestive of demyelination.[146,154,169,170] Somatosensory evoked potential and nerve conduction studies suggest impaired central conduction and varying degrees of peripheral neuropathy, respectively.[146,161,186] Other reported electrophysiologic abnormalities noted in patients with copper deficiency and neurologic manifestations include prolonged visual evoked potentials and impaired central conduction on transcranial magnetic stimulation.[146,149,169,170]

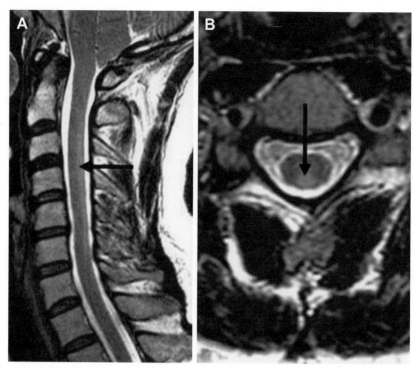

Fig. 4. Cord MRI in copper deficiency myelopathy. Sagittal (*A*) and axial (*B*) T2-weighted magnetic resonance images in a patient with copper deficiency showing increased signal in the paramedian aspect of the dorsal cervical cord (*arrows*).

Management

In patients with copper deficiency caused by excess zinc ingestion, stopping zinc supplementation may suffice.[163] Despite a suspected absorption defect, oral copper supplementation is generally the preferred route of supplementation. A commonly used regimen involves administering 8 mg of elemental copper orally for a week, 6 mg for the second week, 4 mg for the third week, and 2 mg thereafter (see **Table 1**). Periodic assessment of serum copper is essential to determine adequacy of replacement. Because of the need for long-term replacement, parenteral therapy is not preferred and generally not required. If oral therapy does not result in improvement or if there is rapid deterioration or significant hematologic derangement, then 2 mg of elemental copper may be administered intravenously daily for 5 days and periodically thereafter. Initial parenteral administration followed by oral therapy has also been used.[158,162]

Response of the hematologic parameters (including bone marrow findings) is prompt and often complete.[154,157,163,172,174,182,194] Hematologic recovery may be accompanied by reticulocytosis. Recovery of neurologic signs and symptoms is variable. Normalization of serum copper with improvement in neurologic symptoms, electrophysiology, and imaging has been reported but the more common outcome is cessation of progression.[154,157,161–163,165,167,169–172,174,184,187,195] A relapse in the copper-deficient state may not necessarily be accompanied by neurologic deterioration.[170] The initial response to copper replacement may not be sustained over time and a relapse may occur during continued oral treatment.[155]

Vitamin E

Vitamin E comprises a family of tocopherols (α, β, γ, and δ) and tocoretinols (α, β, γ, and δ). In humans α-tocopherol is the active and most important biologic form of vitamin E. The terms vitamin E and α-tocopherol are used simultaneously. Vitamin E supplements contain esters of α-tocopherol such as α-tocopheryl acetate, succinate, or nicotinate. The esters prevent vitamin E oxidation and prolong its shelf life. These esters are readily hydrolyzed in the gut and absorbed in the unesterified form.[196] Vitamin E serves as an antioxidant and prevents the formation of toxic free radical products. It seems to protect cellular membranes from oxidative stress, and inhibits the peroxidation of polyunsaturated fatty acids of membrane phospholipids. **Fig. 5** shows the pathways involved in vitamin E absorption and distribution. Most ingested vitamin E is eliminated by the fecal route.

Causes of deficiency

Because of the ubiquitous distribution of tocopherols in foods, vitamin E deficiency is almost never the consequence of a dietary inadequacy.[197] Vitamin E absorption

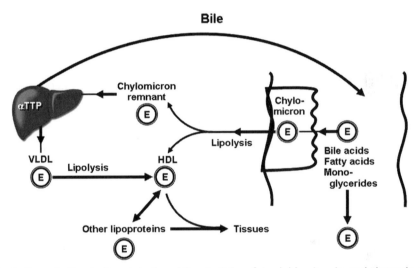

Fig. 5. Normal vitamin E metabolism. Vitamin E is a fat-soluble vitamin and depends on pancreatic esterases and bile salts for its solubilization and absorption in the lumen. Its absorption from the gastrointestinal tract is a nonenergy-requiring diffusion mediated process that requires bile acids, fatty acids, and monoglycerides for micelle formation. Following uptake by enterocytes, all forms of dietary vitamin E are incorporated into chylomicrons. The chylomicrons are secreted into the circulation, where lipolysis by lipoprotein lipase takes place. During lipolysis, various forms of vitamin E are transferred to high-density lipoproteins or other circulating lipoproteins and subsequently to tissues. The chylomicron remnants are taken up by the liver. In the liver the α-tocopherol transfer protein (TTP) incorporates α-tocopherol into VLDLs, which are secreted into plasma. Lipolysis of VLDL results in enrichment of circulating lipoproteins with R,R,R-α-tocopherol which is delivered to peripheral tissue. Most of the vitamin E in the human body is localized in the adipose tissue. Analysis of adipose tissue α-tocopherol content provides a useful estimate of long-term vitamin E intake. More than 2 years are required for adipose tissue α-/γ-tocopherol ratios to reach new steady-state levels in response to changes in dietary intake. Most ingested vitamin E is eliminated by the fecal route. (*Adapted from* Kumar N. Metabolic and toxic myelopathies. Continuum Spinal Cord, Root, and Plexus Disorders 2008;14(3):91–115; with permission.)

requires biliary and pancreatic secretions. Hence vitamin E deficiency is seen with chronic cholestasis and pancreatic insufficiency. Vitamin E deficiency is also seen with other conditions associated with malabsorption such as celiac disease, Crohn disease, cystic fibrosis, biliary atresia, blind loop syndrome, bowel irradiation, and extensive small bowel resection. Vitamin E supplementation in total parenteral nutrition may be inadequate to maintain vitamin E stores.[198]

Vitamin E deficiency may be seen because of genetic defects in α-thiamine triphosphate (TTP; ataxia with vitamin E deficiency [AVED]), in apolipoprotein B (homozygous hypobetalipoproteinemia), or in the microsomal triglyceride transfer protein (abetalipoproteinemia) (**Table 4**). An additional cause is a defect in chylomicron synthesis and secretion (chylomicron retention disease). AVED is an autosomal recessive disorder in which isolated vitamin E deficiency occurs without generalized fat malabsorption or gastrointestinal disease. The defect lies in impaired incorporation of vitamin E into hepatic lipoproteins for tissue delivery.[199] Mutations in the α-TTP gene on chromosome 8q13 are responsible.[200–202] Patients with hypobetalipoproteinemia or abetalipoproteinemia have an inability to secrete chylomicrons or other apolipoprotein B-containing lipoproteins, specifically very low density lipoprotein (VLDL) and low density lipoproteins (LDL).[197] Homozygous hypobetalipoproteinemia patients have a defect in the *apoB* gene. ApoB-containing lipoproteins secreted into the circulation turnover rapidly. In abetalipoproteinemia patients have a genetic defect in microsomal triglyceride transfer protein, which prevents normal lipidation of apoB and the secretion of apoB-containing lipoproteins is nonexistent. In chylomicron retention disease there is impaired assembly and secretion of chylomicrons and chylomicron retention in the intestinal mucosa is present.[203]

Clinical significance
In children with cholestatic liver disease, neurologic abnormalities appear as early as the second year of life. In AVED, hypolipoproteinemia, and abetalipoproteinemia, neurologic manifestations start by the first or second decade. Development of neurologic symptoms in adults with acquired fat malabsorption syndromes takes decades. Many years of malabsorption are required to deplete vitamin E stores.

The neurologic manifestations of vitamin E deficiency include a spinocerebellar syndrome with variable peripheral nerve involvement.[204–206] The phenotype is similar to that of Friedreich ataxia. The clinical features include cerebellar ataxia, hyporeflexia, proprioceptive, and vibratory loss, and an extensor plantar response. Cutaneous sensations may be affected to a lesser degree. Ophthalmoplegia, ptosis, and pigmentary retinopathy may be seen. An associated myopathy, at times with inflammatory infiltrates and rimmed vacuoles, has been described.[207–209] The neuropathy associated with vitamin E deficiency preferentially involves centrally directed fibers of large myelinated neurons. It is rare for vitamin E deficiency to present as an isolated neuropathy; isolated vitamin E deficiency with a demyelinating neuropathy has been reported.[210,211] Loss of myelinated nerve fibers may be seen on sural nerve biopsy before onset of neurologic signs and symptoms.[212] Reduction of peripheral nerve tocopherol may precede the axonal degeneration.[213] Swollen dystrophic axons (spheroids) have been seen in the gracile and cuneate nuclei of the brainstem. Lipofuscin may accumulate in the dorsal sensory neurons and peripheral Schwann cell cytoplasm. The peripheral nerves, posterior columns, and sensory roots show degeneration of large myelinated fibers.

Table 4
Summary of disorders of vitamin E metabolism

Disease	AVED	Homozygous Hypobetalipoproteinemia	Abetalipoproteinemia (Bassen-Kornzweig Disease)	Chylomicron Retention Disease
Source of defect	Mutations in α-TTP gene on chromosome 8q13 (AR)	Defect in apolipoprotein B gene (AD)	Genetic defect in microsomal triglyceride transfer protein (AR)	Chylomicron synthesis and secretion
Consequence of defect	Impaired incorporation of vitamin E into hepatic lipoproteins for tissue delivery	ApoB-containing lipoproteins secreted into the circulation turnover rapidly	Normal lipidation of apoB is prevented and secretion of apoB-containing lipoproteins is virtually nonexistent	Impaired assembly and secretion of chylomicrons with chylomicron retention in intestinal mucosa
Fat malabsorption	Absent	Present	Present	Present
Age of onset	Generally first decade, adult onset described	Early childhood	Early childhood	Early childhood
Other clinical features	Retinitis pigmentosa, skeletal deformities, cardiomyopathy	Retinitis pigmentosa, acanthocytosis, retarded growth, steatorrhea		Impacts growth and has gastrointestinal manifestations but acanthocytes are essentially absent, neuromuscular manifestations are less severe, and ocular manifestations are subclinical
Laboratory findings	Very low serum vitamin E (as low as 1/100th of normal)	Low serum vitamin E and other fat-soluble vitamins, low to nondetectable circulating lipoproteins (apoB, chylomicrons, VLDLs, or LDLs), serum cholesterol and triglycerides are markedly reduced (The ratio of free to esterified cholesterol in plasma is normal in hypolipoproteinemia and elevated in abetalipoproteinemia)		Hypocholesterolemia, normal fasting triglycerides, reduced plasma LDL apoprotein B, absence of chylomicrons after a fat test meal
Treatment	800–1200 mg/d of vitamin E (prompt normalization of plasma α-tocopherol concentration)	100–200 mg/kg of vitamin E	100–200 mg/kg of vitamin E	100–200 mg/kg of vitamin E

Abbreviations: AD, autosomal dominant; AR, autosomal recessive; AVED, ataxia with vitamin E deficiency; LDL, low density lipoprotein; TTP, thiamine triphosphate; VLDL, very low density lipoprotein.

Adapted from Kumar N. Metabolic and toxic myelopathies. Cont Spin Cord Root Plexus Disord 2008;14:91–115; Kumar N. Neurogastroenterology. Cont Neurol Manifest Syst Dis 2008;14:13–52; with permission.

Investigations

Serum vitamin E levels are dependent on the concentrations of serum lipids, cholesterol, and VLDL. Hyperlipidemia or hypolipidemia can independently increase or decrease serum vitamin E without reflecting similar alterations in tissue levels of the vitamin.[214,215] Effective serum α-tocopherol concentrations are calculated by dividing the serum α-tocopherol by the sum of serum cholesterol and triglycerides.[216,217] Serum α-tocopherol concentrations may be in the normal range in patients with α-tocopherol deficiency caused by cholestatic liver disease, a disorder that is also associated with high lipid levels.[215] In patients with neurologic manifestations caused by vitamin E deficiency, serum vitamin E levels are frequently undetectable. Additional markers of fat malabsorption such as increased stool fat and decreased serum carotene levels may be present.

Somatosensory evoked potential studies may show evidence of central delay and nerve conduction studies may show evidence of an axonal neuropathy.[5,8] Spinal MRI in patients with myeloneuropathy related to vitamin E deficiency may show increased signal in the cervical cord dorsal column.[218]

Management

In AVED, supplementation with vitamin E 600 IU twice daily raises plasma concentration to normal and is accompanied by beneficial effects on neurologic function. Because of limited absorption, patients with abetalipoproteinemia may need high doses.[219] With cholestatic liver disease treatment with standard doses of fat-soluble vitamin E may be ineffective because of fat malabsorption. Larger oral doses or intramuscular administration or a water-miscible product (D-α-tocopherol glycol) may be required.[4,220,221] An empiric approach is to start with a lower dose, increase it gradually, and based on the clinical and laboratory response consider a higher dose or parenteral formulation (see **Table 1**). Early diagnosis and treatment of neurologic manifestations caused by vitamin E deficiency may result in dramatic recovery.[147] Supplements of bile salts may be of value in some patients. The free radical scavenger and antioxidant properties of vitamin E has led to its use in conditions such as Alzheimer disease and amyotrophic lateral sclerosis. The use of vitamin E in these conditions is unproven.

Thiamine

The terms vitamin B_1 (B_1) and thiamine (also spelled thiamin) are used interchangeably. Thiamine functions as a coenzyme in the metabolism of carbohydrates, lipids, and branched-chain amino acids. It has a role in energy production by adenosine triphosphate synthesis, in myelin sheath maintenance, and in neurotransmitter production. Following cellular uptake, thiamine is phosphorylated into thiamine diphosphate (TDP), the metabolically active form that is involved in several enzyme systems.[222–224] TDP is a cofactor for pyruvate dehydrogenase (PDH), α-ketoglutarate dehydrogenase (α-KGDH), and transketolase (TK).[222] PDH and α-KGDH are involved in the tricarboxylic acid cycle in oxidative decarboxylation of α-ketoacids such as pyruvate and α-ketoglutarate to acetyl coenzyme A (CoA) and succinate, respectively. TK transfers activated aldehydes in the hexose monophosphate shunt (pentose-phosphate pathway) in the generation of nicotinamide adenine dinucleotide phosphate (NADPH) for reductive biosynthesis. TDP may be further phosphorylated to TTP, which may activate high-conductance chloride channels and have a role in regulating cholinergic and serotonergic neurotransmission.[225] Thiamine deficiency results in reduced synthesis of high-energy phosphates and lactate accumulation. It has been suggested that decreased α-KGDH, rather than decreased PDH complex constitutes "the biochemical lesion" in thiamine deficiency.[226–228] α-KGDH is the rate-limiting enzyme in the tricarboxylic acid cycle. Decreased activity of α-KGDH results in decreased synthesis of amino acid neurotransmitters such as glutamate and γ-aminobutyric acid (GABA).[229] Decreased α-KGDH activity in astrocytes is the earliest biochemical change and has been noted after 4 days of experimental thiamine deficiency (pyrithiamine-induced thiamine deficiency).[228] Reduction in TK activity is noted after 7 days, and reduction in PDH is noted after 10 days. These biochemical events result in reduced cerebral glucose use and impaired cellular energy metabolism.[230] Thiamine-deficient membranes are unable to maintain osmotic gradients. Intracellular and extracellular swelling results and astrocyte-related functions are impaired. These include intracellular and extracellular glutamate concentrations, maintenance of ionic gradients across cell membranes, and blood-brain barrier permeability.[227] Proposed mechanisms that lead to neurotoxicity also include glutamate-mediated excitotoxicity, deoxyribonucleic acid fragmentation, and apoptotic cell death, decreased synaptic transmission, mitochondrial dysfunction, and intracellular oxidative stress with free radical and cytokine production.[222,231–235]

At low concentrations, thiamine is absorbed in jejunum and ileum by an active, carrier-mediated, rate-limited process.[236] At higher concentrations, absorption takes place by passive diffusion. After gastrointestinal uptake, thiamine is transported by portal blood to the liver. Transport of thiamine across the blood-brain barrier occurs by both active and passive mechanisms.[236,237] Because of a short half-life and the absence of significant storage amounts, a continuous dietary supply of thiamine is necessary. A thiamine-deficient diet may result in manifestations of thiamine deficiency in a few days.[238,239] This may occur even earlier in individuals with marginal stores, particularly so if the diet is rich in carbohydrates.[240]

Causes of deficiency

The prerequisite for the development of clinically significant thiamine deficiency is a poor nutritional status, either from reduced intake or reduced absorption or increased metabolic requirement or increased losses or defective transport (**Box 1**). Often multiple contributing factors coexist. Thiamine requirements are highest during periods of high metabolic demand or high glucose intake.[241] Thiamine requirements increase in children, during pregnancy and lactation, and with vigorous exercise. Disorders such as systemic infections, malignancy, and hyperthyroidism are also associated with an increased metabolic demand. Relative thiamine deficiency may be seen in high-risk patients during periods of high-carbohydrate intake as is seen with nasogastric feeding, total parenteral nutrition, or intravenous hyperalimentation.[240,242–249] In these circumstances, a high percentage of calories is derived from glucose, and the amount of corresponding thiamine replacement is inadequate. This is particularly common when there is preceding starvation or where several days of intravenous nutrition without adequate vitamin replacement is followed by oral food intake.[250,251] This "refeeding syndrome" may have been an explanation for sudden death seen in prisoners of war.[252]

The commonest clinical setting for Wernicke encephalopathy (WE) is alcoholism. Thiamine deficiency in alcoholism results from inadequate dietary intake, reduced gastrointestinal absorption, reduced liver thiamine stores, increased demand for thiamine for alcohol metabolism, and impaired phosphorylation of thiamine to TDP.[253] Postulated factors that may predispose to the development of Wernicke-Korsakoff syndrome (WKS) while on a marginal thiamine diet include individual variations in the biochemical activity of TK, variations in TK affinity for thiamine, susceptibility mediated by GABA-A receptor subunit gene cluster, changes in thiamine transport

---

Box 1
Conditions or settings reported to be associated with thiamine deficiency

Increased requirements

Children, pregnancy, lactation, vigorous exercise

Critically ill

Hyperthyroidism

Malignancy, chemotherapy (eg, erbulozole, ifosfamide), bone marrow transplantation

Systemic infection, prolonged febrile illness

Marginal nutritional status (decreased intake or decreased absorption or increased losses)

AIDS

Alcoholism

Anorexia nervosa, dieting, starvation, hunger strike, food refusal, dietary neglect in the elderly

Commercial dietary formula, slimming diets, food fads

Decreased absorption caused by excess use of antacids

Diet: polished rice, foods containing thiaminase or antithiamine compounds

Dietary supplements with herbal preparations

Gastrointestinal surgery (including bariatric surgery)

Inactivation of thiamine in food by excessive cooking of thiaminase-containing foods

Inadequate supplementation in parenteral or enteral nutrition

Thiamine loss related to loop diuretics therapy

Magnesium deficiency

Persistent vomiting (pancreatitis, migraine attacks, hyperemesis gravidarum) or diarrhea

Renal failure, hemodialysis, peritoneal dialysis

Severe gastrointestinal or liver or pancreatic disease

Tolazamide, high-dose nitroglycerine infusion (ethyl alcohol and propylene glycol on thiamine metabolism)

High glucose intake

Intravenous glucose administration

Refeeding after prolonged starvation

Data from Sechi G, Serra A. Wernicke's encephalopathy: new clinical settings and recent advances in diagnosis and management. Lancet Neurol 2007;6(5):442–5; Reuler JB, Girard DE, Cooney TG. Current concepts. Wernicke's encephalopathy. N Engl J Med 1985;312(16):1035–9.

systems, variants in genes encoding enzymes involved in alcohol metabolism, and gene polymorphisms with a potential modifying effect.[235,254–256] Thiamine deficiency is being increasingly identified in nonalcoholics (**Box 1**). **Box 1** lists the conditions that have been associated with thiamine deficiency.[235,252]

Maternal thiamine deficiency may result from eating a staple diet of polished rice with foods containing thiaminase or antithiamine compounds. Commercial dietary formula, slimming diets, and food fads can all cause thiamine deficiency.[257–259] Some dietary supplements have herbal preparations that can interfere with thiamine absorption or act as thiamine antagonists.[260] Certain raw fish and shellfish contain bacteria rich in thiaminases.[261] These can inactivate thiamine in food, as can prolonged cooking, baking of bread, and pasteurization of milk. Antithiamine factors are also present in betel nut, tea, and coffee.[261–263] Excess sulfites can destroy thiamine, and a WE-like syndrome has been reported after prolonged feeding of dogs with sulfite-preserved meats.[264] Excess antacid use can interfere with thiamine absorption.

Clinical Significance

Beriberi has the distinction of being the first human nutritional deficiency disorder to be identified. During the industrial revolution of the nineteenth century, introduction of milled rice was accompanied by epidemics of beriberi. A connection between the consumption of polished rice and beriberi was shown in the latter part of the nineteenth century. In the 1950s, universal enrichment of rice, grains, and flour products with thiamine was successful in achieving significant worldwide control. Carl Wernicke first described WE in 1881 as an acute superior hemorrhagic polioencephalitis ("polioencephalitis hemorrhagica superioris") in 2 alcoholic men and a woman who developed recurrent vomiting as a result of pyloric stenosis related to sulfuric acid ingestion. In the 1940s it was established that WE is caused by thiamine deficiency.[265]

Thiamine deficiency affects the CNS, peripheral nervous system, and cardiovascular system in varying combinations.[235,266] Cardiac involvement may manifest as high-output or low-output cardiac failure. The best characterized human neurologic disorders related to thiamine deficiency are beriberi, WE, and Korsakoff syndrome (KS, also referred to as Korsakoff psychosis). Because of the close relationship between WE and KS, the term WKS is commonly used. WE or KS may be associated with a peripheral neuropathy. WE often results from severe, short-term thiamine deficiency, whereas peripheral neuropathy is more often a consequence of prolonged mild to moderate thiamine deficiency.[235] WE related to alcoholism is more common in men. WE related to bariatric surgery is more commonly reported in women. KS is more likely to occur when WE is a consequence of alcohol abuse.[267] The symptoms of subclinical thiamine deficiency are often vague and nonspecific and include fatigue, irritability, headaches, and lethargy.[235]

The 3 forms of beriberi are dry beriberi, wet beriberi, and infantile beriberi.[224] Dry beriberi is characterized by a sensorimotor, distal, axonal peripheral neuropathy often associated with calf cramps, muscle tenderness, and burning feet.[268,269] Autonomic neuropathy may be present. A rapid progression of the neuropathy may mimic Guillain-Barre syndrome.[269] Pedal edema may be seen as a result of coexisting wet beriberi. Wet beriberi is associated with a high-output congestive heart failure with peripheral neuropathy. This distinction between dry and wet beriberi is of limited significance because the wet form may be converted to the dry form after diuresis. The terms wet and dry beriberi have been used to describe the presence or absence of edema in neuropathic beriberi. "Shoshin" beriberi is the name given to a fulminant form that presents with tachycardia and circulatory collapse. Acute quadriplegia caused by central-pontine myelinolysis has been reported in Shoshin beriberi.[270] Infantile beriberi is seen in infants breastfed by thiamine-deficient asymptomatic mothers or in infants fed on thiamine-deficient diets. It may present with the cardiac, aphonic, or pseudomeningitic forms.[224] Clinical features include cardiomyopathy, vomiting, diarrhea, failure to thrive, irritability, drowsiness, seizures, nystagmus, ophthalmoplegia, and respiratory symptoms.[259] Dyspnea, cyanosis, and signs of heart failure follow and can lead to death. Arytenoid edema and recurrent laryngeal neuropathy can result in hoarseness, dysphonia, and eventually aphonia. The term gastrointestinal beriberi has been used to describe a primary gastrointestinal thiamine deficiency syndrome characterized by abdominal pain, vomiting, and lactic acidosis. Peripheral neuropathy attributable to thiamine deficiency following bariatric surgery has been referred to as "bariatric beriberi."[271]

The clinical features of WE include a subacute onset of the classic triad of ocular abnormalities, gait ataxia, and mental status changes.[8,235,252,272–274] The onset may be gradual, the classic triad is frequently absent, 1 or more components of the triad may be seen later in the course, and some patients may have none of the manifestations related to the classic triad.[252,272,273,275,276] Reliance on the classic triad, not recognizing thiamine deficiency in nonalcoholics, nonspecific or poorly recognized signs and symptoms, all result in missing the diagnosis. Skin changes, tongue redness, and other features of chronic liver disease or nutritional deficiency may be present.

Ocular abnormalities include nystagmus (horizontal more common than vertical), ophthalmoparesis (commonly involving the lateral recti), and conjugate gaze palsies (usually horizontal). Complete ophthalmoplegia is rare. Other reported findings include sluggish pupillary reactivity, anisocoria, miosis, light-near dissociation, optic neuropathy, central scotomas, sudden bilateral blindness, retinal hemorrhages or papilledema, and a Miller-Fisher syndrome-like presentation.[247,276–283] Gait and trunk ataxia is a consequence of cerebellar and vestibular dysfunction. Vestibular dysfunction is an under appreciated feature and may be demonstrable on caloric testing or with the head impulse maneuver.[284–286] Other manifestations of cerebellar involvement such as dysarthria may be present. A coexisting chronic peripheral or acute neuropathy may be an additional contributing factor for the gait difficulty.[269,287] Mental status changes are the most constant component of the disease and include inability to concentrate, apathy, impaired awareness of the immediate situation, spatial disorientation, confusion, delirium, frank psychosis, and coma.[252,275,288–294] It is important to recognize that the intoxicated patient who does not recover fully and spontaneously may be suffering from WE.[236]

Involvement of the hypothalamic and brainstem autonomic pathways may be associated with hypothermia, hypotension, or bradycardia.[289,290,295–299] Other unusual manifestations of thiamine deficiency include seizures, myoclonus, dysphagia, chorea, orthostatic tremor, hypertonia, quadriparesis, tinnitus, or hearing loss.[234,300–309]

Recently thiamine responsive PDH deficiency was reported in an adult with peripheral neuropathy and optic neuropathy.[310] The following signs, often in combination, suggest PDH complex deficiency: Leigh syndrome, fever-induced ataxia or weakness, polyneuropathy, and optic neuropathy. Thiamine responsive megaloblastic anemia syndrome is characterized by diabetes mellitus and deafness in association with anemia. Inadequate thiamine supplementation in these patients may precipitate ketoacidosis.[311]

About 80% of patients with WE who survive develop KS.[236,312] KS is an amnestic-confabulatory syndrome characterized by severe anterograde and retrograde amnesia that follows WE; KS emerges as ocular manifestations and encephalopathy subside.[252,313–317] Rarely, KS may be present without WE or may be present at the time of diagnosis of WE.[318–320] In KS, memory is disproportionately impaired relative to other aspects of cognitive function. Alertness, attention, social behavior, and other aspects of cognitive functioning are generally preserved. A typical finding is a striking loss of working memory and relative preservation of reference memory. Implicit learning is retained, and these patients can learn new motor skills or develop conditioned reactions to stimuli. Disorientation to time and place may be present. Minor executive dysfunction may also be seen.[321] Confabulation becomes less evident with time.[316] Emotional changes may develop and include apathy or mild euphoria. Structural or neurochemical abnormalities within the limbic and diencephalic circuits likely account for anterograde amnesia. Frontal lobe dysfunction possibly underlies the severe retrograde memory loss and emotional changes found in this syndrome.[316,321] A study using functional connectivity MRI scans showed that memory function in patients recovering from WE parallels the level of mammillothalamic functional connectivity.[322]

The frequency of WE in various autopsy studies is far in excess of the level expected from clinical studies.[252,272,275] Thiamine deficiency leads to brain lesions in selective vulnerable areas that have a high thiamine content and turnover (such as the caudal brain and cerebellum).[323] The neuropathologic changes in WE include a symmetric grayish discoloration involving the mammillary bodies, hypothalamus and thalamus, superior cerebellar vermis, brainstem (including the periaqueductal gray matter, pontine tegmentum, and midbrain reticular formation), walls of the third ventricle, and floor of the fourth ventricle.[6,314,324] Associated congestion and pinpoint hemorrhages may be seen. Gross hemorrhage is rare. There can be involvement of the third and sixth nerve nuclei, vestibular nuclei, locus ceruleus, and, rarely, vagal nuclei. Involvement of the colliculi, fornices, septal region, hippocampi, and cerebral cortex is also described. In WE the characteristic finding is mammillary body involvement; patients with KS typically have involvement of the dorsal median nucleus of the thalamus. Microscopically acute lesions are characterized by multiple small hemorrhages with intervening spongiosis and edema without interstitial infiltration or capillary proliferation. Prominent vessels result from hypertrophy and hyperplasia. Extravasated red blood cells and hemosiderin-laden macrophages may be seen. Chronic lesions show loosening of the neuropil accompanied by activated microglia, reactive astrocytes, gliosis, and vascular proliferation. There is relative neuronal and axonal sparing. Pathologic studies of beriberi in nonalcoholics are limited.[5,268,325] Axonal degeneration has been noted in distal nerves. Chromatolysis of dorsal root ganglia neurons and anterior horn cell neurons may be seen as a result of axonal degeneration. Segmental demyelination is rare and likely secondary to axonal degeneration. Severe cases may have involvement of the vagus and phrenic nerves. Degeneration of the posterior columns may be present.

Investigations

Urinary thiamine excretion and serum thiamine levels may be decreased in thiamine deficiency but do not accurately reflect tissue concentrations and are not reliable indicators of thiamine status. A normal serum thiamine level does not exclude WE. The preferred tests are the erythrocyte TK activation assay or measurement of TDP in red blood cell hemolysates using high-performance liquid chromatography (HPLC).[326–329] The erythrocyte TK activation assay is an assay of functional status and is based on measurement of TK activity in hemolysates of red blood cells in the absence of (and in the presence of) added excess cofactor (TDP). Measurement of TDP in human erythrocytes by HPLC has improved reproducibility and is suitable for clinical and research purposes.[328] Because these laboratory abnormalities normalize quickly, a blood sample should be drawn before initiation of treatment. Pyruvate accumulates during thiamine deficiency and elevated serum lactate provides additional confirmation. An anion-gap metabolic acidosis accompanied by a primary respiratory alkalosis may be present.[330]

MRI is the imaging modality of choice.[331] Typical MRI findings include increased T2 or proton density or fluid-attenuated inversion recovery (FLAIR) signal in the paraventricular regions. Involved areas include the thalamus, hypothalamus, mammillary body, periaqueductal midbrain, tectal plate, pons, fourth ventricle floor, medulla, midline cerebellum, and, rarely, in the splenium of the corpus callosum or basal ganglia structures (**Fig. 6**).[234,303,305,308,331–342] Increased signal may involve the hypoglossal, medial vestibular, facial, and dentate nuclei.[343] Involvement of cortical regions on MRI has also been reported and may indicate irreversible lesions and poor prognosis.[301,303,333,336,339,344,345] Contrast enhancement may be present in the early stages.[303,337,338,340,346–349] Mammillary body enhancement on MRI has been reported as being the only imaging abnormality in WE.[347] Hemorrhagic lesions are rare.[346,350] In 1 report, midbrain swelling was accompanied by hydrocephalus that required shunting.[234] The neuropathology corresponding to the T2-signal change is spongy degeneration of the neuropil.[335] The signal abnormalities resolve with treatment, but shrunken mamillary bodies may persist as sequelae. Additional findings in the chronic stages include dilated aqueduct and third ventricles with atrophy of the midbrain tegmentum, paramedian thalamic nuclei, mamillary bodies, and frontal lobes.[331,351,352] Frontal atrophy may also be seen. Diffusion-weighted MRI abnormalities may be seen in the early stages.[338,339,353–357] These may disappear after successful thiamine therapy, suggesting underlying vasogenic edema. Cytotoxic and vasogenic edema may be present concurrently.[341,342] Proton MR spectroscopy may show evidence of lactate accumulation.[358]

A broad spectrum of conditions are included in the differential diagnosis of the MRI changes seen in WE, including paramedian thalamic infarction as seen in the top-of-the-basilar syndrome, CNS lymphoma, Leigh disease, variant Creutzfeldt-Jakob disease, paraneoplastic encephalitis, ventriculoencephalitis, Miller-Fisher syndrome, severe hypophosphatemia, alcoholic pellagra encephalopathy, multiple sclerosis, Behçet disease, Whipple disease and other CNS infections, cerebral hypoxia, and various acute and chronic intoxications.[235,359] Similar MRI lesions have been described in the so-called energy deprivation syndromes, which are toxic, genetic, or nutritional disorders that disrupt enzymes involved in energy-generating metabolic pathways such as glycolysis and pyruvate oxidation. These conditions merit consideration particularly when the response to thiamine is absent or when a predisposing condition is absent.

Management
Intravenous glucose infusion in patients with thiamine deficiency may consume the available thiamine and precipitate an acute WE. At-risk patients should receive

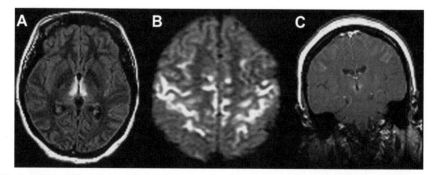

Fig. 6. MRI in WE. (*A*) Axial FLAIR MRI showing bilateral symmetric hyperintense lesions of the periaqueductal gray matter and medial portions of both thalami. (*B*) Diffusion-weighted MRI showing restricted diffusion symmetrically in the motor and premotor cortices. (*C*) Postcontrast coronal T1-weighted MRI with thalamic and cortical contrast enhancement (all images are from the same patient with Wernicke encephalopathy). (*Adapted from* Foster D, Falah M, Kadom N, Mandler R. Wernicke encephalopathy after bariatric surgery: losing more than just weight. Neurology 2005;65:1987; with permission.)

parenteral thiamine before administration of glucose or parenteral nutrition. Patients suspected of having beriberi or WE should promptly receive parenteral thiamine. Adverse effects are rare and include pruritus, transient local irritation, or, rarely, anaphylaxis. Thiamine for parenteral use should be diluted in 100 mL of normal saline or 5% glucose and be infused over 30 minutes.[236,312] The thiamine solution should be freshly prepared. Old solutions exposed to heat may be inactivated.[252] A commonly used thiamine replacement regimen is 100 mg intravenously every 8 hours.[303] Higher doses may be required in WE, particularly when WE occurs in the setting of alcoholism.[235,360] Long-term oral maintenance with 50 to 100 mg of thiamine is commonly used (see **Table 1**). WE often develops in a predisposed individual because of increased metabolic demands related to coexisting conditions, such as an infection, which need independent attention.

In wet beriberi a rapid improvement is seen with clearing of symptoms within days.[268] Improvement in motor and sensory symptoms takes weeks or months.[268,269] Response in WE is variable. Ocular signs improve in a few hours.[361] A fine horizontal nystagmus may persist in 60% of patients. Improvement in gait ataxia and memory is variable and often delayed.[362] Changes in mental status improve over days or weeks. As the global confusional state recedes, some patients are left with KS. Prompt treatment of WE prevents the development of KS. KS does not respond to thiamine therapy. Even with thiamine treatment, the mortality rate is about 20%.[236,275,312,363] Sudden death can occur and may be related to hemorrhagic brainstem lesions.[299,364] Those with KS who do improve do so after a delay of a month or so; occasionally patients may not achieve maximal improvement for more than a year.

Niacin

Niacin in humans is an end product of tryptophan metabolism. Niacin is converted in the body to nicotinamide adenine dinucleotide (NAD) and nicotinamide adenine dinucleotide phosphate (NADP), 2 coenzymes that have a role in carbohydrate metabolism. Niacin and its amide are absorbed through the intestinal mucosa by simple diffusion; 15% to 30% of niacin is protein bound. Complexed and free niacin are taken up by tissues. Niacin and nicotinamide are metabolized by separate pathways. The major metabolite of niacin is nicotinuric acid and the major metabolite of nicotinamide is N^1-methyl-nicotinamide and its oxidized products, 2- and 4-pyridones.

Causes of deficiency
Pellagra is rare in developed countries. Niacin deficiency is predominantly seen in populations dependent on corn as the primary carbohydrate source.[365] Corn lacks niacin and tryptophan. Nonendemic pellagra may be seen with alcoholism and malabsorption. Pellagra may be seen in the carcinoid syndrome because tryptophan is converted to serotonin instead of being used in niacin synthesis. Biotransformation of tryptophan to nicotinic acid requires several vitamins and minerals such as B_2, B_6, iron, and copper. Because tryptophan is necessary for niacin synthesis, vitamin B_6 deficiency can result in secondary niacin deficiency. Isonicotinic acid hydrazide (isoniazid) depletes B_6 and can trigger pellagra. Excess neutral amino acids in the diet such as leucine can compete with tryptophan for uptake and predispose to niacin deficiency by impairing its synthesis from tryptophan. Hartnup syndrome is an autosomal recessive disorder characterized by impaired synthesis of niacin from tryptophan and results in pellagra-like symptoms. Bacterial colonization of the small intestines can lead to conversion of dietary tryptophan to indoles. Nicotinamide deficiency has been described in some disorders of the alimentary tract such as diverticulosis.

Reversible nicotinamide deficiency encephalopathy has been described in a patient with jejunal diverticulosis.

Clinical significance

Pellagra affects the gastrointestinal tract, skin, and nervous system.[365] The classic clinical hallmarks of pellagra have been alluded to by the mnemonic dermatitis, diarrhea, and dementia. The dermatologic and gastrointestinal manifestations are frequently absent, particularly so in nonendemic pellagra. Skin changes include a reddish-brown hyperkeratotic rash, which has a predilection for the face, chest, and dorsum of the hands and feet. Gastrointestinal manifestations include anorexia, abdominal pain, diarrhea, and stomatitis. The neurologic syndrome caused by niacin deficiency has not been well characterized. Reported cases are confounded by the presence of coexisting nutrient deficiencies as is common in alcoholics. Reported manifestations include a confusional state that may progress to coma and be accompanied by spasticity and myoclonus. Unexplained progressive encephalopathy in alcoholics that is not responsive to thiamine should raise the possibility of pellagra.[366] Alcoholics with encephalopathy may receive thiamine and pyridoxine without niacin and this may trigger an encephalopathy caused by niacin deficiency. The peripheral neuropathy seen in pellagra is indistinguishable from the peripheral neuropathy seen with thiamine deficiency. The neuropatholic hallmark of neurologic pellagra is diffuse neuronal chromatolysis.

Investigations

There are no sensitive and specific blood measures of niacin status. It has been suggested that measures of erythrocyte NAD and plasma metabolites of niacin may serve as indirect markers. The more reliable measures of niacin status may be urinary excretion of the methylated metabolites N^1-methyl-nicotinamide and its 2-pyridone derivative (N^1-methyl-2-pyridone-5-carboxamide).

Management

Oral nicotinic acid in a dose of 50 mg 3 times a day or parenteral doses of 25 mg 3 times a day are used for treatment of symptomatic patients (see **Table 1**).[8] Nicotinamide has comparable therapeutic efficacy in pellagra but does not have the vasodilatory and cholesterol-lowering activities of niacin. Advanced stages of pellagra can be cured with intramuscular nicotinamide given in doses of 50 to 100 mg 3 times a day for 3 to 4 days followed by similar quantities orally.[365]

Vitamin B$_6$

The term pyridoxine is generally used synonymously with vitamin B$_6$ (B$_6$). Pyridoxal and pyridoxamine are 2 other naturally occurring compounds that have comparable biologic activity. All 3 compounds are readily converted to pyridoxal phosphate (PLP). PLP serves as a coenzyme in many reactions involved in the metabolism of amino acids, lipids, nucleic acid, 1 carbon units, and in the pathways of gluconeogenesis, and neurotransmitter and heme biosynthesis. The interconversion and metabolism of B$_6$ is dependent on riboflavin, niacin, and zinc. Niacin, carnitine, and folate require B$_6$ for their metabolism. Humans and other mammals cannot synthesize B$_6$ and thus must obtain this micronutrient from exogenous sources via intestinal absorption. B$_6$ uptake by intestinal epithelial cells occurs by a carrier-mediated, pH-dependent mechanism that has saturable and nonsaturable components.[367] B$_6$ (mostly in the form of pyridoxal) enters the portal circulation and is transported bound to albumin in plasma and hemoglobin in red blood cells. Absorbed dietary pyridoxine, pyridoxal, and pyridoxamine are phosphorylated for metabolic trapping. Tissue uptake of B$_6$

from circulation requires dephosphorylation. PLP and pyridoxal are the main circulating forms of B_6.

Causes of deficiency

Most diets are adequate in B_6. Its deficiency is seen with B_6 antagonists such as isonicotinic acid hydrazide, cycloserine, hydralazine, and penicillamine.[368] Neuropathic symptoms in association with pellagra-like dermatitis have been described in association with the use of the B_6 antagonist desoxypyridoxine.[369] Alcohol intake antagonizes B_6 status through production of acetaldehyde, which competes with PLP for binding sites of PLP-dependent enzymes.[370] Individuals at risk of developing B_6 deficiency include pregnant and lactating women and elderly individuals.[371] Plasma PLP levels are reduced in celiac disease, inflammatory bowel disease, and renal disease.

Clinical significance

Dietary deficiency of pyridoxine or congenital dependency on pyridoxine may manifest as infantile seizures. Infantile seizures caused by dietary B_6 deficiency are rare and may be seen in breastfed infants of malnourished mothers from poor socioeconomic backgrounds in underdeveloped countries. Abrupt onset recurrent convulsions may be accompanied by hyperirritability and an exaggerated auditory startle. Another form of pyridoxine-responsive seizures occurs in infants with a hereditary dependency on pyridoxine caused by a mutation of the antiquitin gene.[372] Pyridoxine-dependent epilepsy is caused by a defect of α-amino adipic semialdehyde dehydrogenase (antiquitin) in the cerebral lysine degradation pathway. The accumulating compound, piperideine-6-carboxylic acid (P6C), was shown to inactivate PLP by a Knoevenagel condensation. Pipecolic acid and α-amino adipic semialdehyde are markedly elevated in urine, plasma, and cerebrospinal fluid and thus can be used as biomarkers of the disease. These infants have a normal dietary pyridoxine intake. They develop seizures within days of birth and require high doses of pyridoxine for seizure control. Even after years of treatment with high doses of pyridoxine, seizures reappear within days of pyridoxine withdrawal.

Adults are much more tolerant of pyridoxine deficiency. Even with low levels, symptoms are rare. Up to 50% of slow activators may develop a dose-related peripheral neuropathy when treated with isonicotinic acid hydrazide.[8] Isonicotinic acid hydrazide use has been associated with painful distal paresthesias that can rapidly progress to limb weakness and sensory ataxia.[373] Axonal degeneration and regeneration affect myelinated and unmyelinated fibers.[374] Chronic B_6 deficiency results in a microcytic hypochromic anemia. A form of sideroblastic anemia can be treated with pyridoxine supplementation.[375] Chronic vitamin B_6 deficient patients may develop secondary hyperoxaluria and thus are at higher risk for nephrolithiasis. As with other B vitamin deficiencies, glossitis, stomatitis, cheilosis, and dermatitis may be seen.

Excess consumption of B_6 has been associated with a pure sensory peripheral neuropathy or ganglionopathy.[376,377] It is characterized by sensory ataxia, areflexia, impaired cutaneous and deep sensations, and positive Romberg sign. The site of the lesion is most likely the dorsal root ganglia. The presence of a Lhermitte sign in some patients suggests involvement of the spinal cord also.[4] The risk of developing this increases at doses greater than 100 mg/d. A recent population-based study noted that higher dietary vitamin B_6 intake was associated with a reduced risk of Parkinson disease.[378]

Investigations

Microbiologic assays measure total vitamin B_6. HPLC methods allow estimation of the various forms of vitamin B_6. Vitamin B_6 status can be assessed by measuring its levels in the blood or urine. The most commonly used measure is plasma PLP. A plasma PLP concentration of more than 30 nmol/L has been considered to indicate adequate status.[379] A concentration greater than 20 nmol/L is considered a more conservative cutoff value. Functional indicators of vitamin B_6 status are based on PLP-dependent reactions. The methionine load test is used as a functional indicator of vitamin B_6 status. B_6 deficiency results in a higher homocysteine concentration after methionine load, caused by impairment of the transsulfuration pathway. Vitamin B_6 deficiency has little effect on fasting plasma homocysteine concentration.

Management
Neuropathy induced by isonicotinic acid hydrazide is reversible by drug discontinuation or B_6 supplementation.[377] Vitamin B_6 may be supplemented in a dose of 50 to 100 mg/d to prevent development of the neuropathy (see **Table 1**). In an isolated report, peripheral neuropathy symptoms associated with hemodialysis were ameliorated with supplemental pyridoxine given in a dose of 250 mg/d.[380] The neuropathy caused by vitamin B_6 toxicity may reverse once the supplementation is withdrawn. Patients with pyridoxine-dependent epilepsy develop symptoms despite a normal dietary supplementation of pyridoxine. High doses of B_6 are required and even after years, seizures reappear within days of B_6 withdrawal.

Vitamin A

Vitamin A refers to retinol. The term retinoids refers to vitamin A derivatives such as retinal (vitamin A aldehyde), retinoic acid (vitamin A acid), and the carotenoids. Vitamin A is essential for visual function. Retinol binds with the protein opsin to form rhodopsin, which is responsible for vision at dim illumination. It influences growth and tissue differentiation and is required for maintenance of epithelial cell integrity. In the intestinal mucosa retinol is esterified to retinyl palmitate, which is incorporated into chylomicrons and transported into the general circulation. Vitamin A is stored in the liver in the form of retinyl palmitate and is released from the liver by hydrolysis. It is derived from numerous animal sources such as liver and internal organs; liver of shark, halibut, and polar bear are the highest sources. β-Carotene is present in many plant sources such as carrots, papayas, oranges, and green leafy vegetables. Chronic daily vitamin A consumption of more than 25,000 IU may result in toxicity.

Causes of deficiency
Nutritional deficiency of vitamin A is seen when the diet consists predominantly of rice and wheat (grains lacking β-carotene). Dietary deficiency may be seen in alcoholics, the elderly, and the poor. Vitamin A deficiency is also seen in conditions associated with fat malabsorption such as celiac disease, pancreatitis, sprue, cystic fibrosis, biliary atresia, and cholestatic liver disease.

Clinical significance
Vitamin A deficiency causes night blindness and dryness and keratinization of the cornea and conjunctiva. White, foamy spots on the conjunctiva caused by sloughed cells may be seen (Bitot spots). Other manifestations include impaired taste, follicular hyperkeratosis of the skin, and keratinization of the respiratory, gastrointestinal, and urinary tracts. Rarely vitamin A deficiency in children may manifest with raised intracranial pressure.[381] Excess ingestion of carotenes causes yellow skin pigmentation. Excess vitamin A ingestion causes dry skin, pruritis, chelitis, brittle nails, alopecia, petechiae, bone pain, painful joints, hyperostoses, anorexia, fatigue, nausea, diarrhea, and hepatotoxicity. Neurologic manifestations of vitamin A toxicity include headache, insomnia, irritability, papilledema, and pseudotumor cerebri.

Investigations
Normal vitamin A levels range from 30 to 65 μg/dl. Levels less than 10 μg/dL are clearly low and levels more than 100 μg/dL are suggestive of toxicity.

Management
Prophylactically treating high-risk infants and children with large oral doses of vitamin A prevents development of a deficient state. In the setting of malabsorption-related vitamin A deficiency, oral vitamin A supplementation is undertaken to normalize plasma levels.

Vitamin D

Vitamin D exists in 2 forms: vitamin D_2 (ergocalciferol, produced by plants) and vitamin D_3 (cholecalciferol, derived from 7-dehydrocholesterol when exposed to ultraviolet light in the skin). Vitamin D functions more like a hormone than a vitamin. It acts intracellularly at high affinity nuclear receptors, which, when stimulated, alter gene transcription. Receptors in small bowel enterocytes enhance calcium and phosphorus absorption and bone receptors stimulate mineralization of newly formed bone. Sun-stimulated skin synthesis can provide 100% of the daily requirement from 7-dehydrocholesterol in the absence of oral intake. In the presence of bile salts, orally ingested vitamin D is packaged into micelles and absorbed passively in the small intestine. It is then bound to lipoproteins and transported in chylomicrons to the liver via the lymphatic system. In the liver it is hydroxylated to 25-(OH)-vitamin D. Further hydroxylation occurs in the kidney to 1,25-(OH)-vitamin D, the active form. Vitamin D hydroxylation is increased by parathormone. With replete stores, 25-(OH)-vitamin D is hydroxylated to 24,25-(OH)-vitamin D and is excreted in the bile and urine. Liver (especially fish liver), eggs, and some dairy products are good sources of vitamin D. Routine supplementation of foods such as dairy products makes dietary deficiency rare.

Causes of deficiency
Inadequate sun exposure may cause vitamin D deficiency in chronically ill, institutionalized, or housebound individuals. Vitamin D deficiency can result from dietary insufficiency. Malabsorption as seen in celiac disease, Crohn disease, cholestatic liver disease, and extensive small bowel resection may also cause vitamin D deficiency. Vitamin D deficiency has also been reported following gastric bypass and partial gastrectomy. Pancreatic disease rarely leads to vitamin D deficiency. Advanced liver or kidney disease can decrease the active form of vitamin D. The antiepileptic drugs phenobarbital and phenytoin inhibit vitamin D hydroxylation in the liver and inhibit calcium absorption in the intestines.

Clinical significance
Vitamin D deficiency results in defective mineralization of newly formed bone, and in hypocalcemia with secondary hyperparathyroidism, which further impairs normal bone mineralization. This causes rickets in kids and osteomalacia in adults. Vitamin D deficiency can cause a proximal myopathy that often exists in association with osteomalacia, pathologic fractures, and bone pain.[382] The pelvic and thigh musculature are involved more than the arms. A waddling gait may be present. Neck muscles may be involved; bulbar and ocular muscles are spared. Severe hypocalcemia may result in tetany and may be associated with hypomagnesemia. Vitamin D deficiency has been reported to cause cutaneous hyperalgesia that is resistant to antidepressants and opiates but responds to vitamin D repletion.[383] Hypovitaminosis D has been associated with persistent, nonspecific musculoskeletal pain in some studies

but not in others.[384–386] Studies have also reported an inverse association between vitamin D (both dietary intake and blood levels) and the risk of developing multiple sclerosis.[387–390] In an isolated report parkinsonism and hypocalcemia reversed with vitamin D therapy.[391]

Investigations

Vitamin D deficiency may be accompanied by decreased serum calcium and increased parathormone levels. Because 25-(OH)-vitamin D is hydroxylated to the active form, the level of 1,25-(OH)-vitamin D may be normal although its immediate precursor may be very low. Hence, vitamin D status is best assessed by 25-(OH)-vitamin D levels.[392] Other laboratory abnormalities may include increased alkaline phosphatase of bone origin, hypocalcemia, hypophosphatemia, increased parathormone, reduced urinary calcium excretion, and increased urinary hydroxyproline. Radiological changes of rickets or osteopenia may be present.

Management

Vitamin D can be given orally as vitamin D_2 or vitamin D_3. 400 IU of vitamin D per day is adequate to prevent deficiency in individuals with minimal sun exposure. With clinical deficiency 50,000 IU weekly may be required. Larger oral doses or parenteral administration may be required in the presence of malabsorption. Associated secondary hyperparathyroidism can cause hypercalcemia, hypercalciuria, and nephrolithiasis. This can be prevented by ensuring that there is adequate calcium repletion and thus avoiding parathyroid stimulation. An inappropriately high phosphate level suggests secondary hyperparathyroidism. Laboratory monitoring is required with doses of 50,000 IU 3 times a week. Toxicity includes hypercalcemia, hypercalciuria, and renal failure. Serum and urine calcium and serum 25-(OH)-vitamin D should be monitored and when urinary calcium excretion exceeds 100 mg/24 h the vitamin D dose should be reduced. 25-(OH)-vitamin D (calciferol) can be used when liver dysfunction is present.

NEUROLOGIC COMPLICATIONS RELATED TO BARIATRIC SURGERY
Types of Surgeries

The epidemic of obesity and limited efficacy of its medical treatments has led to increasing use of bariatric surgical procedures for the treatment of medically complicated obesity. Several different surgical procedures have been used.[393–397] The earliest surgical treatments for obesity were malabsorptive procedures such as the jejunocolic shunt and jejunoileal bypass. These operations were abandoned because of severe metabolic derangements and associated malnutrition that frequently necessitated revision surgeries. Gastric restriction procedures have included gastric partitioning, gastroplasty, and vertical-banded gastroplasty. These procedures separate the stomach into a small pouch that empties into the greater stomach through a narrow channel thus restricting the quantity and rate of food ingested without affecting digestion or absorption. However, the weight loss after these procedures has not been found to be sustained either because the surgical technique was not durable or because patients developed maladaptive eating behaviors that circumvented the restriction. Gastric bypass procedures result in weight loss by a more physiologic mechanism. They restrict the volume ingested, cause partial malabsorption of fat, and induce a dumping syndrome with a high-carbohydrate meal thus leading to sustained weight loss. The Roux-en-Y gastric bypass is often the procedure of choice and is often done laparoscopically. Recently, a laparoscopically placed adjustable gastric band has gained popularity. This procedure differs from previous restrictive procedures in that there is adjustment of the band in response to rate of weight loss and absence of an enterotomy or permanent change to the anatomy. Additional procedures that result in greater degrees of maldigestion and malabsorption combined with partial gastric resection have been advocated for the treatment of patients with "super" obesity (body mass index >50 kg/m^2). These include distal gastric bypass, biliopancreatic diversion with duodenal switch modification, partial biliopancreatic bypass, and very, very long limb Roux-en-Y gastric bypass.

Vitamin Deficiencies

B$_{12}$ deficiency is the most common nutritional deficiency noted after bariatric surgery.[16,18,159,398–404] A low B$_{12}$ level has been noted in 70% of patients undergoing gastric bypass surgery and B$_{12}$ deficiency in nearly 40%.[401] Deficiency may result from inadequate intake, impaired hydrolysis of B$_{12}$ from dietary protein, or because of abnormal intrinsic factor and B$_{12}$ interaction.[16,399,400,402] B$_1$ deficiency is also seen frequently following bariatric surgery.[306,398,404–412] Preoperative thiamine deficiency in patients undergoing bariatric surgery has also been recognized.[413,414] B$_1$ deficiency following bariatric surgery may be caused by intractable vomiting, rapid weight loss, inadequate vitamin repletion, parenteral nutrition, glucose administration without thiamine, bacterial overgrowth, and altered gut ecology. Thiamine deficiency has been reported as early as 2 weeks and as late as 20 years after gastrointestinal surgery; most cases are seen 1 to 8 months after surgery. Neurologic complications caused by B$_1$ deficiency such as WE and peripheral neuropathy may be seen as early as 6 weeks after gastric surgery. Other vitamin deficiencies such as folate and vitamin D are also recognized.[398,401,402,415–417] The significance of deficiencies of riboflavin, niacin, pyridoxine, vitamin C, and vitamin E in the bariatric surgery population is less well established.[418]

Mineral Deficiencies

The most commonly identified mineral deficiency following bariatric surgery is iron and may be seen in nearly 50% of patients.[400–402] Aches and pains occurring 1 year after bypass surgery has been called "bypass bone disease" and is believed to be caused by bone demineralization from impaired calcium absorption, often with concurrent vitamin D deficiency.[400] Other identified mineral deficiencies include copper and potassium.[151,153,159,402,419]

Abnormal Fat and Carbohydrate Metabolism

Reports of neurologic disorders following bariatric surgery caused by rapid fat metabolism are of uncertain significance.[420,421] Recurrent spells of encephalopathy with lactic acidosis following high-carbohydrate diets have been reported following jejunoileostomy.[422] The elevated D-lactate level is believed to result from fermentation of carbohydrates in the colon or bypassing a segment of the small bowel. The presence of recurrent hyperammonemia and encephalopathy following bariatric surgery may be caused by previously undetected ornithine transcarbamylase deficiency.[423]

Types, Frequency, and Risk Factors for Neurologic Complications

Complications related to the central and/or peripheral nervous system may be seen in 5% to 16% of patients after surgery for peptic ulcer disease or obesity; not infrequently the precise cause is not determined and a multifactorial nutritional cause is suspected.[159,306,404,405,407,409,420,421,424–427] Complications involving the peripheral nervous system include a polyneuropathy or mononeuropathy and less commonly a lumbar plexopathy or radiculopathy or polyradiculoneuropathy or radiculoplexpathy or myopathy. Compressive neuropathies may accompany dramatic weight loss.

A gastric bypass surgery-like presentation or presentation as a sensory ganglionop-athy have also been reported.[420,427,428] Complications involving the CNS include an encephalopathy or posterolateral myelopathy and less commonly optic neuropathy. Development of a seizure and ischemic stroke 3 months after bariatric surgery were reported in a patient who developed malnutrition and dehydration.[429] The polyneurop-athy may be caused by thiamine or vitamin B_{12} deficiency and the myelopathy may be caused by vitamin B_{12} or copper deficiency. Multiple nutritional deficits may coexist.

Risk factors for neurologic complications include the rate and absolute amount of weight loss, prolonged gastrointestinal symptoms (particularly protracted vomiting), not attending a nutritional clinic after bariatric surgery, less vitamin and mineral supplementation, reduced serum albumin and transferrin, postoperative surgical complications requiring hospitalization, and having jejunoileal bypass.[405,426]

Management

Prevention, diagnosis, and treatment of these disorders are necessary parts of lifelong care after bariatric surgery.[400,430,431] Long-term follow-up with dietary counseling are important. All bariatric surgery patients should have 6-month follow-up laboratory studies that include complete blood count, serum iron, iron-binding capacity, vitamin B_{12}, calcium, and alkaline phosphatase. It is unclear which patients may develop copper deficiency after gastric surgery and if routine screening and supplementation should be considered. Oral supplementation containing the recommended daily allowance for micronutrients can prevent abnormal blood indicators of most vitamins and minerals but are insufficient to maintain normal plasma B_{12} levels in approximately 30% of patients after gastric bypass.[403] Multivitamin plus mineral supplements may not prevent development of iron deficiency or subsequent anemia.[432] Indefinite use of the following daily supplements has been suggested[400]: a multivitamin-mineral combination containing B_{12}, folic acid, vitamin D, and iron; an additional iron tablet preferably with vitamin C; an additional B_{12} tablet of 50 to 100 μg; a calcium supple-ment equivalent to 1 g of elemental calcium.

Preoperative thiamine deficiency in patients undergoing bariatric surgery has also been recognized.[413,414] Thiamine deficiency following bariatric surgery may be caused by small intestinal bacterial overgrowth and altered gut ecology.[412] WE generally occurs 1 to 8 months after surgery. Thiamine deficiency has been reported as early as 2 weeks and as late as 20 years after gastrointestinal surgery.[406,411] Thiamine deficiency is particularly common with rapid weight loss (greater than 7 kg/month). Additional risk factors include inadequate dietary supplementation and recurrent vomiting. Atypical clinical features may be present when WE is seen following bariatric surgery.[306]

NEUROLOGIC PRESENTATIONS OF DEFICIENCY DISEASES SEEN IN THE SETTING OF ALCOHOLISM
Alcoholic Neuropathy

Alcohol displaces food in the diet, increases the demand for B-group vitamins, causes decreased absorption of lipid soluble vitamins caused by pancreatic and hepatic dysfunction, and possibly has a role as a secondary neurotoxin.[6,433] The direct role of alcohol in the pathogenesis of neuropathy related to chronic alcoholism has been a matter of debate. It is likely that in at least a subgroup of patients the direct toxic effects of alcohol are responsible.[434–437] The peripheral neuropathy associated with alcoholism has more commonly been considered to be nutritional in origin.[438] Even though a specific nutrient is often not implicated, the B-group vitamin deficiencies, particularly thiamin, have been suspected. Alcoholic neuropathy is a slowly progressive, distally predominant, painful, symmetric, sensorimotor, axonal neuropathy with preferential small fiber involvement and autonomic dysfunction.[434–437] In contrast, thiamine deficiency-related neuropathy is often a more rapidly progressive, sensorimotor neuropathy with large-fiber predominant sensory loss. Subperineurial edema may be more prominent in neuropathy related to thiamine deficiency, whereas segmental demyelination and remyelination resulting from widening of consecutive nodes of Ranvier may be more frequent in alcoholic neuropathy. Some patients may have a subacute presentation that mimics Guillain-Barré syndrome.[439] The presence of a vagal neuropathy may be associated with a higher mortality.[440] Trophic skin changes and a distal neuropathic arthropathy may be present.

Alcoholic Cerebellar Degeneration

Alcoholic cerebellar degeneration is characterized by early involvement of the anterior and superior parts of the cerebellar vermis and lesser involvement of the cerebellar hemispheres.[441] The Purkinje cells are most affected. Secondary neuronal loss in deep cerebellar nuclei and pathologic changes of WKS may be seen. The neurologic presentation of alcoholic cerebellar degeneration includes a truncal ataxia with a wide-based gait and difficulty with tandem walking. Limb ataxia, if present, is milder and more evident in the lower limbs. Other cerebellar features such as nystagmus, dysarthria, intention tremor, and hypotonia are rare. An accompanying polyneuropathy is common. Vermal atrophy in alcoholic cerebellar degeneration may relate to thiamine deficiency.[442] Positron emission tomography studies in patients with alcoholic cerebellar degeneration have shown hypometabolism involving the superior vermis and medial frontal lobes.[443]

Tobacco-alcohol Amblyopia

Tobacco-alcohol or tobacco-nutritional amblyopia refers to a syndrome of bilateral, progressive, painless visual loss in severe alcoholics caused by damage to the papillomacular bundle of fibers.[444–446] Despite impaired vision the optic discs may be normal or show only mild pallor. Other findings include central or cecocentral scotomas and peripapillary hemorrhages. Multifocal electroretinography suggests that the disorder may involve the macula.[447] Although called tobacco-alcohol amblyopia, neither agent has been proven to be directly responsible. The syndrome is similar to the amblyopia seen in prisoners of war and malnourished individuals. Partial visual recovery may result with an adequate diet and B vitamins, despite continued use of alcohol and tobacco.

Marchiafava-Bignami Disease

The initial descriptions of Marchiafava-Bignami disease were those of selective demyelination of the corpus callosum in Italians who consumed excess amounts of red wine. However, the disorder is not restricted to Italians and consumption of red wine is not an invariable feature. The precise pathophysiology is not known. The commonest clinical presentation includes a frontal lobe syndrome characterized by personality change and psychomotor slowing. Other manifestations include dysarthria, quadriparesis, incontinence, seizures, symptoms of interhemispheric disconnection, and rarely coma.[448,449] The central part of the body of the corpus callosum is preferentially involved by acute demyelination and necrosis. This shows on MRI as areas of low T1 signal intensity and high T2 and FLAIR signal intensity.[448,450] Lesions may be seen in the hemispheric white matter and in the middle cerebellar peduncle. Subcortical U fibers tend to be spared. The extent of involvement seen on diffusion-weighted imaging may be more than that seen on FLAIR.[451] The presence of restricted diffusion, cortical involvement on diffusion-weighted imaging, and greater extent of the callosal lesion may be associated with worse prognosis.[448,451] With chronicity, atrophy and cyst formation may be seen.

NEUROLOGIC DEFICIENCY/NUTRITIONAL DISEASES THAT HAVE A GEOGRAPHIC PREDELICTION
Tropical Myeloneuropathies

"Burning feet" were described first in 1826 by a British medical officer in the Indian army. Entities described later included Strachan's Jamaican neuropathy, Cuban retrobulbar optic neuropathy, and the Cuban "amblyopia of the blockade." Similar disorders were reported among prisoners of war in tropical and subtropical regions during World War II and in victims of the Spanish Civil War. The term "happy feet" was used to describe similar symptoms in prisoners of war in camps in the tropics in World War II. Restoration of a normal diet and vitamin supplementation improved symptoms but often some deficits remained. Lack of multiple dietary components, in particular B-group vitamins was the likely cause. More recently from 1991 to 1994, an epidemic in Cuba affected more than 50,000 persons and caused optic neuropathy, sensorineural deafness, dorsolateral myelopathy, and axonal sensory neuropathy.[452,453] Identified risk factors included irregular diet, weight loss, smoking, alcohol, and excessive sugar consumption. Patients responded to B-group vitamins and folic acid. Overt malnutrition was not present.

There are numerous descriptions of neuropathies and myeloneuropathies from the tropics, particularly from developing countries, for which a nutritional cause has been postulated.[6,454] The term tropical myeloneuropathies has been used to describe these multifactorial conditions. The neurologic manifestations have included polyneuropathy, sensory ataxia, impaired vision, tinnitus, hearing loss, and vertigo in varying combinations. Accompanying cutaneous manifestations are common. Associations have included malnutrition, malabsorption, cyanide intoxication caused by cassava consumption, lathyrism, organophosphate neurotoxicity, and vegetarian diets. Multiple nutritional deficits, in particular B-group vitamins, may coexist. Often the precise cause is unknown.

The term tropical myeloneuropathies includes 2 major groups of conditions: patients with prominent sensory ataxia (tropical ataxic neuropathy [TAN]), and those with prominent spastic paraparesis (tropical spastic paraparesis [TSP]). Although initial used to describe the neurologic manifestations caused by possible cassava toxicity, the term TAN is now more commonly used to describe a broader spectrum of toxic-nutritional myeloneuropathies seen in some developing countries.[454,455] Human T-lymphotropic virus-I myelitis had been called TSP in many equatorial regions and human T-lymphotropic virus-I-associated myelopathy (HAM) in Japan. HAM and TSP are now believed to be identical syndromes.[456] Human T-lymphotropic virus-II is also recognized to cause a chronic myelopathy that resembles TSP, at times with ataxia.[457,458]

Fluorosis

Fluorosis occurs when a large amount of fluoride, naturally present in the earth and water in certain parts of the world, are deposited in bones. The vertebral column is commonly involved. This results in back pain and stiffness with limited spine mobility. Neurologic manifestations are delayed and are seen in 10% of patients with skeletal fluorosis. These include cord compression and less commonly radiculopathy.[459] The spastic paraparesis may be accompanied by some sensory manifestations and lower motor neuron involvement. Sphincter disturbance may be present. A sensory level is not seen. Some patients may have decreased hearing caused by compression of the auditory nerves in the sclerosed auditory canal. Entrapment neuropathies may be seen as a result of bony deformities. The typical radiological findings are osteosclerosis and ligamentous calcification. A characteristic finding is calcification of the interosseous membrane of the forearm. Laboratory studies show increased alkaline phosphatase and parathormone levels with normal calcium and phosphorus. Estimation of urinary fluoride levels is not reliable.

Organophosphate Toxicity

Triorthocresyl phosphate is an organophosphate compound that has been used as an adulterant. In 1930, thousands of Americans developed neurologic deficits after consuming a popular illicit alcoholic beverage (Jamaica ginger extract or "jake") that had been adulterated with triorthocresyl phosphate.[460] Jamaican ginger paralysis was associated with peripheral neuropathy and spastic paraparesis.

An outbreak of acute polyneuropathy occurred in a tea plantation in Sri Lanka during 1977-1978 affecting adolescent girls.[461] The cause was attributed to tri-cresyl phosphate, which was present as a contaminant in a type of cooking oil. Contamination likely occurred when the oil was transported in containers previously used to store mineral oils. A distal axonopathy and pyramidal tract dysfunction with minimal sensory abnormalities were present. Significant improvement was noted over a 3-year period.[462]

The signs and symptoms of acute organophosphate toxicity are caused by acetylcholinesterase inhibition and resulting muscarinic and nicotinic dysfunction. Pralidoxime is a reactivator of inhibited acetylcholinesterase and is the specific antidote for acute organophosphate poisoning. It is used in conjunction with atropine. In some patients an intermediate syndrome develops after resolution of the cholinergic crisis.[463] This is characterized by weakness of neck flexors, proximal limb, and respiratory muscles. This weakness may relate to depolarization blockade at the neuromuscular junction. Organophosphate-induced delayed neurotoxicity is another well-recognized complication of organophosphorus compounds.[464] Organophosphate-induced delayed neurotoxicity is caused by phosphorylation and subsequent aging of a protein neurotoxic esterase in the nervous system.[465] Pathologic studies have shown involvement of the anterior horn cell, corticospinal tracts, and peripheral nerves. Organophosphate-induced delayed neurotoxicity occurs 1 to 3 weeks after acute exposure and after a more uncertain duration after chronic exposure. Organophosphate-induced delayed neurotoxicity may occur in the absence of the cholinergic or intermediate phase. The symptoms include distal paresthesias, progressive leg weakness and wasting, and cramping muscle pain. There may be evidence of upper limb involvement and CNS dysfunction. Sensory loss when present is mild. The red blood cell cholinesterase activity is less rapidly depressed than the serum cholinesterase activity and is a measure of chronic exposure to organophosphates.[466] Most modern organophosphate pesticides do not cause the delayed neurotoxic syndrome. Prevention of organophosphate insecticide toxicity requires good occupational practices including use of gloves and protective clothing.

Lathyrism

Lathyrus sativus (grass pea or chickling pea) is an environmentally tolerant legume that resists drought conditions. Lathyrism is a self-limiting neurotoxic disorder that is endemic in parts of Bangladesh, India, and Ethiopia. It presents as a subacute or insidious onset spastic paraparesis and affects individuals who consume *Lathyrus sativus* as a staple. Studies have suggested that β-*N*-oxalyl-amino-L-alanine (L-BOAA), an excitotoxic amino acid in *Lathyrus sativus* is the toxin responsible.[467] It is a potent agonist of the excitatory neurotransmitter glutamate. The spastic paraparesis seen in lathyrism is associated with greatly increased tone in thigh extensors, thigh adductors, and gastrocnemius leading to a lurching scissoring gait characterized by patients walking on the balls of their feet.[468] Sensory symptoms may be reported at onset in the legs; sensory signs are rare. In severely affected individuals pyramidal signs may also be present in the upper limbs. In the early stages, there may be diffuse and transitory CNS excitation of somatic motor and autonomic function including the presence of bladder symptoms.[468] An early improvement in limb strength is seen and may be substantial. The degree of neurologic deficit has been classified as the "no-stick stage," "1-stick stage," "2-stick stage," and "crawler stage." Some patients stabilize in a subclinical asymptomatic stage with minimal deficits. Electrophysiologic studies suggest subclinical anterior horn cell involvement.[469] Neuropathologic studies have shown loss of axons and myelin in the pyramidal tract in the lumbar cord and mild degeneration of the anterior horn cells at the same level.[470] It has been suggested that neurolathyrism may be prevented by mixing grass pea preparations with cereals or detoxification of grass peas through aqueous leaching.[471,472]

Cassava Toxicity

Weeks of high dietary cyanide exposure caused by consumption of insufficiently processed cassava in parts of Africa, such as Zaire and Tanzania, results in konzo. Konzo is a distinct tropical myelopathy characterized by the abrupt onset of symmetric, nonprogressive, spastic paraparesis.[473,474] Upper limb involvement and central visual field defects may be present. There is absence of sensory or autonomic disturbance. Improvement after onset is seen. Permanent deficits remain. Brain and spinal cord MRI are normal. Motor evoked potentials on magnetic brain stimulation may be absent.[475] Decreased sulfur intake with impaired conversion of cyanide to thiocyanate may be responsible.[474] Drought increases the natural occurrence of cyanogenic glucosides in the cassava roots.[473] Because of food shortages, the processing procedure normally used to remove cyanide before consumption is shortened. Minor improvement in food processing may be preventive.[474] The abrupt onset and nonprogressive course differentiates konzo from HAM/TSP. Lathyrism has clinical similarities to konzo but has a different geographic distribution, is caused by a different diet, may have autonomic dysfunction, and does not have visual involvement. In parts of Africa (eg, Nigeria) a syndrome characterized by slowly progressive ataxia, peripheral neuropathy, and optic atrophy has been described.[476] Years of low dietary cyanide exposure caused by cassava consumption is a likely cause.

Subacute Myelo-Optic Neuropathy

Subacute myelo-optic neuropathy (SMON) is a myeloneuropathy with optic nerve involvement that affected approximately 10,000 individuals in Japan between 1955 and 1970.[477] A similar syndrome has also been rarely reported outside Japan.[478] Epidemiologic studies have suggested that SMON was caused by toxicity from the antiparasitic drug clioquinol. SMON was characterized by subacute onset of lower limb paresthesias and spastic paraparesis with optic atrophy. Tendon hyperreflexia and extensor plantar responses were seen although the ankle jerk was absent at times. Electrophysiologic studies have shown delayed central conduction and normal conduction in peripheral sensory axons.[479] Autopsy studies have shown symmetric axonal degeneration in the corticospinal tracts in the lumbar spine, gracile columns at the cervicomedullary junction, and in the optic tracts.[480] Morphometric studies have shown only slight reduction of large myelinated fibers in the sural nerve.[481]

The precise mechanism of action of clioquinol is unclear. Clioquinol is a copper chelator. Identification of a myelopathy resulting from acquired copper deficiency has led to speculation that clioquinol-induced neurotoxicity could be a consequence of copper deficiency.[178,179]

Protein-Calorie Malnutrition

Protein and calorie deficiency in infants and children in underdeveloped countries results in 2 related disorders: marasmus and kwashiorkor.[482] Marasmus is caused by caloric insufficiency and results in growth failure and emaciation in early infancy. Kwashiorkor presents between 2 and 3 years of age with edema, ascites, hepatomegaly, hair loss, and skin depigmentation. Its underlying cause is protein deficiency. Generalized muscle wasting and weakness with hypotonia and hyporeflexia are seen. Cognitive deficits may be permanent. Autopsy studies show cerebral atrophy and immature neuronal development. During the initial stages of dietary treatment, an encephalopathy may be seen.

Amyotrophic Lateral Sclerosis and Parkinsonism-dementia Complex of Guam

In 1945 a high prevalence of motor neuron disease, clinically and pathologically similar to amyotrophic lateral sclerosis, was reported among the indigenous Chamorro population of Guam. Subsequently it was noted that an atypical Parkinsonian syndrome with mental slowness and mid-life onset was also seen among the Chamorros, at times in the families with individuals afflicted by motor neuron disease or in individuals with the amyotrophic lateral sclerosis syndrome. The parkinsonism-dementia complex of Guam and the amyotrophic lateral sclerosis (ALS) syndrome were linked and considered variants of the same disease process. Follow-up studies on the "ALS and parkinsonism-dementia complex of Guam" has shown a declining incidence, particularly for the amyotrophic lateral sclerosis syndrome.[483,484] Environmental lifestyle and diet have been suspected causes.[485] A traditional food in Guam is a tortilla made from a flour called fadang. Fadang is made from the seeds of *Cycas cicinalis* or *Cycas micronesica* (false sago palm). Major cycad toxins include β-D-glucoside (cycasin) and β-*N*-methyl-amino-L-alanine. The "cycad hypothesis" has been challenged.[486] The disease has persisted despite cessation of fading consumption. Other epidemiologic aspects that go against the "cycad hypothesis" include a familial occurrence, restriction to the Chamorro population, and a regional variation on Guam itself.[486]

REFERENCES

1. Perkin GD, Murray-Lyon I. Neurology and the gastrointestinal system. J Neurol Neurosurg Psychiatr 1998;65(3):291–300.
2. Skeen MB. Neurologic manifestations of gastrointestinal disease. Neurol Clin 2002;20(1):195–225.
3. Murray JA, Ross MA. Malabsorption and neurological disease. In: Quigley EMM, Pfeiffer RF, editors. Neuro-gastroenterology. Philadelphia: Butterworth Heinemann; 2004. p. 203–54.
4. Saperstein DS, Bahron RJ. Polyneuropathy caused by nutritional and vitamin deficiency. In: Dyck PJ, Thomas PK, editors. Peripheral neuropathy. 4th edition. Philadelphia: Elsevier Saunders; 2005. p. 2051–62.
5. Suarez GA. Peripheral neuropathy associated with alcoholism, malnutrition and vitamin deficiencies. In: Noseworthy JN, editor, Neurological therapeutics principles and practice, vol. 3. Abingdon, UK: Informa Healthcare; 2006. p. 2294–306.

6. Roman GC. Nutritional disorders of the nervous system. In: Shils ME, Shike M, Ross AC, et al, editors. Modern nutrition in health and disease. 10th edition. Baltimore (MD): Lippincott Williams and Wilkins; 2006. p. 1362–80.
7. Kumar N. Nutritional neuropathies. Neurol Clin 2007;25(1):209–55.
8. So YT, Simon RP. Deficiency diseases of the nervous system. In: Bradley WG, Daroff RB, Fenichel GM, et al, editors. 4th edition, Neurology in clinical practice, vol. 2. Philadelphia: Elsevier; 2008. p. 1643–55.
9. Kumar N. Metabolic and toxic myelopathies. Continuum Spinal Cord, Root, and Plexus Disorders 2008;14(3):91–115.
10. Kumar N. Neurogastroenterology. Continuum Neurologic Manifestations of Systemic Disease 2008;14(1):13–52.
11. Tefferi A, Pruthi RK. The biochemical basis of cobalamin deficiency. Mayo Clin Proc 1994;69(2):181–6.
12. Green R, Kinsella LJ. Current concepts in the diagnosis of cobalamin deficiency. Neurology 1995;45(8):1435–40.
13. Carmel R. Cobalamin, the stomach, and aging. Am J Clin Nutr 1997;66(4):750–9.
14. Hurwitz A, Brady DA, Schaal SE, et al. Gastric acidity in older adults. JAMA 1997;278(8):659–62.
15. Doscherholmen A, Swaim WR. Impaired assimilation of egg Co 57 vitamin B 12 in patients with hypochlorhydria and achlorhydria and after gastric resection. Gastroenterology 1973;64(5):913–9.
16. Schilling RF, Gohdes PN, Hardie GH. Vitamin B12 deficiency after gastric bypass surgery for obesity. Ann Intern Med 1984;101(4):501–2.
17. Rhode BM, Tamin H, Gilfix BM, et al. Treatment of vitamin B12 deficiency after gastric surgery for severe obesity. Obes Surg 1995;5(2):154–8.
18. Sumner AE, Chin MM, Abrahm JL, et al. Elevated methylmalonic acid and total homocysteine levels show high prevalence of vitamin B12 deficiency after gastric surgery. Ann Intern Med 1996;124(5):469–76.
19. Marcuard SP, Albernaz L, Khazanie PG. Omeprazole therapy causes malabsorption of cyanocobalamin (vitamin B12). Ann Intern Med 1994;120(3):211–5.
20. Ting RZ, Szeto CC, Chan MH, et al. Risk factors of vitamin B(12) deficiency in patients receiving metformin. Arch Intern Med 2006;166(18):1975–9.
21. Rosenblatt DS, Cooper BA. Inherited disorders of vitamin B12 utilization. Bioessays 1990;12(7):331–4.
22. Kieburtz KD, Giang DW, Schiffer RB, et al. Abnormal vitamin B12 metabolism in human immunodeficiency virus infection. Association with neurological dysfunction. Arch Neurol 1991;48(3):312–4.
23. Robertson KR, Stern RA, Hall CD, et al. Vitamin B12 deficiency and nervous system disease in HIV infection. Arch Neurol 1993;50(8):807–11.
24. Di Rocco A, Bottiglieri T, Werner P, et al. Abnormal cobalamin-dependent trans-methylation in AIDS-associated myelopathy. Neurology 2002;58(5):730–5.
25. Deacon R, Lumb M, Perry J, et al. Selective inactivation of vitamin B12 in rats by nitrous oxide. Lancet 1978;2(8098):1023–4.
26. Schilling RF. Is nitrous oxide a dangerous anesthetic for vitamin B12-deficient subjects? JAMA 1986;255(12):1605–6.
27. Marie RM, Le Biez E, Busson P, et al. Nitrous oxide anesthesia-associated myelopathy. Arch Neurol 2000;57(3):380–2.
28. Kinsella LJ, Green R. 'Anesthesia paresthetica': nitrous oxide-induced cobalamin deficiency. Neurology 1995;45(8):1608–10.
29. Layzer RB. Myeloneuropathy after prolonged exposure to nitrous oxide. Lancet 1978;2(8102):1227–30.

30. Sahenk Z, Mendell JR, Couri D, et al. Polyneuropathy from inhalation of N2O cartridges through a whipped-cream dispenser. Neurology 1978;28(5):485–7.
31. Ng J, Frith R. Nanging. Lancet 2002;360(9330):384.
32. Savage D, Lindenbaum J. Relapses after interruption of cyanocobalamin therapy in patients with pernicious anemia. Am J Med 1983;74(5):765–72.
33. Magnus EM. Cobalamin and unsaturated transcobalamin values in pernicious anaemia: relation to treatment. Scand J Haematol 1986;36(5):457–65.
34. Lindenbaum J, Healton EB, Savage DG, et al. Neuropsychiatric disorders caused by cobalamin deficiency in the absence of anemia or macrocytosis. N Engl J Med 1988;318(26):1720–8.
35. Carmel R. Pernicious anemia. The expected findings of very low serum cobalamin levels, anemia, and macrocytosis are often lacking. Arch Intern Med 1988;148(8):1712–4.
36. Healton EB, Savage DG, Brust JC, et al. Neurologic aspects of cobalamin deficiency. Medicine (Baltimore) 1991;70(4):229–45.
37. Savage D, Gangaidzo I, Lindenbaum J, et al. Vitamin B12 deficiency is the primary cause of megaloblastic anaemia in Zimbabwe. Br J Haematol 1994; 86(4):844–50.
38. Carmel R, Melnyk S, James SJ. Cobalamin deficiency with and without neurologic abnormalities: differences in homocysteine and methionine metabolism. Blood 2003;101(8):3302–8.
39. Morris MC, Evans DA, Bienias JL, et al. Dietary folate and vitamin B12 intake and cognitive decline among community-dwelling older persons. Arch Neurol 2005; 62(4):641–5.
40. Tangney CC, Tang Y, Evans DA, et al. Biochemical indicators of vitamin B12 and folate insufficiency and cognitive decline. Neurology 2009;72(4):361–7.
41. Vogiatzoglou A, Refsum H, Johnston C, et al. Vitamin B12 status and rate of brain volume loss in community-dwelling elderly. Neurology 2008;71(11): 826–32.
42. White WB, Reik L Jr, Cutlip DE. Pernicious anemia seen initially as orthostatic hypotension. Arch Intern Med 1981;141(11):1543–4.
43. Eisenhofer G, Lambie DG, Johnson RH, et al. Deficient catecholamine release as the basis of orthostatic hypotension in pernicious anaemia. J Neurol Neurosurg Psychiatr 1982;45(11):1053–5.
44. McCombe PA, McLeod JG. The peripheral neuropathy of vitamin B12 deficiency. J Neurol Sci 1984;66(1):117–26.
45. Kandler RH, Davies-Jones GA. Internuclear ophthalmoplegia in pernicious anaemia. BMJ 1988;297(6663):1583.
46. Benito-Leon J, Porta-Etessam J. Shaky-leg syndrome and vitamin B12 deficiency. N Engl J Med 2000;342(13):981.
47. Morita S, Miwa H, Kihira T, et al. Cerebellar ataxia and leukoencephalopathy associated with cobalamin deficiency. J Neurol Sci 2003;216(1):183–4.
48. Puri V, Chaudhry N, Gulati P. Syringomyelia-like manifestation of subacute combined degeneration. J Clin Neurosci 2004;11(6):672–5.
49. Ahn TB, Cho JW, Jeon BS. Unusual neurological presentations of vitamin B(12) deficiency. Eur J Neurol 2004;11(5):339–41.
50. Saperstein DS, Wolfe GI, Gronseth GS, et al. Challenges in the identification of cobalamin-deficiency polyneuropathy. Arch Neurol 2003;60(9):1296–301.
51. Allen RH, Stabler SP, Savage DG, et al. Diagnosis of cobalamin deficiency I: usefulness of serum methylmalonic acid and total homocysteine concentrations. Am J Hematol 1990;34(2):90–8.

52. Lindenbaum J, Savage DG, Stabler SP, et al. Diagnosis of cobalamin deficiency: II. Relative sensitivities of serum cobalamin, methylmalonic acid, and total homocysteine concentrations. Am J Hematol 1990;34(2):99–107.
53. Stabler SP, Allen RH, Savage DG, et al. Clinical spectrum and diagnosis of cobalamin deficiency. Blood 1990;76(5):871–81.
54. Savage DG, Lindenbaum J, Stabler SP, et al. Sensitivity of serum methylmalonic acid and total homocysteine determinations for diagnosing cobalamin and folate deficiencies. Am J Med 1994;96(3):239–46.
55. Stabler SP. Screening the older population for cobalamin (vitamin B12) deficiency. J Am Geriatr Soc 1995;43(11):1290–7.
56. Carmel R. Current concepts in cobalamin deficiency. Annu Rev Med 2000;51:357–75.
57. Carmel R, Green R, Rosenblatt DS, et al. Update on cobalamin, folate, and homocysteine. Hematology 2003;62–81.
58. Lindenbaum J, Rosenberg IH, Wilson PW, et al. Prevalence of cobalamin deficiency in the Framingham elderly population. Am J Clin Nutr 1994;60(1):2–11.
59. Metz J, Bell AH, Flicker L, et al. The significance of subnormal serum vitamin B12 concentration in older people: a case control study. J Am Geriatr Soc 1996;44(11):1355–61.
60. Waters WE, Withey JL, Kilpatrick GS, et al. Serum vitamin B 12 concentrations in the general population: a ten-year follow-up. Br J Haematol 1971;20(5):521–6.
61. Elwood PC, Shinton NK, Wilson CI, et al. Haemoglobin, vitamin B12 and folate levels in the elderly. Br J Haematol 1971;21(5):557–63.
62. Karnaze DS, Carmel R. Neurologic and evoked potential abnormalities in subtle cobalamin deficiency states, including deficiency without anemia and with normal absorption of free cobalamin. Arch Neurol 1990;47(9):1008–12.
63. Carmel R, Gott PS, Waters CH, et al. The frequently low cobalamin levels in dementia usually signify treatable metabolic, neurologic and electrophysiologic abnormalities. Eur J Haematol 1995;54(4):245–53.
64. Carmel R, Green R, Jacobsen DW, et al. Serum cobalamin, homocysteine, and methylmalonic acid concentrations in a multiethnic elderly population: ethnic and sex differences in cobalamin and metabolite abnormalities. Am J Clin Nutr 1999;70(5):904–10.
65. Carmel R. How I treat cobalamin (vitamin B12) deficiency. Blood 2008;112(6):2214–21.
66. Snow CF. Laboratory diagnosis of vitamin B12 and folate deficiency: a guide for the primary care physician. Arch Intern Med 1999;159(12):1289–98.
67. Bolann BJ, Solli JD, Schneede J, et al. Evaluation of indicators of cobalamin deficiency defined as cobalamin-induced reduction in increased serum methylmalonic acid. Clin Chem 2000;46(11):1744–50.
68. Carmel R, Vasireddy H, Aurangzeb I, et al. High serum cobalamin levels in the clinical setting–clinical associations and holo-transcobalamin changes. Clin Lab Haematol 2001;23(6):365–71.
69. Carmel R. Mild transcobalamin I (haptocorrin) deficiency and low serum cobalamin concentrations. Clin Chem 2003;49(8):1367–74.
70. Solomon LR. Cobalamin-responsive disorders in the ambulatory care setting: unreliability of cobalamin, methylmalonic acid, and homocysteine testing. Blood 2005;105(3):978–85.
71. Kinsella LJ. Megaloblastic anemias – vitamin B12, folate. In: Noseworthy JN, editor. Neurological therapeutics principles and practice. Abingdon, UK: Informa Healthcare; 2006. p. 1478–84.

72. Lindemans J, Schoester M, van Kapel J. Application of a simple immunoadsorption assay for the measurement of saturated and unsaturated transcobalamin II and R-binders. Clin Chim Acta 1983;132(1):53–61.
73. Seetharam B. Receptor-mediated endocytosis of cobalamin (vitamin B12). Annu Rev Nutr 1999;19:173–95.
74. Nexo E, Christensen AL, Hvas AM, et al. Quantification of holo-transcobalamin, a marker of vitamin B12 deficiency. Clin Chem 2002;48(3):561–2.
75. Carmel R. Measuring and interpreting holo-transcobalamin (holo-transcobalamin II). Clin Chem 2002;48(3):407–9.
76. Bor MV, Nexo E, Hvas AM. Holo-transcobalamin concentration and transcobalamin saturation reflect recent vitamin B12 absorption better than does serum vitamin B12. Clin Chem 2004;50(6):1043–9.
77. Hvas AM, Nexo E. Holotranscobalamin–a first choice assay for diagnosing early vitamin B deficiency? J Intern Med 2005;257(3):289–98.
78. Herrmann W, Obeid R, Schorr H, et al. The usefulness of holotranscobalamin in predicting vitamin B12 status in different clinical settings. Curr Drug Metab 2005;6(1):47–53.
79. Miller JW, Garrod MG, Rockwood AL, et al. Measurement of total vitamin B12 and holotranscobalamin, singly and in combination, in screening for metabolic vitamin B12 deficiency. Clin Chem 2006;52(2):278–85.
80. Clarke R, Sherliker P, Hin H, et al. Detection of vitamin B12 deficiency in older people by measuring vitamin B12 or the active fraction of vitamin B12, holotranscobalamin. Clin Chem 2007;53(5):963–70.
81. Carmel R. Macrocytosis, mild anemia, and delay in the diagnosis of pernicious anemia. Arch Intern Med 1979;139(1):47–50.
82. Carmel R. The disappearance of cobalamin absorption testing: a critical diagnostic loss. J Nutr 2007;137(11):2481–4.
83. Carmel R. Pepsinogens and other serum markers in pernicious anemia. Am J Clin Pathol 1988;90(4):442–5.
84. Miller A, Slingerland DW, Cardarelli J, et al. Further studies on the use of serum gastrin levels in assessing the significance of low serum B12 levels. Am J Hematol 1989;31(3):194–8.
85. Rothenberg SP, Kantha KR, Ficarra A. Autoantibodies to intrinsic factor: their determination and clinical usefulness. J Lab Clin Med 1971;77(3):476–84.
86. Fairbanks VF, Lennon VA, Kokmen E, et al. Tests for pernicious anemia: serum intrinsic factor blocking antibody. Mayo Clin Proc 1983;58(3):203–4.
87. Carmel R. Reassessment of the relative prevalences of antibodies to gastric parietal cell and to intrinsic factor in patients with pernicious anaemia: influence of patient age and race. Clin Exp Immunol 1992;89(1):74–7.
88. Fine EJ, Soria E, Paroski MW, et al. The neurophysiological profile of vitamin B12 deficiency. Muscle Nerve 1990;13(2):158–64.
89. Hemmer B, Glocker FX, Schumacher M, et al. Subacute combined degeneration: clinical, electrophysiological, and magnetic resonance imaging findings. J Neurol Neurosurg Psychiatr 1998;65(6):822–7.
90. Timms SR, Cure JK, Kurent JE. Subacute combined degeneration of the spinal cord: MR findings. AJNR Am J Neuroradiol 1993;14(5):1224–7.
91. Larner AJ, Zeman AZ, Allen CM, et al. MRI appearances in subacute combined degeneration of the spinal cord due to vitamin B12 deficiency. J Neurol Neurosurg Psychiatr 1997;62(1):99–100.

92. Ravina B, Loevner LA, Bank W. MR findings in subacute combined degeneration of the spinal cord: a case of reversible cervical myelopathy. AJR Am J Roentgenol 2000;174(3):863–5.
93. Stojsavljevic N, Levic Z, Drulovic J, et al. 44-month clinical-brain MRI follow-up in a patient with B12 deficiency. Neurology 1997;49(3):878–81.
94. Kuker W, Hesselmann V, Thron A, et al. MRI demonstration of reversible impairment of the blood-CNS barrier function in subacute combined degeneration of the spinal cord. J Neurol Neurosurg Psychiatr 1997;62(3):298–9.
95. Locatelli ER, Laureno R, Ballard P, et al. MRI in vitamin B12 deficiency myelopathy. Can J Neurol Sci 1999;26(1):60–3.
96. Bassi SS, Bulundwe KK, Greeff GP, et al. MRI of the spinal cord in myelopathy complicating vitamin B12 deficiency: two additional cases and a review of the literature. Neuroradiology 1999;41(4):271–4.
97. Karantanas AH, Markonis A, Bisbiyiannis G. Subacute combined degeneration of the spinal cord with involvement of the anterior columns: a new MRI finding. Neuroradiology 2000;42(2):115–7.
98. Katsaros VK, Glocker FX, Hemmer B, et al. MRI of spinal cord and brain lesions in subacute combined degeneration. Neuroradiology 1998;40(11):716–9.
99. Su S, Libman RB, Diamond A, et al. Infratentorial and supratentorial leukoencephalopathy associated with vitamin B12 deficiency. J Stroke Cerebrovasc Dis 2000;9(3):136–8.
100. Verhaeverbeke I, Mets T, Mulkens K, et al. Normalization of low vitamin B12 serum levels in older people by oral treatment. J Am Geriatr Soc 1997;45(1):124–5.
101. Rajan S, Wallace JI, Brodkin KI, et al. Response of elevated methylmalonic acid to three dose levels of oral cobalamin in older adults. J Am Geriatr Soc 2002; 50(11):1789–95.
102. Seal EC, Metz J, Flicker L, et al. A randomized, double-blind, placebo-controlled study of oral vitamin B12 supplementation in older patients with subnormal or borderline serum vitamin B12 concentrations. J Am Geriatr Soc 2002;50(1): 146–51.
103. Eussen SJ, de Groot LC, Clarke R, et al. Oral cyanocobalamin supplementation in older people with vitamin B12 deficiency: a dose-finding trial. Arch Intern Med 2005;165(10):1167–72.
104. Lederle FA. Oral cobalamin for pernicious anemia. Medicine's best kept secret? JAMA 1991;265(1):94–5.
105. Berlin H, Berlin R, Brante G. Oral treatment of pernicious anemia with high doses of vitamin B12 without intrinsic factor. Acta Med Scand 1968;184(4): 247–58.
106. Kokkola A, Sjoblom SM, Haapiainen R, et al. The risk of gastric carcinoma and carcinoid tumours in patients with pernicious anaemia. A prospective follow-up study. Scand J Gastroenterol 1998;33(1):88–92.
107. Carmel R, Spencer CA. Clinical and subclinical thyroid disorders associated with pernicious anemia. Observations on abnormal thyroid-stimulating hormone levels and on a possible association of blood group O with hyperthyroidism. Arch Intern Med 1982;142(8):1465–9.
108. Carmel R, Weiner JM, Johnson CS. Iron deficiency occurs frequently in patients with pernicious anemia. JAMA 1987;257(8):1081–3.
109. Stacy CB, Di Rocco A, Gould RJ. Methionine in the treatment of nitrous-oxide-induced neuropathy and myeloneuropathy. J Neurol 1992;239(7):401–3.
110. Di Rocco A, Tagliati M, Danisi F, et al. A pilot study of L-methionine for the treatment of AIDS-associated myelopathy. Neurology 1998;51(1):266–8.

111. Di Rocco A, Werner P, Bottiglieri T, et al. Treatment of AIDS-associated myelopathy with L-methionine: a placebo-controlled study. Neurology 2004;63(7):1270–5.
112. Carmel R. Treatment of severe pernicious anemia: no association with sudden death. Am J Clin Nutr 1988;48(6):1443–4.
113. Skouby AP. Hydroxocobalamin for initial and long-term therapy for vitamin B12 deficiency. Acta Med Scand 1987;221(4):399–402.
114. Tudhope GR, Swan HT, Spray GH. Patient variation in pernicious anaemia, as shown in a clinical trial of cyanocobalamin, hydroxocobalamin and cyanocobalamin–zinc tannate. Br J Haematol 1967;13(2):216–28.
115. Slot WB, Merkus FW, Van Deventer SJ, et al. Normalization of plasma vitamin B12 concentration by intranasal hydroxocobalamin in vitamin B12-deficient patients. Gastroenterology 1997;113(2):430–3.
116. Sirotnak FM, Tolner B. Carrier-mediated membrane transport of folates in mammalian cells. Annu Rev Nutr 1999;19:91–122.
117. Moran RG. Roles of folylpoly-gamma-glutamate synthetase in therapeutics with tetrahydrofolate antimetabolites: an overview. Semin Oncol 1999;26(2 Suppl 6): 24–32.
118. Eichner ER, Pierce HI, Hillman RS. Folate balance in dietary-induced megaloblastic anemia. N Engl J Med 1971;284(17):933–8.
119. Carmel R. Folic acid. In: Shils ME, Shike M, Ross AC, et al, editors. Modern nutrition in health and disease. 10th edition. Baltimore (MD): Lippincott Williams and Wilkins; 2006. p. 470–81.
120. Elsborg L. Malabsorption of folic acid following partial gastrectomy. Scand J Gastroenterol 1974;9(3):271–4.
121. Russell RM, Krasinski SD, Samloff IM, et al. Folic acid malabsorption in atrophic gastritis. Possible compensation by bacterial folate synthesis. Gastroenterology 1986;91(6):1476–82.
122. Russell RM, Golner BB, Krasinski SD, et al. Effect of antacid and H2 receptor antagonists on the intestinal absorption of folic acid. J Lab Clin Med 1988; 112(4):458–63.
123. Lambie DG, Johnson RH. Drugs and folate metabolism. Drugs 1985;30(2): 145–55.
124. Green R, Miller JW. Folate deficiency beyond megaloblastic anemia: hyperhomocysteinemia and other manifestations of dysfunctional folate status. Semin Hematol 1999;36(1):47–64.
125. Diaz-Arrastia R. Homocysteine and neurologic disease. Arch Neurol 2000; 57(10):1422–7.
126. Grant HC, Hoffbrand AV, Wells DG. Folate deficiency and neurological disease. Lancet 1965;2(7416):763–7.
127. Reynolds EH, Rothfeld P, Pincus JH. Neurological disease associated with folate deficiency. Br Med J 1973;2(5863):398–400.
128. Manzoor M, Runcie J. Folate-responsive neuropathy: report of 10 cases. Br Med J 1976;1(6019):1176–8.
129. Lever EG, Elwes RD, Williams A, et al. Subacute combined degeneration of the cord due to folate deficiency: response to methyl folate treatment. J Neurol Neurosurg Psychiatr 1986;49(10):1203–7.
130. Parry TE. Folate responsive neuropathy. Presse Med 1994;23(3):131–7.
131. Shorvon SD, Carney MW, Chanarin I, et al. The neuropsychiatry of megaloblastic anaemia. Br Med J 1980;281(6247):1036–8.
132. Reynolds EH. Benefits and risks of folic acid to the nervous system. J Neurol Neurosurg Psychiatr 2002;72(5):567–71.

133. Toole JF, Malinow MR, Chambless LE, et al. Lowering homocysteine in patients with ischemic stroke to prevent recurrent stroke, myocardial infarction, and death: the Vitamin Intervention for Stroke Prevention (VISP) randomized controlled trial. JAMA 2004;291(5):565–75.

134. Kado DM, Karlamangla AS, Huang MH, et al. Homocysteine versus the vitamins folate, B6, and B12 as predictors of cognitive function and decline in older high-functioning adults: MacArthur studies of successful aging. Am J Med 2005; 118(2):161–7.

135. Zittoun J. Congenital errors of folate metabolism. Baillieres Clin Haematol 1995; 8(3):603–16.

136. Gunter EW, Bowman BA, Caudill SP, et al. Results of an international round robin for serum and whole-blood folate. Clin Chem 1996;42(10):1689–94.

137. Brouwer DA, Welten HT, Reijngoud DJ, et al. Plasma folic acid cutoff value, derived from its relationship with homocysteine. Clin Chem 1998;44(7): 1545–50.

138. Eichner ER, Hillman RS. Effect of alcohol on serum folate level. J Clin Invest 1973;52(3):584–91.

139. Lucock M, Yates Z. Measurement of red blood cell methylfolate. Lancet 2002; 360(9338):1021–2 [author reply 1022].

140. Butterworth CE Jr, Tamura T. Folic acid safety and toxicity: a brief review. Am J Clin Nutr 1989;50(2):353–8.

141. Stabler SP, Marcell PD, Podell ER, et al. Elevation of total homocysteine in the serum of patients with cobalamin or folate deficiency detected by capillary gas chromatography-mass spectrometry. J Clin Invest 1988;81(2):466–74.

142. Williams DM. Copper deficiency in humans. Semin Hematol 1983;20(2):118–28.

143. Spiegel JE, Willenbucher RF. Rapid development of severe copper deficiency in a patient with Crohn's disease receiving parenteral nutrition. JPEN J Parenter Enteral Nutr 1999;23(3):169–72.

144. Fuhrman MP, Herrmann V, Masidonski P, et al. Pancytopenia after removal of copper from total parenteral nutrition. JPEN J Parenter Enteral Nutr 2000; 24(6):361–6.

145. Kumar N, Low PA. Myeloneuropathy and anemia due to copper malabsorption. J Neurol 2004;251(6):747–9.

146. Spinazzi M, De Lazzari F, Tavolato B, et al. Myelo-optico-neuropathy in copper deficiency occurring after partial gastrectomy. Do small bowel bacterial overgrowth syndrome and occult zinc ingestion tip the balance? J Neurol 2007; 254(8):1012–7.

147. Henri-Bhargava A, Melmed C, Glikstein R, et al. Neurologic impairment due to vitamin E and copper deficiencies in celiac disease. Neurology 2008;71(11):860–1.

148. Halfdanarson T, Kumar N, Hogan WJ, et al. Copper deficiency in celiac disease. J Clin Gastroenterol 2009;43(2):162–4.

149. Schleper B, Stuerenburg HJ. Copper deficiency-associated myelopathy in a 46-year-old woman. J Neurol 2001;248(8):705–6.

150. Gregg XT, Reddy V, Prchal JT. Copper deficiency masquerading as myelodysplastic syndrome. Blood 2002;100(4):1493–5.

151. Kumar N, McEvoy KM, Ahlskog JE. Myelopathy due to copper deficiency following gastrointestinal surgery. Arch Neurol 2003;60(12):1782–5.

152. Kumar N, Crum B, Petersen RC, et al. Copper deficiency myelopathy. Arch Neurol 2004;61(5):762–6.

153. Kumar N, Ahlskog JE, Gross JB Jr. Acquired hypocupremia after gastric surgery. Clin Gastroenterol Hepatol 2004;2(12):1074–9.

154. Kumar N, Gross JB Jr, Ahlskog JE. Copper deficiency myelopathy produces a clinical picture like subacute combined degeneration. Neurology 2004;63(1):33–9.
155. Prodan CI, Bottomley SS, Holland NR, et al. Relapsing hypocupraemic myelopathy requiring high-dose oral copper replacement. J Neurol Neurosurg Psychiatr 2006;77(9):1092–3.
156. Weihl CC, Lopate G. Motor neuron disease associated with copper deficiency. Muscle Nerve 2006;34:789–93.
157. Kumar N. Copper deficiency myelopathy (human swayback). Mayo Clin Proc 2006;81(10):1371–84.
158. Everett CM, Matharu M, Gawler J. Neuropathy progressing to myeloneuropathy 20 years after partial gastrectomy. Neurology 2006;66(9):1451.
159. Juhasz-Pocsine K, Rudnicki SA, Archer RL, et al. Neurologic complications of gastric bypass surgery for morbid obesity. Neurology 2007;68(21): 1843–50.
160. Halfdanarson T, Kumar N, Li C-Y, et al. Hematological manifestations of copper deficiency. Eur J Haematol 2008;80(6):523–31.
161. Kumar N, Gross JB Jr, Ahlskog JE. Myelopathy due to copper deficiency. Neurology 2003;61(2):273–4.
162. Rowin J, Lewis SL. Copper deficiency myeloneuropathy and pancytopenia secondary to overuse of zinc supplementation. J Neurol Neurosurg Psychiatr 2005;76(5):750–1.
163. Willis MS, Monaghan SA, Miller ML, et al. Zinc-induced copper deficiency: a report of three cases initially recognized on bone marrow examination. Am J Clin Pathol 2005;123(1):125–31.
164. Sorenson EJ. Copper deficiency misdiagnosed as postpolio syndrome. J Clin Neuromuscul Dis 2006;8(2):70–4.
165. Nations SP, Boyer PJ, Love LA, et al. Denture cream: an unusual source of excess zinc, leading to hypocupremia and neurological disease. Neurology 2008;71(9):639–43.
166. Spain RI, Leist TP, De Sousa EA. When metals compete: a case of copper-deficiency myeloneuropathy and anemia. Nat Clin Pract Neurol 2009;5(2):106–11.
167. Yaldizli O, Johansson U, Gizewski ER, et al. Copper deficiency myelopathy induced by parenteral zinc supplementation during chronic hemodialysis. J Neurol 2006;253(11):1507–9.
168. Hassan HA, Netchvolodoff C, Raufman JP. Zinc-induced copper deficiency in a coin swallower. Am J Gastroenterol 2000;95(10):2975–7.
169. Prodan CI, Holland NR. CNS demyelination from zinc toxicity? Neurology 2000; 54(8):1705–6.
170. Prodan CI, Holland NR, Wisdom PJ, et al. CNS demyelination associated with copper deficiency and hyperzincemia. Neurology 2002;59(9):1453–6.
171. Hedera P, Fink JK, Bockenstedt PL, et al. Myelopolyneuropathy and pancytopenia due to copper deficiency and high zinc levels of unknown origin: further support for existence of a new zinc overload syndrome. Arch Neurol 2003; 60(9):1303–6.
172. Greenberg SA, Briemberg HR. A neurological and hematological syndrome associated with zinc excess and copper deficiency. J Neurol 2004;251:111–4.
173. Harless W, Crowell E, Abraham J. Anemia and neutropenia associated with copper deficiency of unclear etiology. Am J Hematol 2006;81(7):546–9.
174. Goodman BP, Chong BW, Patel AC, et al. Copper deficiency myeloneuropathy resembling B12 deficiency: partial resolution of MR imaging findings with copper supplementation. AJNR Am J Neuroradiol 2006;27(10):2112–4.

175. Hedera P, Brewer GJ. Myeloneuropathy due to copper deficiency or zinc excess? Arch Neurol 2004;61:605.
176. Kumar N, Ahlskog JE. Myelopolyneuropathy due to copper deficiency or zinc excess? Arch Neurol 2004;61(4):604–5 [author reply 605].
177. Lang TF, Glynne-Jones R, Blake S, et al. Iatrogenic copper deficiency following information and drugs obtained over the Internet. Ann Clin Biochem 2004;41(Pt 5):417–20.
178. Kumar N, Knopman DS. SMON, clioquinol, and copper. Postgrad Med J 2005; 81:227.
179. Schaumburg H, Herskovitz S. Copper deficiency myeloneuropathy: a clue to clioquinol-induced subacute myelo-optic neuropathy? Neurology 2008;71: 622–3.
180. Valentine JS, Gralla EB. Delivering copper inside yeast and human cells. Science 1997;278(5339):817–8.
181. Kumar A, Jazieh AR. Case report of sideroblastic anemia caused by ingestion of coins. Am J Hematol 2001;66(2):126–9.
182. Kumar N, Elliott MA, Hoyer JD, et al. "Myelodysplasia," myeloneuropathy, and copper deficiency. Mayo Clin Proc 2005;80(7):943–6.
183. Prodan CI, Holland NR, Wisdom PJ, et al. Myelopathy due to copper deficiency. Neurology 2004;62(9):1655–6, author reply 1656.
184. Kumar N, Ahlskog JE, Klein CJ, et al. Imaging features of copper deficiency myelopathy: a study of 25 cases. Neuroradiology 2005;48:78–83.
185. Kelkar P, Chang SC, Muley S. Response to oral supplementation in copper deficiency myelopathy. Neurology 2007;68(Suppl 1):A104.
186. Goodman BP, Bosch EP, Ross MA, et al. Clinical and electrodiagnostic findings in copper deficiency myeloneuropathy. J Neurol Neurosurg Psychiatr 2009;80: 524–7.
187. Kelkar P, Shereen C, Muley S. Response to oral supplementation in copper deficiency myeloneuropathy. J Clin Neuromuscul Dis 2008;10(1):1–3.
188. Zara G, Grassivaro F, Brocadello F, et al. Case of sensory ataxic ganglionopathy-myelopathy in copper deficiency. J Neurol Sci 2009;277(1–2):184–6.
189. Crum BA, Kumar N. Electrophysiologic findings in copper deficiency myeloneuropathy. Neurology 2005;64(Suppl 1):A123.
190. Prodan CI, Bottomley SS, Vincent AS, et al. Hypocupremia associated with prior vitamin B12 deficiency. Am J Hematol 2007;82(4):288–90.
191. Uauy R, Castillo-Duran C, Fisberg M, et al. Red cell superoxide dismutase activity as an index of human copper nutrition. J Nutr 1985;115(12):1650–5.
192. Milne DB. Assessment of copper nutritional status. Clin Chem 1994;40(8): 1479–84.
193. Kumar N, Butz JA, Burritt MF. Clinical significance of the laboratory determination of low serum copper in adults. Clin Chem Lab Med 2007;45(10):1402–10.
194. Huff JD, Keung YK, Thakuri M, et al. Copper deficiency causes reversible myelodysplasia. Am J Hematol 2007;82(7):625–30.
195. Shahidzadeh R, Sridhar S. Profound copper deficiency in a patient with gastric bypass. Am J Gastroenterol 2008;103(10):2660–2.
196. Cheeseman KH, Holley AE, Kelly FJ, et al. Biokinetics in humans of RRR-alpha-tocopherol: the free phenol, acetate ester, and succinate ester forms of vitamin E. Free Radic Biol Med 1995;19(5):591–8.
197. Traber MG. Vitamin E. In: Shils ME, Shike M, Ross AC, et al, editors. Modern nutrition in health and disease. 10th edition. Baltimore (MD): Lippincott Williams and Wilkins; 2006. p. 396–411.

198. Steephen AC, Traber MG, Ito Y, et al. Vitamin E status of patients receiving long-term parenteral nutrition: is vitamin E supplementation adequate? JPEN J Parenter Enteral Nutr 1991;15(6):647–52.
199. Traber MG, Sokol RJ, Burton GW, et al. Impaired ability of patients with familial isolated vitamin E deficiency to incorporate alpha-tocopherol into lipoproteins secreted by the liver. J Clin Invest 1990;85(2):397–407.
200. Ben Hamida C, Doerflinger N, Belal S, et al. Localization of Friedreich ataxia phenotype with selective vitamin E deficiency to chromosome 8q by homozygosity mapping. Nat Genet 1993;5(2):195–200.
201. Cavalier L, Ouahchi K, Kayden HJ, et al. Ataxia with isolated vitamin E deficiency: heterogeneity of mutations and phenotypic variability in a large number of families. Am J Hum Genet 1998;62(2):301–10.
202. Mariotti C, Gellera C, Rimoldi M, et al. Ataxia with isolated vitamin E deficiency: neurological phenotype, clinical follow-up and novel mutations in TTPA gene in Italian families. Neurol Sci 2004;25(3):130–7.
203. Aguglia U, Annesi G, Pasquinelli G, et al. Vitamin E deficiency due to chylomicron retention disease in Marinesco-Sjogren syndrome. Ann Neurol 2000;47(2):260–4.
204. Harding AE. Vitamin E and the nervous system. Crit Rev Neurobiol 1987;3(1):89–103.
205. Sokol RJ. Vitamin E deficiency and neurologic disease. Annu Rev Nutr 1988;8:351–73.
206. Ben Hamida M, Belal S, Sirugo G, et al. Friedreich's ataxia phenotype not linked to chromosome 9 and associated with selective autosomal recessive vitamin E deficiency in two inbred Tunisian families. Neurology 1993;43(11):2179–83.
207. Tomasi LG. Reversibility of human myopathy caused by vitamin E deficiency. Neurology 1979;29(8):1182–6.
208. Burck U, Goebel HH, Kuhlendahl HD, et al. Neuromyopathy and vitamin E deficiency in man. Neuropediatrics 1981;12(3):267–78.
209. Kleopa KA, Kyriacou K, Zamba-Papanicolaou E, et al. Reversible inflammatory and vacuolar myopathy with vitamin E deficiency in celiac disease. Muscle Nerve 2005;31(2):260–5.
210. Palmucci L, Doriguzzi C, Orsi L, et al. Neuropathy secondary to vitamin E deficiency in acquired intestinal malabsorption. Ital J Neurol Sci 1988;9(6):599–602.
211. Puri V, Chaudhry N, Tatke M, et al. Isolated vitamin E deficiency with demyelinating neuropathy. Muscle Nerve 2005;32(2):230–5.
212. Sokol RJ, Bove KE, Heubi JE, et al. Vitamin E deficiency during chronic childhood cholestasis: presence of sural nerve lesion prior to 2 1/2 years of age. J Pediatr 1983;103(2):197–204.
213. Traber MG, Sokol RJ, Ringel SP, et al. Lack of tocopherol in peripheral nerves of vitamin E-deficient patients with peripheral neuropathy. N Engl J Med 1987;317(5):262–5.
214. Behrens WA, Thompson JN, Madere R. Distribution of alpha-tocopherol in human plasma lipoproteins. Am J Clin Nutr 1982;35(4):691–6.
215. Sokol RJ, Heubi JE, Iannaccone ST, et al. Vitamin E deficiency with normal serum vitamin E concentrations in children with chronic cholestasis. N Engl J Med 1984;310(19):1209–12.
216. Horwitt MK, Harvey CC, Dahm CH Jr, et al. Relationship between tocopherol and serum lipid levels for determination of nutritional adequacy. Ann N Y Acad Sci 1972;203:223–36.

217. Traber MG, Jialal I. Measurement of lipid-soluble vitamins–further adjustment needed? Lancet 2000;355(9220):2013–4.
218. Vorgerd M, Tegenthoff M, Kuhne D, et al. Spinal MRI in progressive myeloneuropathy associated with vitamin E deficiency. Neuroradiology 1996;38(Suppl 1): S111–3.
219. Azizi E, Zaidman JL, Eshchar J, et al. Abetalipoproteinemia treated with parenteral and oral vitamins A and E, and with medium chain triglycerides. Acta Paediatr Scand 1978;67(6):796–801.
220. Sokol RJ, Guggenheim MA, Iannaccone ST, et al. Improved neurologic function after long-term correction of vitamin E deficiency in children with chronic cholestasis. N Engl J Med 1985;313(25):1580–6.
221. Sokol RJ, Butler-Simon N, Conner C, et al. Multicenter trial of d-alpha-tocopheryl polyethylene glycol 1000 succinate for treatment of vitamin E deficiency in children with chronic cholestasis. Gastroenterology 1993;104(6):1727–35.
222. Butterworth RF. Cerebral thiamine-dependent enzyme changes in experimental Wernicke's encephalopathy. Metab Brain Dis 1986;1(3):165–75.
223. Manzo L, Locatelli C, Candura SM, et al. Nutrition and alcohol neurotoxicity. Neurotoxicology 1994;15(3):555–65.
224. Butterworth RF. Thiamin. In: Shils ME, Shike M, Ross AC, et al, editors. Modern nutrition in health and disease. 10th edition. Baltimore (MD): Lippincott Williams and Wilkins; 2006. p. 426–33.
225. Bettendorff L. Thiamine in excitable tissues: reflections on a non-cofactor role. Metab Brain Dis 1994;9(3):183–209.
226. Butterworth RF. Effects of thiamine deficiency on brain metabolism: implications for the pathogenesis of the Wernicke-Korsakoff syndrome. Alcohol Alcohol 1989;24(4):271–9.
227. Hazell AS, Todd KG, Butterworth RF. Mechanisms of neuronal cell death in Wernicke's encephalopathy. Metab Brain Dis 1998;13(2):97–122.
228. Hazell AS, Pannunzio P, Rama Rao KV, et al. Thiamine deficiency results in downregulation of the GLAST glutamate transporter in cultured astrocytes. Glia 2003;43(2):175–84.
229. Butterworth RF, Heroux M. Effect of pyrithiamine treatment and subsequent thiamine rehabilitation on regional cerebral amino acids and thiamine-dependent enzymes. J Neurochem 1989;52(4):1079–84.
230. Hakim AM, Pappius HM. Sequence of metabolic, clinical, and histological events in experimental thiamine deficiency. Ann Neurol 1983;13(4):365–75.
231. McEntee WJ. Wernicke's encephalopathy: an excitotoxicity hypothesis. Metab Brain Dis 1997;12(3):183–92.
232. Todd KG, Butterworth RF. Mechanisms of selective neuronal cell death due to thiamine deficiency. Ann N Y Acad Sci 1999;893:404–11.
233. Todd KG, Hazell AS, Butterworth RF. Alcohol-thiamine interactions: an update on the pathogenesis of Wernicke encephalopathy. Addict Biol 1999;4(3): 261–72.
234. Doss A, Mahad D, Romanowski CA. Wernicke encephalopathy: unusual findings in nonalcoholic patients. J Comput Assist Tomogr 2003;27(2):235–40.
235. Sechi G, Serra A. Wernicke's encephalopathy: new clinical settings and recent advances in diagnosis and management. Lancet Neurol 2007;6(5): 442–55.
236. Thomson AD, Cook CC, Touquet R, et al. Royal College of Physicians L. The Royal College of Physicians report on alcohol: guidelines for managing Wernicke's encephalopathy in the accident and emergency department

[erratum appears in Alcohol Alcohol. 2003;38(3):291]. Alcohol Alcohol 2002; 37(6):513–21.

237. Lockman PR, McAfee JH, Geldenhuys WJ, et al. Cation transport specificity at the blood-brain barrier. Neurochem Res 2004;29(12):2245–50.

238. Schenker S, Henderson GI, Hoyumpa AM Jr, et al. Hepatic and Wernicke's encephalopathies: current concepts of pathogenesis. Am J Clin Nutr 1980; 33(12):2719–26.

239. Singleton CK, Martin PR. Molecular mechanisms of thiamine utilization. Curr Mol Med 2001;1(2):197–207.

240. Koguchi K, Nakatsuji Y, Abe K, et al. Wernicke's encephalopathy after glucose infusion. Neurology 2004;62(3):512.

241. Sauberlich HE, Herman YF, Stevens CO, et al. Thiamin requirement of the adult human. Am J Clin Nutr 1979;32(11):2237–48.

242. Baughman FA Jr, Papp JP. Wernicke's encephalopathy with intravenous hyperalimentation: remarks on similarities between Wernicke's encephalopathy and the phosphate depletion syndrome. Mt Sinai J Med 1976;43(1):48–52.

243. Nadel AM, Burger PC. Wernicke encephalopathy following prolonged intravenous therapy. JAMA 1976;235(22):2403–5.

244. Kramer J, Goodwin JA. Wernicke's encephalopathy. Complication of intravenous hyperalimentation. JAMA 1977;238(20):2176–7.

245. Lonsdale D. Wernicke's encephalopathy and hyperalimentation. JAMA 1978; 239(12):1133.

246. Watson AJ, Walker JF, Tomkin GH, et al. Acute Wernickes encephalopathy precipitated by glucose loading. Ir J Med Sci 1981;150(10):301–3.

247. Pentland B, Mawdsley C. Wernicke's encephalopathy following 'hunger strike'. Postgrad Med J 1982;58(681):427–8.

248. Francini-Pesenti F, Brocadello F, Famengo S, et al. Wernicke's encephalopathy during parenteral nutrition. JPEN J Parenter Enteral Nutr 2007;31(1):69–71.

249. Messina G, Quartarone E, Console G, et al. Wernicke's encephalopathy after allogeneic stem cell transplantation. Tumori 2007;93(2):207–9.

250. Drenick EJ, Joven CB, Swendseid ME. Occurrence of acute Wernicke's encephalopathy during prolonged starvation for the treatment of obesity. N Engl J Med 1966;274(17):937–9.

251. Shikata E, Mizutani T, Kokubun Y, et al. 'Iatrogenic' Wernicke's encephalopathy in Japan. Eur Neurol 2000;44(3):156–61.

252. Reuler JB, Girard DE, Cooney TG. Current concepts. Wernicke's encephalopathy. N Engl J Med 1985;312(16):1035–9.

253. Thomson AD. Mechanisms of vitamin deficiency in chronic alcohol misusers and the development of the Wernicke-Korsakoff syndrome. Alcohol Alcohol Suppl 2000;35(1):2–7.

254. Blass JP, Gibson GE. Abnormality of a thiamine-requiring enzyme in patients with Wernicke-Korsakoff syndrome. N Engl J Med 1977;297(25): 1367–70.

255. Blass JP, Gibson GE. Genetic factors in Wernicke-Korsakoff syndrome. Alcohol Clin Exp Res 1979;3(2):126–34.

256. Leigh D, McBurney A, McIlwain H. Wernicke-Korsakoff syndrome in monozygotic twins: a biochemical peculiarity. Br J Psychiatry 1981;139:156–9.

257. Merkin-Zaborsky H, Ifergane G, Frisher S, et al. Thiamine-responsive acute neurological disorders in nonalcoholic patients. Eur Neurol 2001;45(1):34–7.

258. Sechi G, Serra A, Pirastru MI, et al. Wernicke's encephalopathy in a woman on slimming diet. Neurology 2002;58(11):1697–8.

259. Fattal-Valevski A, Kesler A, Sela BA, et al. Outbreak of life-threatening thiamine deficiency in infants in Israel caused by a defective soy-based formula. Pediatrics 2005;115(2):e233–8.
260. Hilker DM, Somogyi JC. Antithiamins of plant origin: their chemical nature and mode of action. Ann N Y Acad Sci 1982;378:137–45.
261. Vimokesant SL, Hilker DM, Nakornchai S, et al. Effects of betel nut and fermented fish on the thiamin status of northeastern Thais. Am J Clin Nutr 1975; 28(12):1458–63.
262. Murata K, Yamaoka M, Ichikawa A. Reactivation mechanisms of thiamine with thermostable factors. J Nutr Sci Vitaminol (Tokyo) 1976;22(Suppl):7–12.
263. Hilker DM, Clifford AJ. Thiamin analysis and separation of thiamin phosphate esters by high-performance liquid chromatography. J Chromatogr A 1982; 231(2):433–8.
264. Singh M, Thompson M, Sullivan N, et al. Thiamine deficiency in dogs due to the feeding of sulphite preserved meat. Aust Vet J 2005;83(7):412–7.
265. Pearce JMS. Wernicke-Korsakoff encephalopathy. Eur Neurol 2008;59(1-2): 101–4.
266. Donnino MW, Vega J, Miller J, et al. Myths and misconceptions of Wernicke's encephalopathy: what every emergency physician should know. Ann Emerg Med 2007;50(6):715–21.
267. Homewood J, Bond NW. Thiamin deficiency and Korsakoff's syndrome: failure to find memory impairments following nonalcoholic Wernicke's encephalopathy. Alcohol 1999;19(1):75–84.
268. Ohnishi A, Tsuji S, Igisu H, et al. Beriberi neuropathy. Morphometric study of sural nerve. J Neurol Sci 1980;45(2–3):177–90.
269. Koike H, Misu K, Hattori N, et al. Postgastrectomy polyneuropathy with thiamine deficiency. J Neurol Neurosurg Psychiatr 2001;71(3):357–62.
270. Aguiar AC, Costa VM, Ragazzo PC, et al. Mielinolise pontina e extra-pontina associada a Shoshin beriberi em paciente etilista. Arq Neuropsiquiatr 2004; 62(3A):733–6.
271. Gollobin C, Marcus WY. Bariatric beriberi. Obes Surg 2002;12(3):309–11.
272. Harper C. The incidence of Wernicke's encephalopathy in Australia–a neuropathological study of 131 cases. J Neurol Neurosurg Psychiatr 1983;46(7):593–8.
273. Harper CG, Giles M, Finlay-Jones R. Clinical signs in the Wernicke-Korsakoff complex: a retrospective analysis of 131 cases diagnosed at necropsy. J Neurol Neurosurg Psychiatr 1986;49(4):341–5.
274. Caine D, Halliday GM, Kril JJ, et al. Operational criteria for the classification of chronic alcoholics: identification of Wernicke's encephalopathy. J Neurol Neurosurg Psychiatr 1997;62(1):51–60.
275. Torvik A, Lindboe CF, Rogde S. Brain lesions in alcoholics. A neuropathological study with clinical correlations. J Neurol Sci 1982;56(2–3):233–48.
276. Vasconcelos MM, Silva KP, Vidal G, et al. Early diagnosis of pediatric Wernicke's encephalopathy. Pediatr Neurol 1999;20(4):289–94.
277. Mumford CJ. Papilloedema delaying diagnosis of Wernicke's encephalopathy in a comatose patient. Postgrad Med J 1989;65(764):371–3.
278. Majolino I, Caponetto A, Scime R, et al. Wernicke-like encephalopathy after autologous bone marrow transplantation. Haematologica 1990;75(3):282–4.
279. Ming X, Wang MM, Zee D, et al. Wernicke's encephalopathy in a child with prolonged vomiting. J Child Neurol 1998;13(4):187–9.
280. Kulkarni S, Lee AG, Holstein SA, et al. You are what you eat. Surv Ophthalmol 2005;50(4):389–93.

281. Cooke CA, Hicks E, Page AB, et al. An atypical presentation of Wernicke's encephalopathy in an 11-year-old child. Eye 2006;20(12):1418–20.
282. Longmuir R, Lee AG, Rouleau J. Visual loss due to Wernicke syndrome following gastric bypass. Semin Ophthalmol 2007;22(1):13–9.
283. Surges R, Beck S, Niesen WD, et al. Sudden bilateral blindness in Wernicke's encephalopathy: case report and review of the literature. J Neurol Sci 2007; 260(1–2):261–4.
284. Tellez I, Terry RD. Fine structure of the early changes in the vestibular nuclei of the thiamine-deficient rat. Am J Pathol 1968;52(4):777–94.
285. Ghez C. Vestibular paresis: a clinical feature of Wernicke's disease. J Neurol Neurosurg Psychiatr 1969;32(2):134–9.
286. Choi KD, Oh SY, Kim HJ, et al. The vestibulo-ocular reflexes during head impulse in Wernicke's encephalopathy. J Neurol Neurosurg Psychiatr 2007; 78(10):1161–2.
287. Ishibashi S, Yokota T, Shiojiri T, et al. Reversible acute axonal polyneuropathy associated with Wernicke-Korsakoff syndrome: impaired physiological nerve conduction due to thiamine deficiency? J Neurol Neurosurg Psychiatr 2003; 74(5):674–6.
288. Wallis WE, Willoughby E, Baker P. Coma in the Wernicke-Korsakoff syndrome. Lancet 1978;2(8086):400–1.
289. Donnan GA, Seeman E. Coma and hypothermia in Wernicke's encephalopathy. Aust N Z J Med 1980;10(4):438–9.
290. Kearsley JH, Musso AF. Hypothermia and coma in the Wernicke-Korsakoff syndrome. Med J Aust 1980;2(9):504–6.
291. Butterworth RF, Gaudreau C, Vincelette J, et al. Thiamine deficiency and Wernicke's encephalopathy in AIDS. Metab Brain Dis 1991;6(4):207–12.
292. Onishi H, Kawanishi C, Onose M, et al. Successful treatment of Wernicke encephalopathy in terminally ill cancer patients: report of 3 cases and review of the literature. Support Care Cancer 2004;12(8):604–8.
293. Jiang W, Gagliardi JP, Raj YP, et al. Acute psychotic disorder after gastric bypass surgery: differential diagnosis and treatment. Am J Psychiatry 2006; 163(1):15–9.
294. Worden RW, Allen HM. Wernicke's encephalopathy after gastric bypass that masqueraded as acute psychosis: a case report. Curr Surg 2006;63(2):114–6.
295. Birchfield RI. Postural hypotension in Wernicke's disease. A manifestation of autonomic nervous system involvement. Am J Med 1964;36:404–14.
296. Koeppen AH, Daniels JC, Barron KD. Subnormal body temperatures in Wernicke's encephalopathy. Arch Neurol 1969;21(5):493–8.
297. Ackerman WJ. Stupor, bradycardia, hypotension and hypothermia. A presentation of Wernicke's encephalopathy with rapid response to thiamine. West J Med 1974;121(5):428–9.
298. Lipton JM, Payne H, Garza HR, et al. Thermolability in Wernicke's encephalopathy. Arch Neurol 1978;35(11):750–3.
299. Harper C. Wernicke's encephalopathy: a more common disease than realised. A neuropathological study of 51 cases. J Neurol Neurosurg Psychiatr 1979;42(3): 226–31.
300. Sechi GP, Bosincu L, Cossu RP, et al. Hyperthermia, choreic dyskinesias and increased motor tone in Wernicke's encephalopathy. Eur J Neurol 1996;3(Suppl 5):133.
301. Kinoshita Y, Inoue Y, Tsuru E, et al. [Unusual MR findings of Wernicke encephalopathy with cortical involvement]. No To Shinkei 2001;53(1):65–8 [in Japanese].

302. Truedsson M, Ohlsson B, Sjoberg K. Wernicke's encephalopathy presenting with severe dysphagia: a case report. Alcohol Alcohol 2002;37(3):295–6.
303. Foster D, Falah M, Kadom N, et al. Wernicke encephalopathy after bariatric surgery: losing more than just weight. Neurology 2005;65(12):1987 [discussion: 1847].
304. Buscaglia J, Faris J. Unsteady, unfocused, and unable to hear. Am J Med 2005; 118(11):1215–7.
305. Flint AC, Anziska Y, Rausch ME, et al. A clinical and radiographic variant of Wernicke-Korsakoff syndrome in a nonalcoholic patient. Neurology 2006; 67(11):2015.
306. Singh S, Kumar A. Wernicke encephalopathy after obesity surgery. Neurology 2007;68:807–11.
307. Nasrallah KM, Mitsias PD. Orthostatic tremor due to thiamine deficiency. Mov Disord 2007;22(3):440–1.
308. Flabeau O, Foubert-Samier A, Meissner W, et al. Hearing and seeing: unusual early signs of Wernicke encephalopathy. Neurology 2008;71(9):694.
309. Karaiskos I, Katsarolis I, Stefanis L. Severe dysphagia as the presenting symptom of Wernicke-Korsakoff syndrome in a non-alcoholic man. Neurol Sci 2008;29(1):45–6.
310. Sedel F, Challe G, Mayer JM, et al. Thiamine responsive pyruvate dehydroge-nase deficiency in an adult with peripheral neuropathy and optic neuropathy. J Neurol Neurosurg Psychiatr 2008;79(7):846–7.
311. Kurtoglu S, Hatipoglu N, Keskin M, et al. Thiamine withdrawal can lead to dia-betic ketoacidosis in thiamine responsive megaloblastic anemia: report of two siblings. J Pediatr Endocrinol 2008;21(4):393–7.
312. Cook CC, Hallwood PM, Thomson AD. B vitamin deficiency and neuropsychi-atric syndromes in alcohol misuse. Alcohol Alcohol 1998;33(4):317–36.
313. Mair WG, Warrington EK, Weiskrantz L. Memory disorder in Korsakoff's psychosis: a neuropathological and neuropsychological investigation of two cases. Brain 1979;102(4):749–83.
314. Victor M. Deficiency diseases of the nervous system secondary to alcoholism. Postgrad Med 1971;50(3):75–9.
315. McEntee WJ, Mair RG, Langlais PJ. Neurochemical pathology in Korsakoff's psychosis: implications for other cognitive disorders. Neurology 1984;34(5): 648–52.
316. Kopelman MD. The Korsakoff syndrome. Br J Psychiatry 1995;166(2):154–73.
317. Fama R, Pfefferbaum A, Sullivan EV. Visuoperceptual learning in alcoholic Kor-sakoff syndrome. Alcohol Clin Exp Res 2006;30(4):680–7.
318. Blansjaar BA, Van Dijk JG. Korsakoff minus Wernicke syndrome. Alcohol Alcohol 1992;27(4):435–7.
319. Toth C, Voll C, Macaulay R. Primary CNS lymphoma as a cause of Korsakoff syndrome. Surg Neurol 2002;57(1):41–5.
320. Yoneoka Y, Takeda N, Inoue A, et al. Acute Korsakoff syndrome following mam-millothalamic tract infarction. AJNR Am J Neuroradiol 2004;25(6):964–8.
321. Brokate B, Hildebrandt H, Eling P, et al. Frontal lobe dysfunctions in Korsakoff's syndrome and chronic alcoholism: continuity or discontinuity? Neuropsychology 2003;17(3):420–8.
322. Kim E, Ku J, Namkoong K, et al. Mammillothalamic functional connectivity and memory function in Wernicke's encephalopathy. Brain 2009;132(Pt 2):369–76.
323. Rindi G, Patrini C, Comincioli V, et al. Thiamine content and turnover rates of some rat nervous regions, using labeled thiamine as a tracer. Brain Res 1980; 181(2):369–80.

324. Kril JJ. Neuropathology of thiamine deficiency disorders. Metab Brain Dis 1996; 11(1):9–17.
325. Wright H. Changes in neuronal centers in beriberi neuritis. Br Med J 1901;1: 1610–6.
326. Dreyfus PM. Thiamine and the nervous system: an overview. J Nutr Sci Vitaminol (Tokyo) 1976;22(Suppl):13–6.
327. Talwar D, Davidson H, Cooney J, et al. Vitamin B(1) status assessed by direct measurement of thiamin pyrophosphate in erythrocytes or whole blood by HPLC: comparison with erythrocyte transketolase activation assay. Clin Chem 2000;46(5):704–10.
328. Mancinelli R, Ceccanti M, Guiducci MS, et al. Simultaneous liquid chromatographic assessment of thiamine, thiamine monophosphate and thiamine diphosphate in human erythrocytes: a study on alcoholics. J Chromatogr B Analyt Technol Biomed Life Sci 2003;789(2):355–63.
329. Lu J, Frank EL. Rapid HPLC measurement of thiamine and its phosphate esters in whole blood. Clin Chem 2008;54(5):901–6.
330. Donnino MW, Miller J, Garcia AJ, et al. Distinctive acid-base pattern in Wernicke's encephalopathy. Ann Emerg Med 2007;50(6):722–5.
331. Antunez E, Estruch R, Cardenal C, et al. Usefulness of CT and MR imaging in the diagnosis of acute Wernicke's encephalopathy. AJR Am J Roentgenol 1998; 171(4):1131–7.
332. Gallucci M, Bozzao A, Splendiani A, et al. Wernicke encephalopathy: MR findings in five patients. AJR Am J Roentgenol 1990;155(6):1309–14.
333. Victor M. MR in the diagnosis of Wernicke-Korsakoff syndrome. AJR Am J Roentgenol 1990;155(6):1315–6.
334. Maeda M, Tsuchida C, Handa Y, et al. Fluid attenuated inversion recovery (FLAIR) imaging in acute Wernicke encephalopathy. Radiat Med 1995;13(6): 311–3.
335. Suzuki S, Ichijo M, Fujii H, et al. Acute Wernicke's encephalopathy: comparison of magnetic resonance images and autopsy findings. Intern Med 1996;35(10): 831–4.
336. D'Aprile P, Tarantino A, Santoro N, et al. Wernicke's encephalopathy induced by total parenteral nutrition in patient with acute leukaemia: unusual involvement of caudate nuclei and cerebral cortex on MRI. Neuroradiology 2000;42(10):781–3.
337. Shin RK, Galetta SL, Imbesi SG. Wernicke encephalopathy. Arch Neurol 2000; 57(3):405.
338. Bergui M, Bradac GB, Zhong JJ, et al. Diffusion-weighted MR in reversible Wernicke encephalopathy. Neuroradiology 2001;43(11):969–72.
339. Doherty MJ, Watson NF, Uchino K, et al. Diffusion abnormalities in patients with Wernicke encephalopathy. Neurology 2002;58(4):655–7.
340. Weidauer S, Nichtweiss M, Lanfermann H, et al. Wernicke encephalopathy: MR findings and clinical presentation. Eur Radiol 2003;13(5):1001–9.
341. Ueda Y, Utsunomiya H, Fujii A, et al. [Wernicke encephalopathy in a chronic peritoneal dialysis patient–correlation between diffusion MR and pathological findings]. No To Hattatsu 2007;39(3):210–3 [in Japanese].
342. Roh JH, Kim JH, Koo Y, et al. Teaching NeuroImage: diverse MRI signal intensities with Wernicke encephalopathy. Neurology 2008;70(15):e48.
343. Zuccoli G, Motti L. Atypical Wernicke's encephalopathy showing lesions in the cranial nerve nuclei and cerebellum. J Neuroimaging 2008;18(2):194–7.
344. Yamashita M, Yamamoto T. Wernicke encephalopathy with symmetric pericentral involvement: MR findings. J Comput Assist Tomogr 1995;19(2):306–8.

345. Fei GQ, Zhong C, Jin L, et al. Clinical characteristics and MR imaging features of nonalcoholic Wernicke encephalopathy. AJNR Am J Neuroradiol 2008;29(1): 164–9.

346. Schroth G, Wichmann W, Valavanis A. Blood-brain-barrier disruption in acute Wernicke encephalopathy: MR findings. J Comput Assist Tomogr 1991;15(6): 1059–61.

347. Shogry ME, Curnes JT. Mamillary body enhancement on MR as the only sign of acute Wernicke encephalopathy. AJNR Am J Neuroradiol 1994;15(1):172–4.

348. Mascalchi M, Simonelli P, Tessa C, et al. Do acute lesions of Wernicke's encephalopathy show contrast enhancement? Report of three cases and review of the literature. Neuroradiology 1999;41(4):249–54.

349. Kaineg B, Hudgins PA. Images in clinical medicine. Wernicke's encephalopathy. N Engl J Med 2005;352(19):e18.

350. Opdenakker G, Gelin G, De Surgeloose D, et al. Wernicke encephalopathy: MR findings in two patients. Eur Radiol 1999;9(8):1620–4.

351. Charness ME, DeLaPaz RL. Mamillary body atrophy in Wernicke's encephalopathy: antemortem identification using magnetic resonance imaging. Ann Neurol 1987;22(5):595–600.

352. Yokote K, Miyagi K, Kuzuhara S, et al. Wernicke encephalopathy: follow-up study by CT and MR. J Comput Assist Tomogr 1991;15(5):835–8.

353. Tajima Y, Yoshida A, Ura S. [Diffusion weighted MR imaging of Wernicke encephalopathy]. No To Shinkei 2000;52(9):840–1 [in Japanese].

354. Oka M, Terae S, Kobayashi R, et al. Diffusion-weighted MR findings in a reversible case of acute Wernicke encephalopathy. Acta Neurol Scand 2001;104(3): 178–81.

355. Chu K, Kang DW, Kim HJ, et al. Diffusion-weighted imaging abnormalities in Wernicke encephalopathy: reversible cytotoxic edema? Arch Neurol 2002; 59(1):123–7.

356. Hong KS, Kang DW, Cho YJ, et al. Diffusion-weighted magnetic resonance imaging in Wernicke's encephalopathy. Acta Neurol Scand 2002;105(2): 132–4.

357. Chung TI, Kim JS, Park SK, et al. Diffusion weighted MR imaging of acute Wernicke's encephalopathy. Eur J Radiol 2003;45(3):256–8.

358. Rugilo CA, Roca MC, Zurru MC, et al. Diffusion abnormalities and Wernicke encephalopathy. Neurology 2003;60(4):727–8 [author reply 727–8].

359. Johkura K, Naito M. Wernicke's encephalopathy-like lesions in global cerebral hypoxia. J Clin Neurosci 2008;15(3):318–9.

360. Thomson AD, Marshall EJ. The treatment of patients at risk of developing Wernicke's encephalopathy in the community. Alcohol Alcohol 2006;41(2): 159–67.

361. Cole M, Turner A, Frank O, et al. Extraocular palsy and thiamine therapy in Wernicke's encephalopathy. Am J Clin Nutr 1969;22(1):44–51.

362. Salas-Salvado J, Garcia-Lorda P, Cuatrecasas G, et al. Wernicke's syndrome after bariatric surgery. Clin Nutr 2000;19(5):371–3.

363. Lindberg MC, Oyler RA. Wernicke's encephalopathy. Am Fam Physician 1990; 41(4):1205–9.

364. Fried RT, Levy M, Leibowitz AB, et al. Wernicke's encephalopathy in the intensive care patient. Crit Care Med 1990;18(7):779–80.

365. Bourgeois C, Cervantes-Laurean D, Moss J. Niacin. In: Shils ME, Shike M, Ross AC, et al, editors. Modern nutrition in health and disease. 10th edition. Baltimore (MD): Lippincott Williams and Wilkins; 2006. p. 442–51.

366. Serdaru M, Hausser-Hauw C, Laplane D, et al. The clinical spectrum of alcoholic pellagra encephalopathy. A retrospective analysis of 22 cases studied pathologically. Brain 1988;111(Pt 4):829–42.
367. Said HM, Ortiz A, Ma TY. A carrier-mediated mechanism for pyridoxine uptake by human intestinal epithelial Caco-2 cells: regulation by a PKA-mediated pathway. Am J Physiol Cell Physiol 2003;285(5):C1219–25.
368. Bhagavan HN, Brin M. Drug–vitamin B6 interaction. Curr Concepts Nutr 1983; 12:1–12.
369. Vilter RW, Mueller JF. Glazer HSea. The effect of vitamin B6 deficiency induced by desoxypyridoxine in human beings. J Lab Clin Med 1953;42:335–57.
370. Lumeng L. The role of acetaldehyde in mediating the deleterious effect of ethanol on pyridoxal 5'-phosphate metabolism. J Clin Invest 1978;62(2): 286–93.
371. Mackey AD, Davis SR, Gregory JFI. Vitamin B6. In: Shils ME, Shike M, Ross AC, et al, editors. Modern nutrition in health and disease. 10th edition. Baltimore (MD): Lippincott Williams and Wilkins; 2006. p. 452–61.
372. Plecko B, Paul K, Paschke E, et al. Biochemical and molecular characterization of 18 patients with pyridoxine-dependent epilepsy and mutations of the antiquitin (ALDH7A1) gene. Hum Mutat 2007;28(1):19–26.
373. Goldman AL, Braman SS. Isoniazid: a review with emphasis on adverse effects. Chest 1972;62(1):71–7.
374. Victor M, Adams RD. The neuropathology of experimental vitamin B6 deficiency in monkeys. Am J Clin Nutr 1956;4:346–53.
375. Mason DY, Emerson PM. Primary acquired sideroblastic anaemia: response to treatment with pyridoxal-5-phosphate. Br Med J 1973;1(5850):389–90.
376. Schaumburg H, Kaplan J, Windebank A, et al. Sensory neuropathy from pyridoxine abuse. A new megavitamin syndrome. N Engl J Med 1983;309(8):445–8.
377. Parry GJ, Bredesen DE. Sensory neuropathy with low-dose pyridoxine. Neurology 1985;35(10):1466–8.
378. de Lau LM, Koudstaal PJ, Witteman JC, et al. Dietary folate, vitamin B12, and vitamin B6 and the risk of Parkinson disease. Neurology 2006;67(2):315–8.
379. Leklem JE. Vitamin B-6: a status report. J Nutr 1990;120(Suppl 11):1503–7.
380. Okada H, Moriwaki K, Kanno Y, et al. Vitamin B6 supplementation can improve peripheral polyneuropathy in patients with chronic renal failure on high-flux haemadialysis and human recombinant erythropoietin. Nephrol Dial Transplant 2000;15(9):1410–3.
381. Keating JP, Feigin RD. Increased intracranial pressure associated with probable vitamin A deficiency in cystic fibrosis. Pediatrics 1970;46(1):41–6.
382. Russell JA. Osteomalacic myopathy. Muscle Nerve 1994;17(6):578–80.
383. Gloth FM 3rd, Lindsay JM, Zelesnick LB, et al. Can vitamin D deficiency produce an unusual pain syndrome? Arch Intern Med 1991;151(8):1662–4.
384. Plotnikoff GA, Quigley JM. Prevalence of severe hypovitaminosis D in patients with persistent, nonspecific musculoskeletal pain. Mayo Clin Proc 2003; 78(12):1463–70.
385. Mouyis M, Ostor AJ, Crisp AJ, et al. Hypovitaminosis D among rheumatology outpatients in clinical practice. Rheumatology (Oxford) 2008;47(9):1348–51.
386. Warner AE, Arnspiger SA. Diffuse musculoskeletal pain is not associated with low vitamin D levels or improved by treatment with vitamin D. J Clin Rheumatol 2008;14(1):12–6.
387. Munger KL, Zhang SM, O'Reilly E, et al. Vitamin D intake and incidence of multiple sclerosis. Neurology 2004;62(1):60–5.

388. Munger KL, Levin LI, Hollis BW, et al. Serum 25-hydroxyvitamin D levels and risk of multiple sclerosis. JAMA 2006;296(23):2832–8.
389. Torkildsen O, Knappskog PM, Nyland HI, et al. Vitamin D-dependent rickets as a possible risk factor for multiple sclerosis. Arch Neurol 2008;65(6):809–11.
390. Kragt J, van Amerongen B, Killestein J, et al. Higher levels of 25-hydroxyvitamin D are associated with a lower incidence of multiple sclerosis only in women. Mult Scler 2009;15(1):9–15.
391. Derex L, Trouillas P. Reversible parkinsonism, hypophosphoremia, and hypocalcemia under vitamin D therapy. Mov Disord 1997;12(4):612–3.
392. Seamans KM, Cashman KD. Existing and potentially novel functional markers of vitamin D status: a systematic review. Am J Clin Nutr 2009;89(6):1997S–2008S.
393. Brolin RE. Bariatric surgery and long-term control of morbid obesity. JAMA 2002;288(22):2793–6.
394. Buchwald H, Buchwald JN. Evolution of operative procedures for the management of morbid obesity 1950–2000. Obes Surg 2002;12(5):705–17.
395. Deitel M, Shikora SA. The development of the surgical treatment of morbid obesity. J Am Coll Nutr 2002;21(5):365–71.
396. Livingston EH. Obesity and its surgical management. Am J Surg 2002;184(2):103–13.
397. Presutti RJ, Gorman RS, Swain JM. Primary care perspective on bariatric surgery. Mayo Clin Proc 2004;79(9):1158–66 [quiz 1166].
398. MacLean LD, Rhode BM, Shizgal HM. Nutrition following gastric operations for morbid obesity. Ann Surg 1983;198(3):347–55.
399. Crowley LV, Olson RW. Megaloblastic anemia after gastric bypass for obesity. Am J Gastroenterol 1983;78(7):406–10.
400. Crowley LV, Seay J, Mullin G. Late effects of gastric bypass for obesity. Am J Gastroenterol 1984;79(11):850–60.
401. Amaral JF, Thompson WR, Caldwell MD, et al. Prospective hematologic evaluation of gastric exclusion surgery for morbid obesity. Ann Surg 1985;201(2):186–93.
402. Halverson JD. Micronutrient deficiencies after gastric bypass for morbid obesity. Am Surg 1986;52(11):594–8.
403. Provenzale D, Reinhold RB, Golner B, et al. Evidence for diminished B12 absorption after gastric bypass: oral supplementation does not prevent low plasma B12 levels in bypass patients. J Am Coll Nutr 1992;11(1):29–35.
404. Koffman BM, Greenfield LJ, Ali II, et al. Neurologic complications after surgery for obesity. Muscle Nerve 2006;33(2):166–76.
405. Abarbanel JM, Berginer VM, Osimani A, et al. Neurologic complications after gastric restriction surgery for morbid obesity. Neurology 1987;37(2):196–200.
406. Shimomura T, Mori E, Hirono N, et al. Development of Wernicke-Korsakoff syndrome after long intervals following gastrectomy. Arch Neurol 1998;55(9):1242–5.
407. Chaves LC, Faintuch J, Kahwage S, et al. A cluster of polyneuropathy and Wernicke-Korsakoff syndrome in a bariatric unit. Obes Surg 2002;12(3):328–34.
408. Sola E, Morillas C, Garzon S, et al. Rapid onset of Wernicke's encephalopathy following gastric restrictive surgery. Obes Surg 2003;13(4):661–2.
409. Berger JR. The neurological complications of bariatric surgery. Arch Neurol 2004;61(8):1185–9.
410. Sanchez-Crespo NE, Parker M. Wernicke's encephalopathy: a tragic complication of gastric bypass. J Hosp Med 2006;1(Suppl 2):72.

411. Al-Fahad T, Ismael A, Soliman MO, et al. Very early onset of Wernicke's encephalopathy after gastric bypass. Obes Surg 2006;16(5):671–2.
412. Lakhani SV, Shah HN, Alexander K, et al. Small intestinal bacterial overgrowth and thiamine deficiency after Roux-en-Y gastric bypass surgery in obese patients. Nutr Res 2008;28(5):293–8.
413. Carrodeguas L, Kaidar-Person O, Szomstein S, et al. Preoperative thiamine deficiency in obese population undergoing laparoscopic bariatric surgery. Surg Obes Relat Dis 2005;1(6):517–22 [discussion: 522].
414. Flancbaum L, Belsley S, Drake V, et al. Preoperative nutritional status of patients undergoing Roux-en-Y gastric bypass for morbid obesity. J Gastrointest Surg 2006;10(7):1033–7.
415. Banerji NK, Hurwitz LJ. Nervous system manifestations after gastric surgery. Acta Neurol Scand 1971;47(4):485–513.
416. Marinella MA. Ophthalmoplegia: an unusual manifestation of hypocalcemia. Am J Emerg Med 1999;17(1):105–6.
417. Alvarez-Leite JI. Nutrient deficiencies secondary to bariatric surgery. Curr Opin Clin Nutr Metab Care 2004;7(5):569–75.
418. Marinella MA. Anemia following Roux-en-Y surgery for morbid obesity: a review. Southampt Med J 2008;101(10):1024–31.
419. Hayton BA, Broome HE, Lilenbaum RC. Copper deficiency-induced anemia and neutropenia secondary to intestinal malabsorption. Am J Hematol 1995;48(1): 45–7.
420. Feit H, Glasberg M, Ireton C, et al. Peripheral neuropathy and starvation after gastric partitioning for morbid obesity. Ann Intern Med 1982;96(4):453–5.
421. Paulson GW, Martin EW, Mojzisik C, et al. Neurologic complications of gastric partitioning. Arch Neurol 1985;42(7):675–7.
422. Dahlquist NR, Perrault J, Callaway CW, et al. D-Lactic acidosis and encephalopathy after jejunoileostomy: response to overfeeding and to fasting in humans. Mayo Clin Proc 1984;59(3):141–5.
423. Hu WT, Kantarci OH, Merritt JL 2nd, et al. Ornithine transcarbamylase deficiency presenting as encephalopathy during adulthood following bariatric surgery. Arch Neurol 2007;64(1):126–8.
424. Banerji NK. Acute polyneuritis cranialis with total external ophthalmoplegia and areflexia. Ulster Med J 1971;40(1):14–6.
425. Hoffman PM, Brody JA. Neurological disorders in patients following surgery for peptic ulcer. Neurology 1972;22:450.
426. Thaisetthawatkul P, Collazo-Clavell ML, Sarr MG, et al. A controlled study of peripheral neuropathy after bariatric surgery. Neurology 2004;63(8):1462–70.
427. Chang CG, Adams-Huet B, Provost DA. Acute post-gastric reduction surgery (APGARS) neuropathy. Obes Surg 2004;14:182–9.
428. Chang CG, Helling TS, Black WE, et al. Weakness after gastric bypass. Obes Surg 2002;12(4):592–7.
429. Choi JY, Scarborough TK. Stroke and seizure following a recent laparoscopic Roux-en-Y gastric bypass. Obes Surg 2004;14(6):857–60.
430. Brolin RE. Gastric bypass. Surg Clin North Am 2001;81(5):1077–95.
431. Mason ME, Jalagani H, Vinik AI. Metabolic complications of bariatric surgery: diagnosis and management issues. Gastroenterol Clin North Am 2005;34(1): 25–33.
432. Brolin RE, Gorman RC, Milgrim LM, et al. Multivitamin prophylaxis in prevention of post-gastric bypass vitamin and mineral deficiencies. Int J Obes 1991;15(10): 661–7.

433. D'Amour ML, Butterworth RF. Pathogenesis of alcoholic peripheral neuropathy: direct effect of ethanol or nutritional deficit? Metab Brain Dis 1994;9(2):133–42.
434. Behse F, Buchthal F. Alcoholic neuropathy: clinical, electrophysiological, and biopsy findings. Ann Neurol 1977;2:95–110.
435. Monforte R, Estruch R, Valls-Sole J, et al. Autonomic and peripheral neuropathies in patients with chronic alcoholism. A dose-related toxic effect of alcohol. Arch Neurol 1995;52(1):45–51.
436. Koike H, Mori K, Misu K, et al. Painful alcoholic polyneuropathy with predominant small-fiber loss and normal thiamine status. Neurology 2001;56(12):1727–32.
437. Koike H, Iijima M, Sugiura M, et al. Alcoholic neuropathy is clinicopathologically distinct from thiamine-deficiency neuropathy. Ann Neurol 2003;54(1):19–29.
438. Victor M, Adams RD. On the etiology of alcoholic neurologic disease with special reference to the role of nutrition. Am J Clin Nutr 1961;9:379–97.
439. Tabaraud F, Vallat JM, Hugon J, et al. Acute or subacute alcoholic neuropathy mimicking Guillain-Barre syndrome. J Neurol Sci 1990;97(2–3):195–205.
440. Johnson RH, Robinson BJ. Mortality in alcoholics with autonomic neuropathy. J Neurol Neurosurg Psychiatr 1988;51(4):476–80.
441. Yokota O, Tsuchiya K, Terada S, et al. Alcoholic cerebellar degeneration: a clinicopathological study of six Japanese autopsy cases and proposed potential progression pattern in the cerebellar lesion. Neuropathology 2007;27(2):99–113.
442. Maschke M, Weber J, Bonnet U, et al. Vermal atrophy of alcoholics correlate with serum thiamine levels but not with dentate iron concentrations as estimated by MRI. J Neurol 2005;252(6):704–11.
443. Gilman S, Adams K, Koeppe RA, et al. Cerebellar and frontal hypometabolism in alcoholic cerebellar degeneration studied with positron emission tomography. Ann Neurol 1990;28(6):775–85.
444. Victor M. Tobacco-alcohol amblyopia. A critique of current concepts of this disorder, with special reference to the role of nutritional deficiency in its causation. Arch Ophthalmol 1963;70:313–8.
445. Samples JR, Younge BR. Tobacco-alcohol amblyopia. J Clin Neuroophthalmol 1981;1(3):213–8.
446. Krumsiek J, Kruger C, Patzold U. Tobacco-alcohol amblyopia neuro-ophthalmological findings and clinical course. Acta Neurol Scand 1985;72(2):180–7.
447. Behbehani R, Sergott RC, Savino PJ. Tobacco-alcohol amblyopia: a maculopathy? Br J Ophthalmol 2005;89(11):1543–4.
448. Heinrich A, Runge U, Khaw AV. Clinicoradiologic subtypes of Marchiafava-Bignami disease. J Neurol 2004;251(9):1050–9.
449. Raina S, Mahesh DM, Mahajan J, et al. Marchiafava-Bignami disease. J Assoc Physicians India 2008;56:633–5.
450. Helenius J, Tatlisumak T, Soinne L, et al. Marchiafava-Bignami disease: two cases with favourable outcome. Eur J Neurol 2001;8(3):269–72.
451. Menegon P, Sibon I, Pachai C, et al. Marchiafava-Bignami disease: diffusion-weighted MRI in corpus callosum and cortical lesions. Neurology 2005;65(3):475–7.
452. Roman GC. An epidemic in Cuba of optic neuropathy, sensorineural deafness, peripheral sensory neuropathy and dorsolateral myeloneuropathy. J Neurol Sci 1994;127(1):11–28.
453. Epidemic optic neuropathy in Cuba – clinical characterization and risk factors. TheCuba Neuropathy Field Investigation Team. N Engl J Med 1995;333:1176–82.

454. Roman GC, Spencer PS, Schoenberg BS. Tropical myeloneuropathies: the hidden endemias. Neurology 1985;35(8):1158–70.
455. Osuntokun BO. An ataxic neuropathy in Nigeria. A clinical, biochemical and electrophysiological study. Brain 1968;91(2):215–48.
456. Roman GC, Osame M. Identity of HTLV-I-associated tropical spastic paraparesis and HTLV-I-associated myelopathy. Lancet 1988;1(8586):651.
457. Jacobson S, Lehky T, Nishimura M, et al. Isolation of HTLV-II from a patient with chronic, progressive neurological disease clinically indistinguishable from HTLV-I-associated myelopathy/tropical spastic paraparesis. Ann Neurol 1993; 33(4):392–6.
458. Harrington WJ Jr, Sheremata W, Hjelle B, et al. Spastic ataxia associated with human T-cell lymphotropic virus type II infection. Ann Neurol 1993;33(4): 411–4.
459. Misra UK, Nag D, Husain M, et al. Endemic fluorosis presenting as cervical cord compression. Arch Environ Health 1988;43(1):18–21.
460. Morgan JP, Penovich P. Jamaica ginger paralysis. Forty-seven-year follow-up. Arch Neurol 1978;35(8):530–2.
461. Senanayake N, Jeyaratnam J. Toxic polyneuropathy due to gingili oil contaminated with tri-cresyl phosphate affecting adolescent girls in Sri Lanka. Lancet 1981;1(8211):88–9.
462. Senanayake N. Tri-cresyl phosphate neuropathy in Sri Lanka: a clinical and neurophysiological study with a three year follow up. J Neurol Neurosurg Psychiatr 1981;44(9):775–80.
463. Senanayake N, Karalliedde L. Neurotoxic effects of organophosphorus insecticides. An intermediate syndrome. N Engl J Med 1987;316(13):761–3.
464. Weiner ML, Jortner BS. Organophosphate-induced delayed neurotoxicity of triarylphosphates. Neurotoxicology 1999;20(4):653–73.
465. Lotti M, Becker CE, Aminoff MJ. Organophosphate polyneuropathy: pathogenesis and prevention. Neurology 1984;34(5):658–62.
466. Jaga K, Dharmani C. Sources of exposure to and public health implications of organophosphate pesticides. Rev Panam Salud Publica 2003;14(3): 171–85.
467. Spencer PS, Roy DN, Ludolph A, et al. Lathyrism: evidence for role of the neuroexcitatory aminoacid BOAA. Lancet 1986;2(8515):1066–7.
468. Ludolph AC, Hugon J, Dwivedi MP, et al. Studies on the aetiology and pathogenesis of motor neuron diseases. 1. Lathyrism: clinical findings in established cases. Brain 1987;110(Pt 1):149–65.
469. Drory VE, Rabey MJ, Cohn DF. Electrophysiologic features in patients with chronic neurolathyrism. Acta Neurol Scand 1992;85(6):401–3.
470. Striefler M, Cohn DF, Hirano A, et al. The central nervous system in a case of neurolathyrism. Neurology 1977;27(12):1176–8.
471. Getahun H, Lambein F, Vanhoorne M, et al. Food-aid cereals to reduce neurolathyrism related to grass-pea preparations during famine. Lancet 2003; 362(9398):1808–10.
472. Spencer PS, Palmer VS. Lathyrism: aqueous leaching reduces grass-pea neurotoxicity. Lancet 2003;362(9398):1775–6.
473. Howlett WP, Brubaker GR, Mlingi N, et al. Konzo, an epidemic upper motor neuron disease studied in Tanzania. Brain 1990;113(Pt 1):223–35.
474. Tylleskar T, Banea M, Bikangi N, et al. Cassava cyanogens and konzo, an upper motoneuron disease found in Africa. [erratum appears in Lancet 1992;339(8790):440]. Lancet 1992;339(8787):208–11.

475. Tylleskar T, Howlett WP, Rwiza HT, et al. Konzo: a distinct disease entity with selective upper motor neuron damage. J Neurol Neurosurg Psychiatr 1993; 56(6):638–43.
476. Osuntokun BO. Cassava diet, chronic cyanide intoxication and neuropathy in the Nigerian Africans. World Rev Nutr Diet 1981;36:141–73.
477. Konagaya M, Matsumoto A, Takase S, et al. Clinical analysis of longstanding subacute myelo-optico-neuropathy: sequelae of clioquinol at 32 years after its ban. J Neurol Sci 2004;218(1–2):85–90.
478. Baumgartner G, Gawel MJ, Kaeser HE, et al. Neurotoxicity of halogenated hydroxyquinolines: clinical analysis of cases reported outside Japan. J Neurol Neurosurg Psychiatr 1979;42(12):1073–83.
479. Shibasaki H, Kakigi R, Ohnishi A, et al. Peripheral and central nerve conduction in subacute myelo-optico-neuropathy. Neurology 1982;32(10):1186–9.
480. Konno H, Takase S, Fukui T. Neuropathology of longstanding subacute myelo-optico-neuropathy (SMON): an autopsy case of SMON with duration of 28 years. No To Shinkei 2001;53(9):875–80.
481. Shiraki H. The neuropathology of subacute myelo-optico-neuropathy, "SMON", in the humans: –with special reference to the quinoform intoxication. Jpn J Med Sci Biol 1975;28(Suppl):101–64.
482. Muller O, Krawinkel M. Malnutrition and health in developing countries. CMAJ 2005;173(3):279–86.
483. Garruto RM, Yanagihara R, Gajdusek DC. Disappearance of high-incidence amyotrophic lateral sclerosis and parkinsonism-dementia on Guam. Neurology 1985;35(2):193–8.
484. McGeer PL, Schwab C, McGeer EG, et al. Familial nature and continuing morbidity of the amyotrophic lateral sclerosis-parkinsonism dementia complex of Guam. Neurology 1997;49(2):400–9.
485. Borenstein AR, Mortimer JA, Schofield E, et al. Cycad exposure and risk of dementia, MCI, and PDC in the Chamorro population of Guam. Neurology 2007;68(21):1764–71.
486. Steele JC, McGeer PL. The ALS/PDC syndrome of Guam and the cycad hypothesis. Neurology 2008;70(21):1984–90.

Neurologic Presentations of Systemic Vasculitides

Alireza Minagar, MD, FAAN[a],*, Marjorie Fowler, MD[b],
Meghan K. Harris, MD[a], Stephen L. Jaffe, MD[a]

KEYWORDS

• Vasculitis • Arteritis • Cryoglobulinemia • Purpura

Vasculitis or angiitis refers to a group of inflammatory disorders of the blood vessels that cause structural damage to the affected vessel, including thickening and weakening of the vessel wall, narrowing of its lumen, and, usually, vascular necrosis.[1] Proposed pathogenetic mechanisms for development of vasculitis include immune complex formation and deposition in the vessel wall; invasion of endothelial cells and perivascular spaces and alteration of endothelial cell functions by infectious microorganisms, underlying neoplastic or autoimmune process (such as systemic lupus erythematosus), or toxins; granuloma formation; presence of autoantibodies, such as antiendothelial cell antibodies or antineutrophil cytoplasmic antibodies (ANCA); and orchestrated action of cellular and molecular immune responses involving proinflammatory cytokines and adhesion molecules.[2–4]

The overall annual incidence of the systemic vasculitides (excluding giant cell arteritis) is approximately at 39 per 1,000,000.[5] Systemic vasculitis is classified according to vessel size and histopathologic and clinical features. Vasculitides with small vessel involvement typically include Henoch-Schönlein purpura and cryoglobulinemia. Polyarteritis nodosa and Wegener granulomatosis are small- and medium-sized vessel vasculitides, whereas temporal arteritis (TA) and Takayasu arteritis involve large vessels. Because of the complex and heterogeneous nature of vasculitic syndromes and diffuse organ distribution, diagnosis and treatment of these disorders pose a formidable challenge to clinicians. The authors of this article review the neurologic presentations of the major systemic vasculitides.

[a] Department of Neurology, Louisiana State University Health Sciences Center, 1501 Kings Highway, Shreveport, LA 71130, USA
[b] Department of Pathology, Louisiana State University Health Sciences Center, 1501 Kings Highway, Shreveport, LA 71130, USA
* Corresponding author.
E-mail address: aminag@lsuhsc.ed (A. Minagar).

Neurol Clin 28 (2010) 171–184
doi:10.1016/j.ncl.2009.09.015
0733-8619/09/$ – see front matter © 2010 Published by Elsevier Inc.

neurologic.theclinics.com

TEMPORAL ARTERITIS

TA, also known as giant cell arteritis (GCA), is a systemic disease that almost exclusively affects individuals older than 50 years, with a mean age of onset of 70 years and a range of 50 to more than 90 years of age. Its estimated occurrence is 15 to 25 per 100,000 individuals.[6,7] TA may cause permanent blindness in one or both eyes in 25% to 50% of affected individuals; therefore, timely diagnosis and aggressive treatment is of obvious significance. Women are affected more frequently,[8] and it is more common in Caucasians than African Americans. Postmortem studies have demonstrated that TA is more frequent than is clinically apparent.[9] TA primarily, but not exclusively, affects the cranial branches of the arteries that originate from the arch of the aorta. Transmural inflammation of the affected arteries and intimal hyperplasia cause luminal occlusion. The initial presentation of TA may be insidious or sudden. Certain presentations, such as visual loss and neurologic impairments, are usually acute, whereas systemic manifestations, such as fatigue, anorexia, weight loss, arthralgia, myalgia, low-grade fever, anemia, and leukocytosis, may be present weeks or months before the time of clinical diagnosis. Alterations of mental status characterized by delusional thinking, confusion, insomnia, lack of attention, and cognitive decline may occur with TA. Many patients complain of headache with a lancinating quality, commonly localized to the areas along the affected arteries of the scalp. The headache associated with TA is persistent and usually unilateral. Indeed, development of a new headache or prominent alteration of the pattern of a chronic headache in an elderly patient is the most frequent symptom of TA and should alert the physician to the possibility of this diagnosis. Diffuse tenderness of the scalp or face which stems from the inflammatory ischemic changes associated with widespread arteritis of the extracranial arteries, presents along with the headache, and is usually present over the temporal or occipital arteries. Jaw pain and claudication and oral mucosa or scalp ulceration can also be presentations of TA.

Other neurologic presentations of TA, which occur in at least 30% of affected individuals, consist of peripheral neuropathy, transient ischemic attack, and stroke.[10] Peripheral neuropathy in patients with TA can occur as a mono- or polyneuropathy and may affect upper or lower extremities. Although the median nerve is the most commonly affected peripheral nerve, other nerves, such as ulnar, radial, tibial, sciatic, spinal, and trigeminal nerve, may also be involved in the pathologic process. On electromyographic and nerve conduction studies, one observes abnormalities of action potential amplitudes and conduction velocities of the affected nerves, indicative of axonal damage and demyelination. Angiographic and neuropathologic examinations reveal that diffuse arteritis of the vessels supplying the damaged nerves plays a significant role in pathogenesis of the peripheral neuropathy in TA.

Cranial neuropathies are also significant presentations of TA. The optic nerve is the most frequently affected cranial nerve; and based on clinical observations over the past 3 decades, up to 23% of affected patients develop permanent visual loss because of anterior ischemic optic neuropathy (AION).[11,12] Indeed, visual loss is the most significant symptom of TA and may be temporary or permanent, monocular or binocular. Transient visual loss experienced with TA is similar to that in patients with atherosclerotic cerebrovascular disease, except in rare instances of TA, where it may alternate between the two eyes. In patients with TA, the most common site of optic nerve involvement is the anterior optic nerve, resulting from posterior ciliary arteritis. Less frequently, ophthalmoscopic examination may reveal retrobulbar optic neuropathy without papillitis. Patients with acute AION develop an altitudinal visual field defect. Other ocular complications of TA include uni- or bilateral central retinal artery occlusion. Although most of these patients develop sudden and permanent visual loss, some may experience transient visual loss in 1 eye before the visual loss becomes permanent. Compromise of the blood circulation through the ophthalmic or central retinal arteries due to inflammation or thrombosis in TA seems to cause the retinal ischemia. Vasculitis of the vessels supplying the optic chiasm is associated with bitemporal visual field defects, whereas vasculitis of the vascular system of the retrochiasmal visual sensory pathway can cause homonymous visual field defects. Some patients with bilateral blindness due to TA may experience visual hallucinations originating from loss of visual input to the cerebral cortex.

Patients with TA may develop diplopia caused by vasculitis affecting the ocular motor system. The oculomotor nerve is commonly affected, and the presence of a combination of ophthalmoparesis and ptosis raises the possibility of oculomotor nerve ischemic infarction. In such cases, paralysis usually does not affect the pupil. Other ocular abnormalities that may be observed in patients with TA include uni- or bilateral internuclear ophthalmoplegia and pupillary disturbances, such as tonic pupils and light-near pupillary dissociation.

Other neurologic presentations of TA, although fairly uncommon, include vertigo and hearing loss, tinnitus, transient hemianesthesia of the tongue, lingual paralysis, and facial pain. Between 10% and 20% of patients with TA have carotid bruits that are commonly bilateral and indicate carotid artery involvement. Almost 40% of these patients develop some form of ischemic ocular or cerebral syndrome.

Histopathologically, TA shows transmural inflammation of the media, intima, and adventitia. Lymphocytes, macrophages, and multinucleated giant cells are present in the arterial wall in a patchy distribution. Arterial narrowing is thought to be caused by mural hyperplasia resulting in occlusive ischemia (**Fig. 1** A and B).[13,14] Similar inflammatory changes are observed in the related disease, polymyalgia rheumatica (PR). Symptoms of PR are more widespread and systemic than TA and include pain, fever, malaise, stiff muscles, and weight loss. There is a significant relationship between the 2 diseases, and it has been proposed that they may be different symptomatic manifestations of the same underlying disease process.[15] Almost 50% of patients with TA present with PR and 10% of patients with PR develop TA.[16]

A diagnosis of TA should be considered in any patient older than 50 years who presents with new-onset headache, jaw claudication, ear pain, scalp tenderness, unexplained fever, anemia, double vision, and visual loss. Patients with TA usually have normochromic normocytic anemia, markedly high erythrocyte sedimentation rate (ESR>40 mm/h), and elevated C-reactive protein. On 4-vessel cerebral angiography, vasculitic changes appear as alternating stenotic segments or complete occlusion of the affected vessels. Biopsy of the temporal artery is performed to confirm the diagnosis before aggressive treatment. However, the pitfall of this procedure, due to the patchy nature of the underlying inflammation, is that biopsy achieves a sensitivity of up to 70%, and thus, a considerable number of patients with TA may have a negative biopsy result. Based on the 1990 American College of Rheumatology[17] criteria for classification of TA, at least three of the following 5 items must be present (sensitivity 93.5%, specificity 91.2%):

1. Age of onset greater than 50 years
2. New-onset headache or localized head pain
3. Temporal artery tenderness to palpation or reduced pulsation
4. ESR greater than 50 mm/h
5. Abnormal arterial biopsy (necrotizing vasculitis with granulomatous proliferation and infiltration)

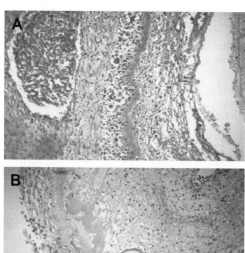
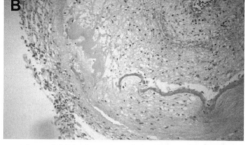

Fig. 1. Neuropathology of TA. (*A*) Early lesion of a large muscular artery. Necrosis, inflammation and giant cell formation can be noted immediately adjacent to the internal elastic lamina, which is undergoing degenerative changes. There is some intimal proliferation (hematoxylin and eosin [H&E], original magnification ×100). (*B*) In this more advanced lesion, there is complete segmental destruction of the internal elastic lamina and virtually the entire media. Marked intimal proliferation has nearly occluded the lumen. Few inflammatory cells remain (H&E, original magnification ×50). (*Courtesy of* William E. Ballinger, MD, Gainesville, FL; *From* Nadeau SE. Neurologic manifestations of systemic vasculitis. Neurol Clin 2002 Feb;20(1):123–50; with permission.)

Once a clinician suspects a diagnosis of TA in an elderly patient on clinical grounds, treatment should be initiated to save the patient's vision. The mainstay of treatment is systemic corticosteroids. Treatment begins immediately with prednisone at a dosage of 40 mg/day to 80 mg/day. This high dose treatment plan is maintained for up to a month and then prednisone dosage should be tapered by 50% during one month and then after slowly reduced by no more than 1 mg/month. The oral prednisone should be tapered slowly to prevent relapses, with the tapering periods as long as 2 years. To lessen corticosteroid-associated osteoporosis, concurrent treatment with alendronate should be initiated.

TAKAYASU ARTERITIS

Takayasu arteritis, also called pulseless disease, is a systemic necrotizing vasculitis that may result in postinflammatory stenosis or occlusion of the entire aorta, the abdominal aorta, the ascending aorta, or just the aortic arch and its proximal branches. The innominate, common carotid, and subclavian arteries and the celiac, mesenteric, renal, pulmonary, iliac, and coronary arteries are frequently affected. Currently, the exact cause and cure for Takayasu disease are unknown. Takayasu disease occurs worldwide, most of the patients are women, and the age of onset is between 10 and 30 years. It seems that hypoperfusion of the affected organ due to the underlying arterial occlusive process causes the clinical manifestations of Takayasu disease. For example, systemic hypertension occurs because of narrowing of the aorta, renal artery stenosis, decreased elasticity of the aortic wall, or a combination of these effects.

Systemic presentations of Takayasu disease are divided into 3 clinical stages: (1) the acute stage, characterized by nonspecific systemic manifestations, such as low-grade fever, fatigue, malaise, anorexia, nocturnal sweating, and widespread aching; (2) the stage of acute inflammation of the affected vessels, characterized by the presence of vascular bruits, diminished or absent pulses, and tenderness; and (3) the chronic obliterative phase due to vascular occlusion, identified by decreased pulses, development of vascular bruits, claudication, and even development of ischemic ulcers in affected extremities. Frequently, neurologic involvement occurs and sometimes, this may be the initial presentation of the disease process. Occlusion of the vertebral or carotid arteries may cause ischemic stroke; and patients may present with headache, syncope, and blurred vision. Patients with Takayasu disease may also develop intracranial aneurysms, with symptoms originating from either ruptured or unruptured aneurysms. Pathologically, Takayasu disease manifests with granulomatous inflammation of the vessel adventitia and the outer part of the media, with infiltration of lymphocytes, plasma cells, histiocytes, and multinucleated giant cells. Diagnosis of Takayasu disease rests on clinical suspicion in any young patient, particularly women, with clinical manifestations of vascular ischemia and the presence of bruits, decrease or absence of pulses, ischemic ulcers, or a combination of these findings. The American College of Rheumatology 1990 criteria for the classification of Takayasu arteritis is presented in **Box 1**.[18] Aortic angiography confirms the diagnosis and one may observe occlusion or dilatation of vascular segments, stenotic segments, aneurysm formation, and increased collateral circulation. Treatment of

---

Box 1
1990 criteria for the classification of Takayasu arteritis[a]

1. Age at disease onset less than 40 years

   Development of symptoms or findings related to Takayasu arteritis at 40 years or younger

2. Claudication of extremities

   Development and worsening of fatigue and discomfort in muscles of one or more extremities while in use, especially the upper extremities

3. Decreased brachial artery pulse

   Decreased pulsation of one or both brachial arteries

4. Blood pressure (BP) difference greater than 10 mm Hg

   Difference of more than 10 mm Hg in systolic blood pressure between arms

5. Bruit over subclavian arteries or aorta

   Bruit audible on auscultation over one or both subclavian arteries or abdominal aorta

6. Arteriogram abnormality

   Arteriographic narrowing or occlusion of the entire aorta, its primary branches, or large arteries in the proximal upper or lower extremities, not due to arteriosclerosis, fibromuscular dysplasia, or similar causes; with changes usually focal or segmental.

[a] For purposes of classification, a patient shall be said to have Takayasu arteritis if at least 3 of these 6 criteria are present. The presence of any 3 or more criteria yields a sensitivity of 90.5% and a specificity of 97.8%. BP = blood pressure (systolic; difference between arms). (*Data from* Arend WP, Michel BA, Bloch DA, et al. The American College of Rheumatology 1990 criteria for the classification of Takayasu arteritis. Arthritis Rheum 1990;33(8):1129–34.)

Takayasu disease with systemic corticosteroids, prednisone 1 mg/kg/d for 3 months, is followed by a gradual tapering regimen based on suppression of the systemic manifestations. Takayasu disease does have a prolonged, relapsing, and remitting course; in cases of unsuccessful treatment with corticosteroids, treatment with cytotoxic agents, such as cyclophosphamide or methotrexate, should be considered. Certain patients may benefit from surgical procedures, such as bypass of the obstructed arteries or percutaneous transluminal angioplasty.

WEGENER GRANULOMATOSIS

Wegener granulomatosis (WG) is a vasculitic disorder of small- and medium-sized vessels that produces necrotizing granulomatous lesions of the upper and/or lower respiratory tract and kidney (necrotizing glomerulonephritis), and disseminated vasculitis. WG develops in association with antineutrophil cytoplasmic antibodies (ANCA) and is a member of the family of ANCA-associated vasculitides (AAV).[1] It is more common in men, and the age range varies from 8 to 80 years, with a mean age of 40 years. In many patients, WG initially presents with granulomatous lesions of the upper respiratory tract. Systemic manifestations of WG consist of chronic sinusitis, chronic rhinitis, nasal ulceration, epistaxis, upper respiratory serosanguineous discharge, serous otitis media, cough and hemoptysis, and dyspnea. Other presentations include fever, weight loss, anorexia, and arthralgia. Clinically, ocular involvement presents with orbital pseudotumor, scleritis, and uveitis, and renal involvement manifests with proteinuria, hematuria, and renal failure.

At any stage of the disease process, up to 50% of patients develop neurologic complications affecting both peripheral and central nervous systems. Almost half of those with neurologic complications suffer from recurrent mononeuropathies, mononeuritis multiplex, or symmetric polyneuropathy. Patients with CNS involvement present with cranial neuropathies, most frequently cranial nerves II, VI, and VII and nonspecific evidence of cerebral vasculitis, such as hemiparesis, seizures, aphasia, and visual field defects. Ischemic strokes, encephalopathy, granulomatous basilar meningitis, pachymeningitis, and myelitis are other CNS manifestations of WG that occur less frequently.

Although the exact cause of WG remains unknown, existing evidence indicates involvement of hypersensitivity mechanisms. Diagnosis of WG can be based on the combination of the clinical picture along with the presence of classical antineutrophil cytoplasmic antibodies (C-ANCA) in the serum and the demonstration of necrotizing vasculitis on histopathologic examination. On neuroimaging, the spectrum of brain computed tomographic (CT) and magnetic resonance (MR) abnormalities in WG include dural thickening and enhancement, and abnormal signals within the brainstem and white matter (Fig. 2 A, B, and C).[19] Before the 1960s, WG was a lethal disorder and most patients succumbed to the progressive renal insufficiency. Administration of systemic corticosteroids may be associated with clinical improvement in only some of the treated patients but does reduce the overall mortality rate. Various immunosuppressive agents, such as cyclophosphamide, azathioprine, methotrexate, chlorambucil, and nitrogen mustard, have been used for treatment of corticosteroid failures. Of these, cyclophosphamide has improved the prognosis for these patients significantly. In many instances, patients are treated with a combination of prednisone and cyclophosphamide. However, one should recognize that although this combination improves 5-year prognosis of the treated patients remarkably, the cumulative toxicity and side effects of these medications over several years are fairly high, and even under this therapeutic regimen, between 10% and 50% of patients relapse.[20] The regimen of

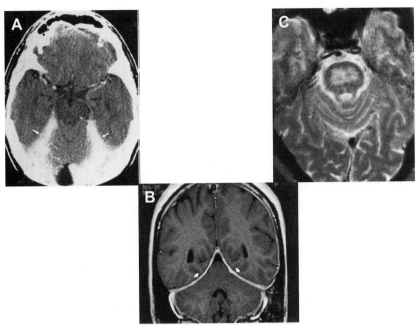

Fig. 2. Neuroimaging findings of Wegener's granulomatosis- (*A*) Contrast-enhanced axial CT scan of brain at the level of the tentorium of a 35-year-old male patient with new-onset headache, which demonstrates dural thickening with contrast enhancement (*arrows*). (*B*) Contrast-enhanced coronal T1-weighted MR image (500/11/1) of a 41-year-old man with severe daily headaches, which reveals dural enhancement (*arrows*). (*C*) T2-weighted axial MR image (2500/80/2) of a 56-year-old man with multiple cranial neuropathies, which shows hyperintense signal throughout much of the pons. (*From* Provenzale JM, Allen NB. Wegener granulomatosis: CT and MR findings. AJNR Am J Neuroradiol 1996;17:785–92; with permission.)

prednisone and cyclophosphamide should be continued until systemic presentations improve, and then it should be slowly tapered. The therapeutic response can be measured by serial clinical assessment and a declining pattern of the ESR, serum C-reactive protein, and C-ANCA.

CRYOGLOBULINEMIA

Cryoglobulins are serum proteins that precipitate at 4°C and re-dissolve after warming to 37°C, and they occur in patients with various clinical conditions. These serum proteins are mainly immunoglobulins and are usually composed of either IgG or IgM. Alternatively, they can be mixed, being composed of 2 different immunoglobulins, most commonly a combination of IgG and IgM. Cryoglobulins, which have a single monoclonal immunoglobulin, are most commonly associated with lymphoproliferative disorders, such as multiple myeloma, lymphomas and leukemias. Mixed cryoglobulins are frequently detected in patients with connective tissue diseases, systemic vasculitic syndromes, and infections such as hepatitis C viral infection; and this condition is called essential mixed cryoglobulinemia (EMC).

Clinically, EMC, which affects mainly middle-aged women, presents with purpura, arthralgia, weakness, and mixed cryoglobulinemia. Patients with EMC develop cutaneous vasculitis and progressive renal insufficiency because of glomerulonephritis. Similar to many other hypersensitivity vasculitides, EMC seems to occur due to deposition of immune complexes in small vessels. In any patient with the combination of hypocomplementemia, cutaneous vasculitis, and elevated liver function tests, a diagnosis of mixed cryoglobulinemia must be considered. A vasculitic motor and sensory peripheral neuropathy commonly occurs in patients with EMC at some point during their disease course. Sensory-motor mononeuritis multiplex is another form of neuropathy that may be present in these patients. CNS complications of mixed cryoglobulinemia are rare and include diffuse encephalopathic syndromes with focal signs, seizures, myelopathy, and sometimes, ischemic stroke.[21–24] The pathogenetic mechanisms of neuropathy include immune-mediated demyelination and nerve ischemia due to occlusion of the vasa nervorum by cryoglobulins or vasculitis.

HENOCH-SCHÖNLEIN PURPURA

Henoch-Schönlein purpura (HSP) is one of the most common forms of systemic vasculitis seen in children, and it is recognized by a combination of nonthrombocytopenic purpura, arthralgia, and abdominal pain. Certain conditions, such as malignancies and infections, and certain drugs are associated with HSP. Systemic complaints include fever, malaise, and edema; nephritis occurs in 40% of affected patients. Although the underlying vasculitis is leukocytoclastic, the exact cause of HSP remains unknown. Neurologic manifestations of HSP consist of headache, encephalopathy, intracranial and intraparenchymal hemorrhage, nonhemorrhagic vasculitic involvement of cerebral tissue, peripheral neuropathy, and entrapment neuropathy due to focal edema. The presence of elevated serum IgA or IgA deposits in the vascular wall indicate that HSP is due to IgA-mediated inflammation. In 1990, the classification criteria for HSP were proposed by the American College of Rheumatology (**Table 1**).[25] The clinical diagnosis is further supported by detection of leukocytoclastic vasculitis on skin biopsy and IgA immunofluorescence in small vessels of skin and renal glomeruli. Differential diagnosis of HSP includes infectious endocarditis, systemic lupus erythematosus, meningococcemia, disseminated intravascular coagulation, and Waldenström hyperglobulinemic purpura. Although there is no specific treatment for HSP, these patients benefit from supportive therapy and brief courses of corticosteroids.

Table 1	
1990 criteria for classification of Henoch-Schönlein purpura	
Criterion	**Definition**
Probable purpura	Slightly raised "palpable" hemorrhagic skin lesions, not related to thrombocytopenia
Age ≤20 years	Patient 20 years or younger at onset of first symptoms
Bowel angina	Diffuse abdominal pain, worse after meals, or the diagnosis of bowel ischemia, usually including bloody diarrhea
Wall granulocyte on biopsy	Histologic changes showing granulocytes in the walls of arterioles or venules

For purposes of classification, a patient shall be said to have Henoch-Schönlein purpura if at least 2 of these 4 criteria are present. The presence of any 2 or more criteria yields a sensitivity of 87.1% and a specificity of 87.7%. (*Data from* Mills JA, Michel BA, Bloch DA, et al. The American College of Rheumatology 1990 criteria for the classification of Henoch-Schönlein purpura. Arthritis Rheum 1990;33(8):1114–21.)

NERVOUS SYSTEM VASCULITIS ASSOCIATED WITH DRUG ABUSE

Drugs, particularly sympathomimetics, have been associated with several neurologic disorders, including cerebral ischemic infarcts and intracerebral and subarachnoid hemorrhage. The most commonly abused drugs that are associated with these neurologic complications include cocaine, heroin, ephedrine, phenylpropanolamine, and amphetamines. These illicit drugs may be taken orally or intravenously or may be snorted. Ischemic or hemorrhagic complications usually affect younger individuals. A brain MR imaging case-controlled study of individuals who were cocaine dependent demonstrated the presence of multiple, small, silent, subcortical ischemic lesions.[26] Cerebral angiography in many cases of illicit drug use has demonstrated vasculitic changes of CNS vessels, including widespread segmental narrowing of the affected vessels with a beading pattern. Some of these illicit drugs are capable of causing vasospasm, and thus, the mechanism behind vascular insufficiency within the CNS may be a vasculopathy rather that true vasculitis. A compounding issue in making a clear-cut diagnosis of illicit drug-induced CNS vasculitis is that there are usually multiple exposures to multiple illicit substances and coexisting infections present, such as syphilis, hepatitis C, and AIDS. Treatment of these patients rests on identification and discontinuation of the offending drug, search for other concurrent infections, particularly human immunodeficiency virus (HIV), control of hypertension when present, and supportive treatment. Administration of systemic corticosteroids or immunosuppressive therapy is not recommended unless diagnosis of CNS vasculitis is supported by histopathologic examination.

MEDICATION-INDUCED VASCULITIS

Vasculitic syndromes may occur in association with use of prescribed drugs and the most common drug-associated vasculitis is usually restricted to the skin. This form of skin vasculitis presents with a maculopapular or vesicular rash, and, less frequently, as palpable purpura. Rarely, vasculitis is widespread and presents with fever; arthralgia; evidence of cardiac, hepatic, or renal dysfunction; and eosinophilia. The pathophysiology of this form of vasculitis is hypothesized to involve the attachment of the drug to proteins, generating haptens that are able to elicit potent immune responses. Neurologically, the central and peripheral nervous system and muscles may be involved. The list of offending drugs that may cause vasculitis contains several general types, antibiotics being a major type. The penicillins are probably the best known members of this group. Treatment of drug-related vasculitis begins with immediate discontinuation of the offending drug followed by use of corticosteroids (prednisone 1 mg/kg/d for up to 30 days).

POLYARTERITIS NODOSA

Polyarteritis nodosa (PAN), also called periarteritis nodosa, is a rare inflammatory necrotizing vasculitis that affects small- to medium-sized arteries. Although it is often idiopathic, it can be associated with other disorders, such as cryoglobulinemia, leukemia, arthritis, Sjogren syndrome, hepatitis C, hepatitis B, and HIV infection.[27] PAN is a systemic disease and may affect any organ; however, the skin, kidney, peripheral nerves, and gastrointestinal tract are most commonly involved. The annual incidence of PAN is about 0.2 to 0.7 per 100,000 and it affects men more than women.[28] PAN is more common in individuals 40 to 60 years of age. PAN affects the central and peripheral nervous systems. The classification scheme proposed by the American College of Rheumatology for PAN is presented in **Table 2**.[29]

Table 2
American College of Rheumatology 1990 criteria for the classification of Polyarteritis Nodosa

	Criterion	Definition
(1)	Weight loss >4 kg	Loss of 4 kg or more body weight since illness began, not due to dieting or other factor
(2)	Livedo reticularis	Mottled reticular pattern over the skin of portions of the extremities or torso
(3)	Testicular pain or tenderness	Pain or tenderness of the testicles, not due to the infection, trauma, or other causes
(4)	Myalgias, weakness, or polyneuropathy	Diffuse myalgias (excluding shoulder and hip girdle) or weakness of muscles or tenderness of leg muscles
(5)	Mononeuropathy or polyneuropathy	Development of mononeuropathy, multiple mononeuropathies, or polyneuropathy
(6)	Diastolic BP>90 mm Hg	Development of hypertension with diastolic BP >90 mm Hg
(7)	Elevated blood urea nitrogen or creatinine	Elevation of blood urea nitrogen >40 mg/dL (14.3 μmol/L) or creatinine >1.5/dL (132 μmol/L), not due to dehydration or obstruction
(8)	Hepatitis B virus	Presence of hepatitis B surface antigen or antibody in serum
(9)	Arteriographic abnormality	Arteriogram showing aneurysm or occlusion of the visceral arteries, not due to arteriosclerosis, fibromuscular dysplasia, or other noninflammatory causes
(10)	Biopsy of small- or medium-sized artery containing polymorphonuclear cells	Histologic changes showing the presence of granulocytes and mononuclear leukocytes in the artery wall

For classification purposes, a patient with vasculitis is diagnosed with PAN if at least 3 criteria of the above criteria are met. (*Data from* Lightfoot RW Jr, Michel BA, Bloch DA, et al. The American College of Rheumatology 1990 criteria for the classification of polyarteritis nodosa. Arthritis Rheum 1990;33(8):1088–93.)

Between 23% and 53% of patients with PAN develop CNS pathology. CNS involvement is less common than that of the peripheral nervous system and usually presents late in the course of disease. The two most frequent central neurologic pictures of PAN include diffuse encephalopathy and focal or multifocal disturbances of the brain or spinal cord. Diffuse encephalopathy associated with PAN presents with rapid decline in level of consciousness and with seizures. Focal neurologic deficits, which may occur suddenly, are due to ischemic stroke affecting the cerebral cortex, brainstem, or cerebellum. Patients with PAN may develop anterior optic neuropathy and posterior (retrobulbar) optic neuropathy; and they tend to experience acute and painless visual loss. These forms of optic neuropathy stem from vasculitis-induced ischemia in the distribution of the posterior ciliary arteries, or inflammation of the optic nerve. Cranial nerve III, IV, VI, VII, and VIII involvement rarely occurs. Rarely, patients with PAN may experience intracranial hemorrhage. Mononeuritis multiplex is common in the context of PAN and presents with asymmetric motor and sensory findings that mainly affect the lower extremities, particularly the sciatic, peroneal, or tibial nerves. Less commonly, the radial, cubital, and median nerves may be affected. The onset of mononeuritis multiplex in these patients is usually sudden, whereas the distal symmetric peripheral neuropathy in these patients develops slowly. Examination of the cerebrospinal fluid may not reveal any diagnostic abnormalities.

Histopathologically, PAN manifests with focal but pan-mural necrotizing inflammatory lesions that affect small- and medium-sized arteries (**Fig. 3**). Further examination of these inflammatory lesions reveals disruption of the normal infrastructure of the vessel wall, fibrinoid necrosis, and pleomorphic cellular infiltration with mainly polymorphonuclear cells and a variable number of lymphocytes and eosinophils.

Diagnosis of PAN is made based on clinical suspicion when a patient presents with constitutional symptoms, such as fever, chills, weight loss, fatigue, and multisystem dysfunction. Anemia, elevated ESR, and evidence of thrombosis further support the diagnosis of PAN. Brain CT and MR neuroimaging illustrates infarctions in the cortical and subcortical regions of the cerebral hemispheres, basal ganglia, internal capsule, brainstem, and cerebellum (**Fig. 4** A and B).[30] Arteriography may reveal the presence of arterial saccular or fusiform aneurysms and narrowing and tapering of the affected vessels. Histopathologic examination of affected tissue, such as skin, sural nerve, muscle, or kidney, confirms the clinical diagnosis.

Treatment of PAN consists of the administration of systemic corticosteroids along with cytotoxic agents, such as cyclophosphamide or azathioprine. If a patient does not tolerate this regimen's side effects, other therapeutic interventions that need to be considered include plasma exchange, intravenous immune globulin, mycophenolate mofetil, and rituximab.

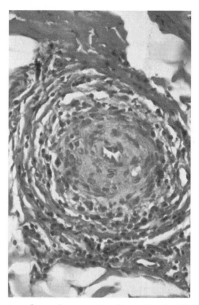

Fig. 3. A small muscular artery from the muscle of a patient with PAN, which illustrates the proliferative phase in which neutrophils have been replaced by chronic inflammatory cells and there is evidence of necrosis of the media, early intimal proliferation, and fibrosis (H&E, original magnification ×250). (*Courtesy of* William E. Ballinger, MD, Gainesville, FL; *From* Nadeau SE. Neurologic manifestations of systemic vasculitis. Neurol Clin 2002 Feb;20(1):123–50; with permission.)

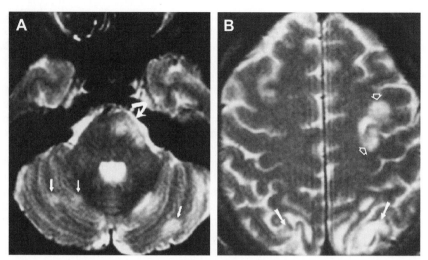

Fig. 4. Case 4: 40-year-old man with multiple cerebral, cerebellar, and brain stem infarctions related to PAN. (*A*) Axial T2-weighted (2200/80/0.75) MR image shows multiple sites of hyperintense signal within the cerebellum (*straight arrows*) and pons (*curved arrow*). (*B*) Axial T2-weighted (2200/80/0.75) MR image reveals bilateral parietal (*solid arrows*) and left frontal (*open arrows*) areas of hyperintense signal within brain cortex. (*From* Provenzale JM, Allen NB. Neuroradiologic findings in polyarteritis nodosa. AJNR Am J Neuroradiol 1996;17(6):1119–26; with permission.)

MICROSCOPIC POLYANGIITIS

Microscopic polyangiitis (MPA) is another member of AAV that predominantly affects small vessels (capillaries, venules, and arterioles). In MPA, granulomata are not present. In MPA, ANCA is directed against myeloperoxidase.[2] MPA is associated with rapidly progressive focal segmental necrotizing glomerulonephritis. The average age of onset is 50 years and men are more often affected than women. Savage and colleagues[31] observed that MPA may have an indolent course before clinical diagnosis. Systemic symptoms, such as arthralgia and hemoptysis, may be present long before the explosive phase of the disease occurs. Peripheral neuropathy is less common in MPA than PAN, whereas pulmonary involvement occurs more frequently. Diagnostic workup for MPA reveals the presence of serum ANCA and absence of surface hepatitis B antigen or antibody. Histopathologic examination of a biopsied specimen from the kidney reveals the presence of focal segmental thrombosing and necrotizing glomerulonephritis. Treatment of MPA is based on immunosuppression with the combination of systemic corticosteroids and cyclophosphamide. Potential therapies under clinical investigation include intravenous immune globulin and rituximab.

REFERENCES

1. Jayne D. Treatment of ANCA-associated systemic small-vessel vasculitis. APMIS Suppl 2009;127:3–9.
2. Holle JU, Gross WL. ANCA-associated vasculitides: pathogenetic aspects and current evidence-based therapy. J Autoimmun 2009;32(3–4):163–71.

3. Pankhurst T, Savage CO, Little MA. Review article: leukocyte-endothelial dysregulation in systemic small vessel vasculitis. Nephrology (Carlton) 2009;14(1): 3–10.
4. Ojeda VJ. Polyarteritis nodosa affecting the spinal cord arteries. Aust N Z J Med 1983;13:287–9.
5. Watts RA, Carruthers DM, Scott DG. Epidemiology of systemic vasculitis: changing incidence or definition? Semin Arthritis Rheum 1995;25(1):28–34.
6. Hunder GG. Epidemiology of giant-cell arteritis. Cleve Clin J Med 2002;69(Suppl 2):SII79–82.
7. Baldursson O, Steinsson K, Björnsson J, et al. Giant cell arteritis in Iceland. An epidemiologic and histopathologic analysis. Arthritis Rheum 1994;37(7):1007–12.
8. Nordborg C, Nordborg E, Petursdottir V. Giant cell arteritis. Epidemiology, etiology and pathogenesis. APMIS 2000;108(11):713–24.
9. Ostberg G. Temporal arteritis in a large necropsy series. Ann Rheum Dis 1971; 30(3):224–35.
10. Weyand CM, Goronzy JJ. Medium- and large-vessel vasculitis. N Engl J Med 2003;349(2):160–9.
11. Caselli RJ, Hunder GG, Whisnant JP. Neurologic disease in biopsy-proven giant cell (temporal) arteritis. Neurology 1988;38(3):352–9.
12. Koorey DJ. Cranial arteritis. A twenty-year review of cases. Aust N Z J Med 1984; 14(2):143–7.
13. Eberhardt RT, Dhadly M. Giant cell arteritis: diagnosis, management, and cardiovascular implications. Cardiol Rev 2007;15(2):55–61.
14. Nadeau SE. Neurologic manifestations of systemic vasculitis. Neurol Clin 2002; 20(1):123–50.
15. Cantini F, Niccoli L, Storri L, et al. Are polymyalgia rheumatica and giant cell arteritis the same disease? Semin Arthritis Rheum 2004;33(5):294–301.
16. Epperly TD, Moore KE, Harrover JD. Polymyalgia rheumatica and temporal arthritis. Am Fam Physician 2000;62(4):789–96, 801.
17. Hunder GG, Bloch DA, Michel BA, et al. The American College of rheumatology 1990 criteria for the classification of giant cell arteritis. Arthritis Rheum 1990; 33(8):1122–8.
18. Arend WP, Michel BA, Bloch DA, et al. The American College of rheumatology 1990 criteria for the classification of Takayasu arteritis. Arthritis Rheum 1990; 33(8):1129–34.
19. Provenzale JM, Allen NB. Wegener granulomatosis: CT and MR findings. AJNR Am J Neuroradiol 1996;17:785–92.
20. de Groot K, Reinhold-Keller E, Tatsis E, et al. Therapy for the maintenance of remission in sixty-five patients with generalized Wegener's granulomatosis. Methotrexate versus trimethoprim/sulfamethoxazole. Arthritis Rheum 1996;39: 2052–61.
21. Abramsky O, Slavin S. Neurologic manifestations in patients with mixed cryoglobulinemia. Neurology 1974;24(3):245–9.
22. Petty GW, Duffy J, Houston J 3rd. Cerebral ischemia in patients with hepatitis C virus infection and mixed cryoglobulinemia. Mayo Clin Proc 1996;71(7): 671–8.
23. Reik L Jr, Korn JH. Cryoglobulinemia with encephalopathy: successful treatment by plasma exchange. Ann Neurol 1981;10(5):488–90.
24. Ristow SC, Griner PF, Abraham GN, et al. Reversal of systemic manifestations of cryoglobulinemia. Treatment with melphalan and prednisone. Arch Intern Med 1976;136(4):467–70.

25. Mills JA, Michel BA, Bloch DA, et al. The American College of rheumatology 1990 criteria for the classification of Henoch-Schönlein purpura. Arthritis Rheum 1990; 33(8):1114–21.
26. Bartzokis G, Beckson M, Hance DB, et al. Magnetic resonance imaging evidence of "silent" cerebrovascular toxicity in cocaine dependence. Biol Psychiatry 1999; 45(9):1203–11.
27. Lhote F, Guillevin L. Polyarteritis nodosa, microscopic polyangiitis, and Churg-Strauss syndrome: clinical aspects and treatment. Rheum Dis Clin North Am 1995;21:911–47.
28. Kurland LT, Hauser WA, Ferguson RH, et al. Epidemiologic features of diffuse connective tissue disorders in Rochester, Minn., 1951 through 1967, with special reference to systemic lupus erythematosus. Mayo Clin Proc 1969;44(9):649–63.
29. Lightfoot RW Jr, Michel BA, Bloch DA, et al. The American College of rheumatology 1990 criteria for the classification of polyarteritis nodosa. Arthritis Rheum 1990;33(8):1088–93.
30. Provenzale JM, Allen NB. Neuroradiologic findings in polyarteritis nodosa. AJNR Am J Neuroradiol 1996;17(6):1119–26.
31. Savage CO, Winearls CG, Evans DJ, et al. Microscopic polyarteritis: presentation, pathology and prognosis. Q J Med 1985;56(220):467–83.

Neurologic Presentations of Sarcoidosis

Barney J. Stern, MD[a],*, Allen Aksamit, MD[b], David Clifford, MD[c],
Thomas F. Scott, MD[d] for the Neurosarcoidosis Study Group

KEYWORDS

- Sarcoidosis • Neurology • Immunosuppression • Diagnosis

Neurologic presentations complicate the course of sarcoidosis in approximately 5% to 26% of patients.[1–3] A neurologic illness suggestive of neurosarcoidosis (NS) can develop in a patient with known systemic sarcoidosis or without previously documented sarcoidosis. In the former scenario, the physician needs to verify that the neurologic manifestations are attributable to sarcoidosis and, in the latter scenario, the cause of the neurologic illness and its potential relationship to sarcoidosis must be discovered. Therefore, the clinician must be familiar with the many manifestations of NS, the diagnostic considerations, and, ultimately, the treatment strategies.

Sarcoidosis occurs worldwide and has an incidence of approximately 1 to 40 per 100,000 population.[4] Neurologic disease is the presenting feature of sarcoidosis in approximately one-half to three-quarters of patients ultimately found to have NS.[1,5] When categorizing the neurologic manifestations of sarcoidosis, it is observed that one-third to one-half of patients can have more than one type of neurologic presentation.[1]

The diagnosis of sarcoidosis is most secure if the patient has documented multisystem disease, including a biopsy consistent with sarcoidosis from at least one site. A discussion of the extensive differential diagnosis of sarcoidosis[6,7] is beyond the scope of this article; the differential diagnosis of NS is also vast but selected disorders are highlighted in **Box 1**. It is particularly important to eliminate infection and malignancy as masqueraders of NS. However, because neural tissue is often not

[a] Department of Neurology, University of Maryland School of Medicine, 3-N-139, 110 South Paca Street, Baltimore, MD 21201, USA
[b] Department of Neurology, Mayo College of Medicine, Mayo Clinic, 200 First Street SW, Rochester, MN 55905, USA
[c] Department of Neurology, Washington University in St Louis, Box 8111, 660 South Euclid, St Louis, MO 63110, USA
[d] Department of Neurology, Drexel University College of Medicine, 420 East North Avenue, Suite 206, Pittsburgh, PA 15212, USA
* Corresponding author.
E-mail address: bstern@som.umaryland.edu (B.J. Stern).

Neurol Clin 28 (2010) 185–198
doi:10.1016/j.ncl.2009.09.012
0733-8619/09/$ – see front matter © 2010 Elsevier Inc. All rights reserved.
neurologic.theclinics.com

Box 1
Selected differential diagnosis of NS

- Multiple sclerosis
- Neuromyelitis optica
- Central nervous system (CNS) lymphoma
- Leptomeningeal metastasis
- Fungal meningitis (histoplasmosis and others)
- Tuberculous meningitis
- Tuberculoma
- Wegener granulomatosis
- Sjögren syndrome-related vasculitis
- CNS lupus
- Primary CNS angiitis
- Behçet disease
- Vogt-Koyanagi-Harada disease
- Toxoplasmosis
- Neurobrucellosis
- CNS Whipple disease
- Germ cell tumors
- Craniopharyngioma
- Isolated CNS angiitis
- Primary CNS neoplasia
- Lymphocytic hypophysitis
- Idiopathic pachymeningitis
- Rosai-Dorfman disease
- Intracranial hypotension with dural enhancement
- Neurosyphilis
- Neuroborreliosis
- Human immunodeficiency virus infection
- Cytomegalovirus ventriculitis or polyradiculopathy

---

readily available for pathologic examination, it is helpful to categorize the certainty of the diagnosis of NS. This encourages the clinician to keep an open mind as to the patient's "true" diagnosis and helps inform management strategies. The following definitions are adapted from Zajicek and colleagues[8]:

- Possible NS: The clinical syndrome and diagnostic evaluation suggest NS. Infection and malignancy are not excluded or there is no pathologic confirmation of systemic sarcoidosis.
- Probable NS: The clinical syndrome and diagnostic evaluation suggest NS. Alternate diagnoses are excluded. There is pathologic confirmation of systemic sarcoidosis.

- Definite NS: The clinical presentation is suggestive of NS, other diagnoses are excluded, and there is supportive nervous system pathology or the criteria for "probable" NS are met and the patient has had a beneficial response to immunotherapy over a 1-year observation period.

Because tissue sampling of the nervous system is rarely possible, much of what is known about the pathogenesis and treatment of NS is extrapolated from studies of systemic sarcoidosis, especially pulmonary disease. This shortage of evidence directly related to NS may be especially troubling if one acknowledges the possibility that these are not simply alternate manifestations of the same disease. Differences in response and course of NS as compared with systemic sarcoidosis leave open the concern that this necessary extrapolation may be hazardous. Even the validity of using a cerebrospinal fluid (CSF) angiotensin converting enzyme (ACE) assay to diagnose CNS disease is questioned,[9] as opposed to the acceptance of a serum ACE assay to aid in the diagnosis of systemic disease.[4] In part, the problem stems from the justified reluctance to obtain CNS tissue samples from all but a few, highly selected patients with presumptive CNS sarcoidosis. Furthermore, given the heterogeneity of the neurologic presentations and the low incidence and prevalence of NS in general, and specific manifestations in particular, it has been extremely challenging to initiate rigorous clinical trials. To attempt to rectify this situation, the Neurosarcoidosis Study Group has been formed to (1) investigate the pathophysiology of NS; (2) develop a diagnostic approach to the disease; and (3) define optimal therapeutic strategies. This article represents a consensus statement from this group.

PATHOPHYSIOLOGY

The signature pathologic finding in sarcoidosis is the noncaseating granuloma. (Iannuzzi)[4] Granulomas are made up of epithelioid cells, giant cells, central CD4+ cells, and peripheral CD8+ cells and B lymphocytes.[10] There is increased production of interleukin-2, interferon-γ, and tumor necrosis factor α (TNF-α). Ultimately fibrosis associated with production of interleukin-4, -10, and -13 can develop.

Although there can be familial aggregation of sarcoidosis, to date there is no defined genetic basis for the disease. One large study found that patients with sarcoidosis had a 5-fold increased likelihood of having parents or siblings with sarcoidosis.[11] A recent genome-wide association study identified variants in the annexin A11 gene as risk factors for sarcoidosis; annexin A11 is involved in apoptosis and cellular proliferation.[12] The current thinking is that susceptibility to sarcoidosis is polygenic and complex.[13]

CLINICAL MANIFESTATIONS
General Approach to the Diagnosis of Sarcoidosis

The most common systemic manifestations of sarcoidosis include pulmonary, lymph node, ocular, and skin lesions.[4] Therefore, these sites should be monitored to "stage" the disease and define a potential biopsy site. Virtually any organ system can be afflicted by the granulomatous process, including the heart, spleen, and kidneys. Asymptomatic muscle granulomas are fairly common in sarcoidosis patients.[14] Other clues to the diagnosis of sarcoidosis include abnormal liver function tests, elevated serum ACE assay, hypercalcemia, hypercalciuria, elevated immunoglobulin levels, and evidence of anergy.

Diagnostic tests for systemic disease include chest radiograph; chest and abdominal computed tomographic (CT) scan; pulmonary function tests with diffusing capacity; ophthalmologic examination, including a slit lamp examination; endoscopic assessment of the nose and sinuses; gallium scan; fluorodeoxyglucose positron emission tomographic scan[15]; and thigh muscle magnetic resonance imaging (MRI). Biopsy should be obtained from sites most readily accessible, such as a skin or conjunctival lesion, or from lung tissue via a transbronchial biopsy.

Diagnosis of central or peripheral nervous system sarcoidosis requires a subacute clinical neurologic syndrome compatible with NS; unfortunately no single finding is diagnostic. The imaging procedure of choice to evaluate CNS disease is brain MRI with and without gadolinium administration. The presence of meningeal, especially subpial, enhancement is suggestive of CNS sarcoidosis. A CSF evaluation is helpful in looking for an inflammatory pattern of reaction and in doing specific microbiologic tests for evaluation of CNS infection and cytology for malignancy. The CSF profile of CNS sarcoidosis is not specific: a moderate mononuclear cell pleocytosis; a normal or moderately elevated total protein; in the minority, a low glucose level; and the occasional presence of oligoclonal bands and an elevated IgG index. The CSF ACE assay has not proven to be a reliable marker for CNS sarcoidosis; it can be normal in patients with definite disease and elevated in patients with infection or malignancy.[9]

Peripheral nervous system sarcoidosis can be assessed using nerve conduction studies and electromyography. A muscle or nerve biopsy can document granulomatous inflammation in patients with an appropriate presentation. Muscle has been regarded as often involved by sarcoidosis systemically, and it is so in autopsy series. However, when there is no symptomatic myopathy, blind muscle biopsy does not seem warranted. In the Mayo Clinic experience, none of the 6 blind muscle biopsies performed in patients later proven to have NS had diagnostic tissue by this means.[16]

Tissue biopsy, either systemically or in the nervous system, is recommended for proof of diagnosis before treatment is initiated. Biopsy of proven cases is not always diagnostic on first attempt (**Table 1**). Skin biopsy with quantitative sensory nerve terminal assessment is useful when evaluating patients with painful feet and impaired pain sensitivity and temperature appreciation.[17] Skin nodules can also be useful in identifying systemic disease. However, the visible changes of sarcoidosis involvement of the skin are highly nonspecific and skin biopsy is required. Bone marrow can be diagnostic, and in patients with NS who were sampled in this way, 28% had granulomas identified as diagnostic of systemic sarcoid. Because of its relative innocuous

Table 1 NS Mayo Clinic cases confirmed by biopsy	
Targeted Biopsy	Diagnostic in Cases
Meningeal	8/12 (67%)
Brain parenchyma	6/10 (60%)
Lung	19/27 (70%)
Lymph node	22/27 (81%)
Skin	5/8 (62%)
Blind biopsy	Diagnostic in cases
Conjunctiva	10/26 (38%)
Bone marrow	2/7 (28%)
Muscle	0/6 (0%)

From Aksamit AJ, Norona F. Neurosarcoidosis without systemic sarcoid. Ann Neurol 1999;46:471.

nature and fairly high yield, the best option for blind biopsy is conjunctival biopsy.[18] Conjunctival biopsy performed on patients with CNS sarcoidosis in the Mayo Clinic series showed that 10 of 26 patients (38%) had a positive conjunctival biopsy result, diagnostic of systemic sarcoidosis. These patients either had no eye findings or nonspecific ones. Therefore, the presence of conjunctival nodules or overt uveitis is not required to give a positive biopsy result by this means. The pathologic changes seen in conjunctival biopsy or at other sites are non-necrotizing (noncaseating) granulomatous inflammation.

Cranial Neuropathies

Any cranial nerve can be compromised by sarcoidosis, in isolation or in combination with other cranial nerves or other manifestations. The inflammatory process can be intra-axial and involve the cranial nerve nucleus or proximal fibers, subarachnoid or parameningeal, or can be outside the CNS. One or more cranial nerves can be dysfunctional in a patient.

The most common cranial neuropathy is a peripheral facial nerve palsy, accounting for perhaps 50% of all of the neurologic presentations of sarcoidosis.[1] Facial nerve palsies can be unilateral or bilateral, simultaneous or sequential, or recurrent. Patients tend to recover well, although residual weakness may remain.

Altered olfaction is common and can be caused by olfactory nerve compromise or granulomatous sinus inflammation. Therefore, an ear, nose, and throat evaluation is indicated in the appropriate setting.

Perhaps the most serious cranial neuropathies involve the optic nerves and cranial nerve VIII. Optic nerve presentations include optic disc edema, retrobulbar optic neuropathy, and optic atrophy.[3,19] Cranial nerve VIII involvement can compromise hearing or vestibular function.[3,20] Sarcoidosis involvement of cranial nerves II and VIII can be fairly refractory to treatment and cause much functional impairment for the patient. Bilateral cranial nerve VII and VIII dysfunction is suggestive of CNS sarcoidosis in the proper setting.

Trigeminal neuropathies are associated with numbness and paresthesias as well as hyperpathia and dysesthesia. A painful trigeminal neuropathy may be the cause of chronic headaches; hydrocephalus and acute or chronic (sarcoidosis-associated) meningitis should also be considered in patients with headache.

Meningitis with or Without Hydrocephalus

Meningitis without hydrocephalus

Meningeal inflammation with concomitant CSF abnormalities is one of the most common manifestations of NS. NS should be considered in the evaluation of subacute or chronic meningitis, in patients presenting with subacute neurologic complaints, such as cranial neuropathies, headache, constitutional symptoms, cognitive complaints, and symptoms related to cranial neuropathies in the setting of a CSF pleocytosis. The evaluation normally includes MRI with and without contrast to assess the extent of meningeal and parenchymal involvement. CSF studies may need to be extensive to exclude alternative diagnoses (see **Box 1**). Listed in **Table 2** are the protean abnormalities of CSF encountered in NS, along with key studies addressing the differential diagnosis.

Although the chronic meningitis seen in NS is often treated with corticosteroids alone, serious associated problems, including intraparenchymal disease, vasculopathy with encephalopathy, and hydrocephalus, generally require more aggressive therapy. Also, the authors have occasionally seen malignant increased intracranial pressure (ICP), even without frank hydrocephalus; they routinely warn their patients

Table 2 CSF in NS		
Test	Expected Result	Comments
Protein	Normal or high	Sometimes very high (>100 mg/d)
Cells	Normal or moderately high	Usually lymphocytic, sometimes PMNs
Glucose	Normal or sometimes low	
ACE	Normal or elevated	Does not easily cross the blood brain barrier
IgG studies and oligoclonal bands	Normal or increased	Consider "IgG index"
Viral PCRs	Negative	Rule out herpes family primarily
Fungal and TB stains and cultures	Negative	Rule out infection
Cytology	Negative	Rule out carcinomatous meningitis

Abbreviations: PCR, polymerase chain reaction; PMN, polymorphonuclear leukocytes; TB, tuberculosis.

and caregivers to report to them increasing headaches, especially in the setting of worsening cognitive function. Meningitis due to NS should only rarely be confused with acute bacterial or acute viral meningitis, given the lack of fever, encephalopathy, meningismus, and other features more typical of NS.

Meningitis with hydrocephalus
NS can present with typical nonspecific signs of increased ICP, often with hydrocephalus found on imaging, which may be noncommunicating with ventricular system obstruction due to a mass or inflammatory adhesions or may be communicating, presumably due to arachnoid villi dysfunction in the setting of very high CSF protein levels and inflammatory changes.[21] Patients with known NS are also at risk of developing hydrocephalus, especially when mass lesions are present in the posterior fossa or when chronic meningitis is present.

Ventricular drainage is likely to be lifesaving in some cases. Patients with rapidly developing lethargy should receive urgent ventricular drainage; it is probably reasonable to emergently treat with high-dose corticosteroids, in an effort to stabilize the patient pending surgery. Less rarely encountered are patients with incomplete improvement following high-dose corticosteroid therapy who then undergo ventriculoperitoneal shunting (3 of 48 in one large series[22]).

CNS Parenchymal Disease
Inflammation can develop in any part of the brain and spinal cord. In patients with CNS parenchymal disease, the presence of associated leptomeningeal inflammation (especially pial inflammation best seen in the area of the ventral pons) should raise suspicion of sarcoidosis, although infection and malignancy can also cause meningeal enhancement. Probably the most common site for CNS disease is in the diencephalon.[23] The most common hypothalamic presentation is excessive thirst; diabetes insipidus and the syndrome of inappropriate secretion of antidiuretic hormone can occur. Any component of the endocrine axis can be compromised; the possibility of hypothalamic hypothyroidism needs to be investigated. Other vegetative symptoms, such as sleep disturbances, altered appetite, and fever, can develop.

Signs and symptoms of brain dysfunction depend on the location of lesions. Single or multiple mass lesions can develop and a mass lesion can masquerade as a glioma. Patients can demonstrate multiple (enhancing) nodules that probably represent inflammation within the Virchow Robin spaces. Diffuse white and gray matter changes can occur, suggesting a diffuse encephalopathy/vasculopathy. Nonspecific deep and superficial white matter lesions are common.[3]

Simple and complex partial seizures can occur as can generalized motor seizures. Seizure control is generally not too difficult if the underlying inflammation can be controlled.[24]

Strokes can develop from various causes, including intracranial large artery inflammation and perivascular small artery inflammation. Cardiac emboli may result from arrhythmias associated with granulomatous inflammation and a sarcoidosis-associated cardiomyopathy.[25]

Spinal cord disease can present with an extradural or intradural granulomatous mass lesion or a diffuse or fairly discrete intramedullary lesion. With time, spinal cord atrophy can develop.[26] Patients can also have cauda equine syndrome or multiple inflammatory radiculopathies.

Peripheral Neuropathy

Sarcoidosis can cause a mononeuritis, a mononeuritis multiplex, or a generalized sensory, motor, or sensorimotor polyneuropathy. The generalized polyneuropathies can be predominantly demyelinating or axonal, and there are reports of a Guillain-Barré syndrome-type presentation. A predominantly small fiber neuropathy can cause loss of pain and temperature sensibility and can be painful.[17] Occasionally, an autonomic neuropathy can develop. Documentation of a small fiber neuropathy is facilitated with skin biopsies with quantitative nerve fiber analysis and is most informative in patients without diabetes mellitus.

Myopathy

Asymptomatic muscle granulomas are found in approximately 50% of patients with sarcoidosis. They can serve as a biopsy site to confirm systemic disease. MRI can highlight muscle granulomas and potentially guide a biopsy. A polymyositis-like presentation and generalized muscle atrophy can occur. Discrete granulomatous nodules can develop.

Isolated Syndromes

Isolated CNS sarcoidosis

Although there have been dozens of individual reports of biopsy-proven NS apparently limited to the CNS, the existence of isolated CNS sarcoidosis (ICNSS) is yet to be codified with any specific criteria. Case studies of isolated peripheral nerve sarcoidosis are even more rarely reported, but many of the same concepts apply. There are now 4 large series[5,8,22,27] that characterize approximately 10% of NS patients as ICNSS, with at least a few years of follow-up. Systemic sarcoidosis rarely emerged from clinical or laboratory measures during the follow-up period in most of these patients. Kveim test results have been inconsistent in the setting of ICNSS but sometimes are positive.[8,27] CNS biopsy for ICNSS is most often obtained when lesions mimic brain tumors, an obvious ascertainment bias occurring in this setting.[8] Long-term outcomes tend to be affected by the burden and extent of intracranial disease, with patients exhibiting multifocal intraparenchymal lesions, encephalopathy, and hydrocephalus faring worse. Outcome in patients with myelopathy due to ICNSS also varies.

Outcomes are perhaps most favorable in patients with single extra-axial lesions (pseudomeningiomas), and minimal preoperative deficits.

Neuropathologic differential diagnosis

In ICNSS, we have the advantage of a tissue diagnosis ruling out, by definition, other diseases that are often in the differential diagnosis radiographically or clinically. However, a differential diagnosis that should be considered based on the presence of granulomatous inflammation found in CNS tissues includes the following:

1. Wegener granulomatosis usually demonstrates more necrotizing changes, with pathology showing significant vasculitic changes and less prominent granulomatous changes. Wegener granulomatosis occurs in the meninges, parenchyma, or as a mass or infarct. An abnormal antineutrophil cytoplasmic antibody assay and sinus lesions helps make this the likely diagnosis.
2. Idiopathic intracranial pachymeningitis usually reveals prominent fibrous tissue with minimal granulomatous features.
3. Tolosa-Hunt syndrome is characterized by granulomatous inflammation limited to the cavernous sinus and nearby adjacent tissues. Within the context of painful ophthalmoplegia, the preferred diagnostic designation is Tolosa-Hunt syndrome, although the relationship between Tolosa-Hunt syndrome and NS has not been elucidated. Patients presenting with classical Tolosa-Hunt syndrome are not expected to develop systemic sarcoidosis.
4. Other meningeal processes that should be considered in the setting of extensive meningeal inflammation (by MRI) include granulomatous disease associated with rheumatoid arthritis, mycoses, tuberculosis (TB), germinoma with granulomatous inflammation, acanthamoeba, mycobacterium, and foreign material.

TREATMENT STRATEGIES

Neurosarcoidosis is a difficult condition to manage. The diagnosis may be difficult to establish, the clinical course is variable, the markers for disease activity are scarce and nonspecific, and the disease can be refractory to aggressive therapeutic efforts. Consequently, the treatment is best managed by specialists with experience with NS, with the use of immunosuppressive agents, and with the care of patients who are immunosuppressed. Biopsy proof of granulomatous inflammation from systemic or nervous system sites is strongly recommended before treatment is initiated.

Because the clinical presentation and anatomic localization of the granulomatous inflammation that cause symptoms in NS varies throughout the nervous system, a simple algorithm for management is not possible. Local peripheral lesions generally are less threatening to global function, and they may be treated along with systemic sarcoidosis symptoms, which may require only modest corticosteroid therapy. Lesions may remit with transient therapy or even spontaneously. However, when NS affects the brain, spinal cord, or pachymeninges, the neurologic disability may be severe and the course progressive or relapsing. In a minority of patients, NS may be refractory even to high-dose corticosteroid therapy. Early use of more potent or more focused immunosuppressive strategies seems important in obtaining optimal outcomes.

It is regrettable that to date, there are no randomized controlled trials to guide therapy for NS. Present recommendations are based on limited case series and on knowledge of clinicians with more substantial experience in the management of this condition.

Goals of Therapy

Clinical symptom control and neurologic function preservation are the key goals of therapeutics in NS. No therapy is known to be curative for this idiopathic disorder, although disease remissions are well known. Sustained remission following an initial prolonged course (at least 6 months) of immunosuppressive therapy occurs in 70% of patients, based on anecdotal clinical experience. Even after remission occurs, clinical vigilance is warranted because signs and symptoms may reappear months or years after clearing. Relapses must be carefully assessed because they cannot be assumed to be NS, and other viable considerations, including new opportunistic infections or development of malignancy, especially lymphoma, must always be considered.

In general, the most important goal of therapy is to target a symptom or set of symptoms seeking maximal reversal of deficit, or at the very least, stabilization and prevention of further progression. In this context, recognizing the reversible component of the neurologic deficit related to inflammation and distinguishing it from irreversible injury is difficult at the initiation of treatment. Therefore expectations of clinical improvement need to be tempered. The absence of clinical progression during treatment, coupled with improvement in markers of inflammation, may be all that can be anticipated with successful treatment. On the other hand, in some cases, therapy can be gratifyingly restorative of neurologic dysfunction as inflammation subsides. Because some clinical deficits may be difficult to measure, concurrent monitoring of imaging evidence of disease activity may be a useful surrogate marker. Often successful therapy results in substantial regression of imaging and CSF inflammatory manifestations, especially a reduction of contrast enhancing abnormalities on MRI or CT scanning suggestive of active inflammatory disease. However, concordance of imaging and clinical responses is not uniformly seen, and clinical judgment is required for treatment decisions.

In addition to clinical and imaging manifestations, CSF abnormalities may also provide evidence of disease activity . Active inflammation reflected by elevated nucleated cells and high protein or low glucose levels in CSF may provide additional surrogate markers suggesting ongoing disease activity with risk of further neurologic impairment. Although these are helpful, rarely should normalization of these markers be a primary therapeutic goal. With successful treatment, normalization of CSF glucose levels occurs initially, followed by reduction in cell count. Spinal fluid protein levels routinely diminish, but in severe disease, complete normalization is unusual. The persistence of elevated protein values presumably represents persistent defects in the blood-brain barrier following permanent CNS injury after resolution of active CNS sarcoidosis.

Corticosteroids

The mainstay of therapy is corticosteroids. These drugs have potent broad-spectrum anti-inflammatory and immunosuppressive effects, reducing lymphocyte, monocyte, and macrophage numbers and function. These effects are achieved through suppression of multiple soluble and cellular factors generating the inflammatory responses. Because neurologic disease is serious and subacutely progressive, aggressive corticosteroid therapy is required for treatment of NS. Oral therapy is used, with doses equivalent to 0.5 to 1 mg/kg/d of prednisone at initiation. Some practitioners initiate therapy with 3 to 5 days of 1 g/d (or 20 mg/kg/d) of intravenous methylprednisolone, but this is generally reserved for profoundly disabling neurologic disease, such as severe myelopathy, mass effect-associated intraparenchymal CNS lesions, or hydrocephalus with increased intracranial pressure. Because prolonged therapy is required for parenchymal or severe leptomeningeal disease, after bolus therapy, a sustained oral course of prednisone is recommended, while monitoring disease manifestations closely to avoid relapse. One approach is to plan for prednisone 60 mg/d for 6 months, or with a slow dose-tapering over this time interval, with explicit instructions to reassess clinically and radiographically at 6 months and, if biologic activity of disease is in doubt, to consider repeating CSF analysis. Many patients will relapse if therapy is tapered off or discontinued too early. For sustained remission, some patients require 12 or more months of therapy.

Given the severe side effects of sustained daily corticosteroid therapy, transition to an alternate-day therapy by tapering the alternate-day dose to zero is a reasonable goal. In cases of significant neurologic deficit, this commits the patient to at least 12 months of therapy in most cases. Transition to alternate-day therapy, however, may not maintain clinical stability. Even with maximally tolerated doses of corticosteroids, remission of neurologic signs is often elusive.

The risks of corticosteroid therapy used over months to years must be recognized, with complications of behavioral changes, cushingoid changes in fat distribution, skin changes, glucose intolerance, weight gain, muscle loss, and ultimately, risks of osteoporosis and cataracts. These complications must be anticipated and managed by an experienced treating physician to obtain optimal outcomes.

Cytotoxic Therapy

Severe NS, optimal treatment often requires more aggressive therapies. Case series suggest that when CNS disease due to NS is encountered, it has a poor prognosis, and early intensive therapy should be considered.[5,22] Lack of controlled trials makes it impossible to determine the optimal drugs for this indication. Case series and reports and the authors' experience include use of cyclophosphamide,[22,28–31] mycophenolate mofetil,[32,33] azathioprine,[4,34–37] methotrexate,[8,22,30,31] cyclosporine,[28,38] chlorambucil,[35] and hydroxychloroquine.[4,8]

The observations that TNF-α may play a critical role in driving the inflammatory response has resulted in trials of infliximab as an intervention for NS.[39–45] This monoclonal antibody binding and inhibiting the action of TNF-α has been widely used for rheumatoid arthritis and inflammatory bowel disease. Clinical trials for pulmonary sarcoidosis have supported use of infliximab, whereas etanercept seems to be less efficacious.[36,40] Recent case reports support the probability that infliximab is effective in many cases, and may be an important agent to compare with the most effective cytotoxic therapy for severe NS. Aksamit and Utz[46] reported that 13 of 14 patients treated with infliximab 5 mg/kg had a beneficial clinical response. Later, the combination of infliximab and mycophenolate was used successfully to treat 7 refractory NS patients.[34] This report reinforces the observation that combination therapies may be required, because many clinicians have experienced an inability to control NS with single-agent therapy, most often relying on some degree of corticosteroid therapy. The possibility of TNF-α antagonists being especially effective for NS is further supported by a report of a patient with corticosteroid-resistant disease being promptly responsive to thalidomide.[47] This agent is a TNF-α antagonist through enhancing TNF-α mRNA degradation. Although use of infliximab or similar agents seems to be a fruitful avenue for therapy of NS, the development of sarcoidosis while on therapy with TNF-α antagonist therapy has been reported, emphasizing that there is no uniformly effective therapy for this complicated disease. Discovery of prognostic biomarkers remains an important improvement in therapeutics.[36] High costs and acknowledged toxicity of infliximab suggest that the systematic evaluation of this approach to therapy should occur to establish its place in NS therapeutics.

Radiation Therapy

Although pharmacotherapy is generally preferred for refractory CNS cases or for those in whom the side effects of therapy exceed apparent benefits, radiation therapy has been tried. In general, the frequency of its use has precluded clear analysis of risk-to-benefit responses.[28,35,38,48] Responses may be long-term and obviate further use of corticosteroids or immunosuppressive therapy, although in a sizable proportion of cases subsequent immunotherapy is necessary. However, given the unpredictable course of disease and the complicated medical therapy preceding radiation, in most cases, it is difficult to assign outcomes to the effect of radiation alone.

Indications for Surgery

At times, surgical decompression of CNS sarcoidosis mass lesions seems necessary, but in general, this is not a surgical disease and aggressive surgical interventions have rarely provided sustained benefit.[37] Surgery is frequently required to establish the diagnosis, where no clear peripheral diagnosis of sarcoidosis is made. The chronic and risky therapy that is required by many patients with NS emphasizes the importance of establishing the diagnosis as early in management as possible. CNS lesions of sarcoidosis can masquerade as infectious granulomatous diseases, such as TB and cryptococcal disease. These diseases would be exacerbated by the therapy required for sarcoidosis. Consequently, if the diagnosis is not otherwise established and the CNS lesion is surgically accessible, brain biopsy should be considered.

A fairly frequent reason for neurosurgical intervention is the development of hydrocephalus. Avoidance of this complication through appropriate aggressive medical therapy is ideal, but recognizing the complication and arranging for ventricular drainage or shunting is critical for the symptomatic patient.

RESEARCH OPPORTUNITIES

Research initiatives directed at a better understanding of the pathophysiology of NS are important for learning more about this disease. Establishing a tissue and CSF sample bank and a DNA repository from patients with probable and definite disease would enable more systematic study of the disease with modern techniques and provide a sufficient number of patients to be informative. Questions that should be answered include determining if the granulomatous process in the CNS is similar to that in other organ systems; determining if there are CSF markers that distinguish CNS sarcoidosis from other CNS inflammatory diseases, such as multiple sclerosis; and probing for genetic variants that distinguish patients with NS from patients with systemic sarcoidosis or those from the general population. [Smith][13] Accumulation of a substantial tissue archive should allow consideration of whether there are genetic variants that are associated with particular presentations of NS and, eventually, might enable a genome-wide association study to provide information that might guide insights into pathophysiology, diagnosis, and treatment.

On a practical level, the establishment of a consortium of expert clinicians allows a more systematic approach to management questions, including targeted treatments for specific neurologic presentations, use of daily or alternate-day corticosteroid therapy, timing for the initiation of novel therapeutic agents, interventions for refractory disease, and determinants for the duration of therapies. As an understanding of the pathophysiology of NS evolves, novel interventions should be studied in defined patient populations. These management studies must make it a priority to evaluate and define outcome measures, which provide critical tools in future therapeutic development. Patient assessment tools that are valid across as broad a range of clinical scenarios as possible should be developed.

Because NS has been an orphan disease, it has been particularly difficult to study. Given the rarity of this disorder, a multi-center approach is necessary, potentially with worldwide contributors. Development of referral centers with special expertise would allow study of more patients at major centers and accumulation of more sophisticated care and management applied to this challenging clinical disease. The National Institute of Neurological Disorders and Stroke Clinical Research Collaboration could represent a contributing infrastructure to access patients throughout the neurologic community. The authors plan to seek resources allowing establishment of a neurosarcoidosis registry and biologic sample repository to initiate this critical project, with a shared data management system allowing coordinated research on this entity at dedicated academic sites with expertise and interest in addressing the challenges of NS.[49]

SUMMARY

Neurosarcoidosis is a diagnostic consideration in diverse clinical settings. Efforts should be made to secure pathologic confirmation of systemic sarcoidosis; only rarely is CNS pathologic confirmation available. CNS infection and malignancy should be reasonably excluded before making a diagnosis of CNS sarcoidosis. Corticosteroid therapy alone may not be sufficient to treat NS; adjunct immunosuppressive agents are increasingly used to achieve an optimal clinical outcome.

REFERENCES

1. Stern BJ, Krumholz A, Johns C, et al. Sarcoidosis and its neurological manifestations. Arch Neurol 1985;42:909–17.
2. Allen RKA, Stellars RE, Sandstrom PA. A prospective study of 32 patients with neurosarcoidosis. Sarcoidosis Vasc Diffuse Lung Dis 2003;20:118–25.
3. Pawate S, Moses H, Sriram S. Presentations and outcomes of neurosarcoidosis: a study of 54 cases. Q J Med. Published online April 20, 2009. Available at: http://qjmed.oxfordjournals.org/cgi/content/abstract/hcp042. Accessed April 25, 2009.
4. Iannuzzi MC, Rybicki BA, Teirstein AS. Sarcoidosis. N Engl J Med 2007;357: 2153–65.
5. Ferriby D, de Seze J, Stojkovic T, et al. Long-term follow-up of neurosarcoidosis. Neurology 2001;57:927–9.
6. Hunninghake GW, Costable U, Ando M, et al. Statement on sarcoidosis. Joint Statement of the American Thoracic Society (ATS), the European Respiratory Society (ERS) and the World Association of Sarcoidosis and Other Granulomatous Disorders (WASOG) adopted by the ATS Board of Directors and by the ERS Executive Committee, February 1999. Am J Respir Crit Care Med 1999; 160:736–55.
7. Nowak DA, Widenka DC. Neurosarcoidosis: a review of its intracranial manifestation. J Neurol 2001;248:363–72.
8. Zajicek JP, Scolding NJ, Foster O, et al. Central nervous system sarcoidosis - diagnosis and management. Q J Med 1999;92:103–17.
9. Khoury J, Wellik KE, Demaerschalk BM, et al. Cerebrospinal fluid angiotensin-converting enzyme for diagnosis of central nervous system sarcoidosis. Neurologist 2009;15:108–11.

10. Ma Y, Gal A, Koss MN. The pathology of pulmonary sarcoidosis: update. Semin Diagn Pathol 2007;24:150–61.
11. Rybicki BA, Iannuzzi MC, Frederick MM, et al. Familial aggregation of sarcoidosis: a case-control etiologic study of sarcoidosis (ACCESS). Am J Respir Crit Care Med 2001;164:2085–91.
12. Hofmann S, Franke A, Fischer A, et al. Genome-wide association study identifies ANXA11 as a new susceptibility locus for sarcoidosis. Nat Genet 2008;40: 1103–6.
13. Smith G, Brownell I, Sanchez M, et al. Advances in the genetics of sarcoidosis. Clin Genet 2008;73:401–12.
14. Johns CJ, Michele TM. The clinical management of sarcoidosis. A 50-year experience at the Johns Hopkins Hospital. Medicine 1999;78:65–111.
15. Teirstein AS, Machac J, Almeida O, et al. Results of 188 whole-body fluorodeoxyglucose positron emission tomography (PET) scans in the identification of occult biopsy sites and reversible granulomatous disease in patients with sarcoidosis. Chest 2007;132:1949–53.
16. Aksamit AJ, Norona F. Neurosarcoidosis without systemic sarcoid. Ann Neurol 1999;46:471.
17. Hoitsma E, Marziniak M, Faber CG, et al. Small fibre neuropathy in sarcoidosis. Lancet 2002;359:2085–6.
18. Leavitt JA, Campbell RJ. Cost-effectiveness in the diagnosis of sarcoidosis: the conjunctival biopsy. Eye 1998;12:959–62.
19. Stern BJ, Corbett J. Neuro-ophthalmologic manifestations of sarcoidosis. Curr Treat Options Neurol 2007;9:63–71.
20. Colvin IB. Audiovestibular manifestations of sarcoidosis: a review of the literature. Laryngoscope 2006;116:75–82.
21. Scott TF. Cerebral herniation after lumbar puncture in sarcoid meningitis. Clin Neurol Neurosurg 2000;102:26–8.
22. Scott TF, Yandora K, Valeri A, et al. Aggressive therapy for neurosarcoidosis long-term follow-up of 48 treated patients. Arch Neurol 2007;64:691–6.
23. Bihan H, Christozova V, Dumas JL, et al. Sarcoidosis: clinical, hormonal, and magnetic resonance imaging (MRI) manifestations of hypothalamic-pituitary disease in 9 patients and review of the literature. Medicine 2007;86(5):259–68.
24. Krumholz A, Stern BJ, Stern EG. Clinical implications of seizures in neurosarcoidosis. Arch Neurol 1991;48:842–4.
25. Olugemo OA, Stern BJ. Stroke and neurosarcoidosis. In: Caplan LR, editor. Uncommon causes of stroke. 2nd edition. New York: Cambridge University Press; 2008. p. 75–80.
26. Junger SS, Stern BJ, Levine SR, et al. Intramedullary spinal sarcoidosis: clinical and magnetic resonance imaging characteristics. Neurology 1993;43:333–7.
27. Oksanen V. Neurosarcoidosis: clinical presentations and course in 50 patients. Acta Med Scand 1986;73:283–90.
28. Agbogu BN, Stern BJ, Sewell C, et al. Therapeutic considerations in patients with refractory neurosarcoidosis. Arch Neurol 1995;52:875–9.
29. Doty JD, Mazur JE, Judson MA. Treatment of corticosteroid-resistant neurosarcoidosis with a short-course cyclophosphamide regimen. Chest 2003;124:2023–6.
30. Lower EE, Broderick JP, Brott TG, et al. Diagnosis and management of neurological sarcoidosis. Arch Intern Med 1997;157:1864–8.
31. Lower EE, Weiss KL. Neurosarcoidosis. Clin Chest Med 2008;29:475–92.
32. Kouba DJ, Mimouni D, Rencic A, et al. Mycophenolate mofetil may serve as a steroid-sparing agent for sarcoidosis. Br J Dermatol 2003;148:147–8.

33. Moravan M, Segal BM. Treatment of CNS sarcoidosis with infliximab and myco-phenolate mofetil. Neurology 2009;72:337–40.
34. Petropoulos IK, Zuber JP, Guex-Crosier Y. Heerfordt syndrome with unilateral facial nerve palsy: a rare presentation of sarcoidosis. Klin Monatsbl Augenheilkd 2008;225:453–6.
35. Gelwan MJ, Kellen RI, Burde RM, et al. Sarcoidosis of the anterior visual pathway: successes and failures. J Neurol Neurosurg Psychiatr 1988;51:1473–80.
36. Baughman RP, Costabel U, du Bois RM. Treatment of sarcoidosis. Clin Chest Med 2008;29:533–48.
37. Cahill DW, Salcman M. Neurosarcoidosis: a review of the rarer manifestations. Surg Neurol 1981;15:204–11.
38. Chapelon C, Ziza JM, Piette JC, et al. Neurosarcoidosis: signs, course and treat-ment in 35 confirmed cases. Medicine 1990;69:261–76.
39. Kumar G, Kang CA, Giannini C. Neurosarcoidosis presenting as a cerebellar mass. J Gen Intern Med 2007;22:1373–6.
40. Denys BG, Bogaerts Y, Coenegrachts KL, et al. Steroid-resistant sarcoidosis: is antagonism of TNF-a the answer. Clin Sci 2007;112:281–9.
41. Pettersen JA, Zochodne DW, Bell RB, et al. Refractory neurosarcoidosis respond-ing to infliximab. Neurology 2002;59:1660–1.
42. Katz JM, Bruno MK, Winterkorn JMS, et al. The pathogenesis and treatment of optic disc swelling in neurosarcoidosis. A unique therapeutic response to inflixi-mab. Arch Neurol 2003;60:426–30.
43. Sollberger M, Fluri F, Baumann T, et al. Successful treatment of steroid-refractory neurosarcoidosis with infliximab. J Neurol 2004;251:760–1.
44. Doty JD, Mazur JE, Judson MA. Treatment of sarcoidosis with infliximab. Chest 2005;127:1064–71.
45. Toth C, Martin L, Morrish W, et al. Dramatic MRI improvement with refractory neu-rosarcoidosis treated with infliximab. Acta Neurol Scand 2007;116:259–62.
46. Aksamit AJ, Utz JP. Infliximab treatment of neurosarcoidosis. Neurology 2006;66: A166.
47. Hammond ER, Kaplin AI, Kerr DA. Thalidomide for acute treatment of neurosar-coidosis. Spinal Cord 2007;45:802–3.
48. Motta M, Alongi F, Bolognesi A, et al. Remission of refractory neurosarcoidosis treated with brain radiotherapy. A case report and a literature review. Neurologist 2008;14:120–4.
49. Available at: http://ninds.nih.gov/funding/research/clinical_research/crc.htm. Accessed July 20, 2008.

Neurologic Aspects of Drug Abuse

Harold W. Goforth, MD[a,b,c,*], Reed Murtaugh, MD[d],
Francisco Fernandez, MD[d]

KEYWORDS

• Addiction • Neurobiology • Neurotoxicity • Epidemiology

Neurologic aspects of drug abuse vary. This article explains the general nature of drug abuse, identifies the physiologic effects of certain drugs, and briefly describes the neurobiology of addiction. This article also reviews available treatment options for those addicted to substances of abuse, and clarifies common misconceptions, including the differences between tolerance, abuse, and addiction.

GENERAL EPIDEMIOLOGY

The epidemiology of substance use varies widely and differs according to the specific substance discussed.

Alcohol

Alcohol abuse and dependence pose significant threats across a variety of areas, including risk of teratagenicity, impairments to cognition, and trauma. Birth defects secondary to alcohol abuse are well documented and include facial anomalies, prenatal and postnatal growth retardation, and functional or structural central nervous system abnormalities. The consequences are life-long with marked behavioral and learning difficulties that appear disproportionate to the degree of neurocognitive impairment. Fetal alcohol spectrum disorders may affect up to 1% of the United States population, and are more strongly associated with higher levels of alcohol consumption.[1,2] Even though these disorders are entirely preventable by abstinence from alcohol while pregnant, data suggest that approximately 10% of women between 18 and 44 years of age used alcohol during pregnancy and that 2% engaged in "binge drinking" (ie, five or more drinks on one occasion).[3]

In addition to fetal alcohol spectrum conditions, states of intoxication and withdrawal (**Table 1**), cognitive impairment, ataxia, cerebellar atrophy, and peripheral neuropathy

[a] Duke University Medical Center, Durham, NC 27705, USA
[b] Consultation-Liaison Psychiatry Service, Durham Veterans Affairs Medical Center, Durham, NC 27705, USA
[c] GRECC, Durham Veterans Affairs Medical Center, Durham, NC 27705, USA
[d] University of South Florida, Tampa, FL 33612, USA
* Corresponding author. Duke University Medical Center, Durham, NC 27705.
E-mail address: harold.goforth@duke.edu (H.W. Goforth).

Neurol Clin 28 (2010) 199–215
doi:10.1016/j.ncl.2009.09.010
0733-8619/09/$ – see front matter. Published by Elsevier Inc.

neurologic.theclinics.com

Table 1
States of intoxication and withdrawal

Clinical Diagnosis	Clinical Appearance
Alcohol intoxication	Incoordination Anxiolysis Cognitive changes Ataxia Nausea, vomiting Stupor
Alcohol withdrawal	Tremor Heightened anxiety Diaphoresis Tachycardia Tachypnea Seizures Delirium (delirium tremens), death
Wernicke-Korsakoff syndrome	Confusion Ophthalmoplegia Ataxia Anterograde amnesia Confabulation Hallucinatory phenomena
Marijuana intoxication	Mild euphoria Relaxation Time distortion Infectious laughter, talkativeness Increased appetitive drive (hunger, sex) Anxiety Phobic reactions Psychomotor slowing Psychotic reactions (paranoia)
Marijuana withdrawal	Restlessness Anorexia Irritability Insomnia
Stimulant (amphetamine, methamphetamine, cocaine) intoxication	Increased arousal, decreased fatigue Euphoria Increased sexual drive Dyskinesias Agitation, irritability Psychosis, paranoia Formication Chest pain, palpitations Mydriasis Hyperthermia Hypertension Tachycardia
Stimulant withdrawal	Excessive sleeping Increased appetite Depression Anxiety

(continued on next page)

Table 1 (continued)	
Clinical Diagnosis	**Clinical Appearance**
Opiate intoxication	Depressed consciousness, stupor, coma
	Drowsiness
	Conjunctival injection
	Euphoria
	Acute mental status changes, delirium
	Seizures
	Bradypnea, hypopnea
	Pruritis
Opiate withdrawal	Agitation, anxiety
	Insomnia
	Lacrimation
	Diaphoresis
	Goose-flesh
	Yawning
	Abdominal cramping, diarrhea
	Miosis
	Nausea, vomiting
Sedative (benzodiazepines, barbiturates) intoxication	Anxiolysis
	Depressed consciousness, stupor, coma
	Nystagmus
	Ataxia
	Respiratory depression
	Death
Sedative (benzodiazepines, barbiturates) withdrawal	Anxiety
	Insomnia
	Restlessness
	Diaphoresis
	Tachycardia
	Tachypnea
	Seizures
	Delirium (delirium tremens), death

Data from Saddock BJ, Saddock VA, Ruiz P, editors. Kaplan's and Saddock's Comprehensive Textbook of Psychiatry. 9th Edition. Volume I, Section 11 "Substance-Related Disorders", Chapters 11.1–11.13; p: 1237–431. 2009 by Lippincott Williams and Wilkins, Philadelphia, PA 19106 USA.

are all associated with chronic alcohol abuse. Ataxia and ocular motility dysfunction are not uncommon. The ataxia seems to spare the upper extremities and is associated with loss of Purkinje cells and the anterior and superior aspects of the vermis as well as adjacent parts of the lobes of the cerebellum. Neuroimaging findings reveal these characteristic changes (**Fig. 1**). Wernicke-Korsakoff syndrome has been clearly linked with nutritional deficiency of thiamine as occurs in alcoholism due to dietary neglect. Neuroimaging findings are consistent with the neuropathological changes (**Fig. 2**). The syndrome appears to have a low prevalence (0.4%–2.8% of reported autopsies), but the disorder is highly underreported and underdiagnosed.[4] Available data suggest only 20% to 25% of cases are correctly diagnosed in life when compared with autopsy results. An estimated 25% of Wernicke-Korsakoff syndrome cases were missed where the brains were not examined microscopically. Another study found that only 20% of clinical Wernicke-Korsakoff syndrome diagnoses were made correctly in life when compared with autopsy results,[5] which illustrates the necessity of a high index of clinical suspicion when dealing with this disease process.

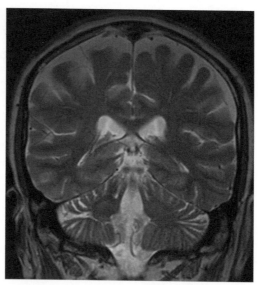

Fig. 1. Coronal high-resolution inversion recovery MRI sequences demonstrating the prominence of the cerebellar hemispheric folia in alcoholic cerebellar atrophy.

Trauma remains highly correlated with alcohol use as well, especially in young adults. Recent data demonstrate that for the time period 1999 to 2005, the proportions of college students ages 18 to 24 who consumed five or more drinks on at least one occasion in the past month increased from 41.7% to 44.7%. Also, the proportion of college students who drove under the influence of alcohol in the past year increased from 26.5% to 28.9%. These rates suggest a national epidemic for patterns of alcohol abuse in this age group, and data illustrate that in 2001, 599,000 (10.5%) full-time 4-year college students were injured because of drinking, 696,000 (12%) were hit or

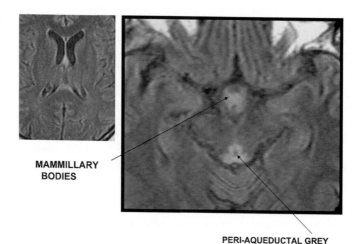

MAMMILLARY
BODIES

PERI-AQUEDUCTAL GREY

Fig. 2. Wernicke-Korsakoff amnestic syndrome. Axial fluid attenuation inversion recovery (FLAIR) MRI images demonstrate the subtle subependymal cytotoxic edema lining the hypothalamic structures of the third ventricle and the aqueduct of Sylvius, including the mammillary bodies. These findings are typical of thiamine deficiency.

assaulted by another drinking college student, and 97,000 (2%) were victims of alcohol-related sexual assault or date rape.[6]

Marijuana

Among illicit drugs, marijuana intoxication and withdrawal are common (see **Table 1**). Recent data confirm a high prevalence of both marijuana and cocaine use among samples sent to forensic laboratories, and these two were the most frequently identified drugs in 16 of 19 reporting areas.[7] Similarly, treatment admission data for the first half of 2007 reveal that treatment admissions for primary cocaine/crack (excluding primary alcohol admissions), ranked first in frequency in 6 of the 15 areas for which treatment data were reported.[7] It has been noted that cocaine is often reported as a secondary or tertiary drug among treatment admissions and that cocaine is used frequently in conjunction with other substances, including marijuana and opiates. Crack remains the predominant form of cocaine used by those entering treatment.[7]

Stimulants

Clinically, states of intoxication and withdrawal (see **Table 1**) are commonly seen in United States emergency services, especially in cardiac and stroke programs. The ongoing high use of cocaine has important medical implications, including premature comorbidities and teratogenicity.

Cocaine abuse most commonly causes seizures, cerebral infarcts, intracerebral hemorrhages, and vasculitis. The neuropsychological complications include attentional deficits and impaired short-term memory. There is no defined neuropathology, but white matter changes are common, suggestive of a vasculopathy (**Fig. 3**).

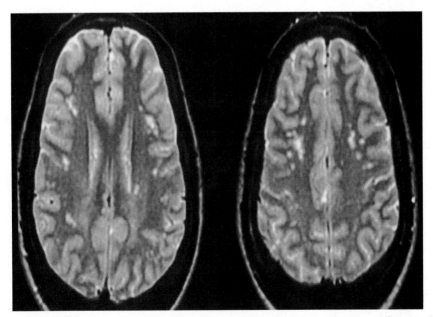

Fig. 3. Stimulant- and cocaine-abuse vasculitis. Peripheral microvascular areas of cytotoxic edema represent end-artery microinfarcts.

Maternal cocaine use has been associated with lower gestational age and decreased growth parameters at birth.[8,9] Similarly, regular cocaine use has been associated with an increased likelihood of myocardial infarction in younger patients, and appears to account for up to one of every four nonfatal myocardial infarctions in persons aged 18 to 45 years.[10] A large epidemiologic study of Texas hospitals demonstrated that risk of stroke significantly increased in amphetamine and cocaine abusers. Amphetamine abuse was associated with hemorrhagic but not ischemic stroke, whereas cocaine abuse was associated with both hemorrhagic and ischemic stroke.[11] Stroke and cocaine use have also been demonstrated to correlate with fatal cerebrovascular accidents and poor outcome following stroke.[12]

Opiates

Heroin remains popular as a primary drug in substance-abuse treatment admissions in the northeastern United States, and injection use remains the most commonly reported route of heroin administration among primary treatment admissions.[7] Clinical states of intoxication and withdrawal are common (see **Table 1**). The continued persistence of injecting behavior is worrisome because of the high likelihood of contracting infections via shared needles or skin contamination. Both HIV and hepatitis C virus are efficiently transmitted via the intravenous route with the sharing of needles. Both are essentially incurable infections that eventually result in death, although some variable successes at treating hepatitis C virus have been demonstrated, depending upon the viral strain. Other infectious complications of intravenous drug abuse include endocarditis, septicemia, and joint infections.

Recent abuse indicators for other opiates are increasing because of diversion and theft of pharmaceutical supplies.[7] Recent abuse indicators for oxycodone, hydrocodone, methadone, and fentanyl suggest increased rates of drug diversion and abuse of prescription opiates—especially oxycodone and hydrocodone—while the prevalence of heroin use has appeared to remain relatively stable. Diversion of buprenorphine to street use has been reported in Chicago, Cincinnati, and Maine, where it has been noted to be increasingly common among heroin users for avoiding withdrawal symptoms from heroin.[7]

TERMINOLOGY

The terms *abuse* and *dependence* were initially separated to provide increasing specificity regarding patterns of misuse in the *Diagnostic and Statistical Manual of Mental Disorders, Third Edition* (*DSM-III*), and the category of dependence was further expanded with the revised edition, *Diagnostic and Statistical Manual of Mental Disorders, Revised Third Edition* (*DSM-IIIR*). Abuse became a residual category for diagnosing those individuals who did not meet the criteria for dependence but who nevertheless used substances despite physical, social, psychological, or occupational consequences, or who drank in physically hazardous situations.

The terms *tolerance*, *sensitization*, and *withdrawal* are incorporated into the *DSM* concept of substance dependence and are important to understanding these diagnoses as an entity. Tolerance generally refers to the concept that, over time and with increased and continued use of a specific substance, one will need markedly increased amounts of the substance to achieve a desired effect, or will use the same amount of the substance with markedly diminished effect. Sensitization, the opposite of tolerance, occurs when repeated stable doses of the drug elicit escalating effects. Withdrawal is a clinical phenomenon that includes a characteristic syndrome, including either physiologic or psychological components for a particular substance following abrupt discontinuation. Intoxication is the physiologic state produced by a poison or other toxic substance.

The current *DSM-IV* criteria for abuse are: A maladaptive pattern of substance use leading to clinically significant impairment or distress, as manifested by one or more of the following, occurring within a 12-month period:

1. Recurrent substance use resulting in a failure to fulfill major role obligations at work, school, home (eg, repeated absences or poor work performance related to substance use; substance-related absences, suspensions, or expulsions from school; neglect of children or household)
2. Recurrent substance use in situations in which it is physically hazardous (eg, driving an automobile or operating a machine when impaired by substance use)
3. Recurrent substance-related legal problems (eg, arrests for substance-related disorderly conduct)
4. Continued substance use despite having persistent or recurrent social or interpersonal problems caused or exacerbated by the effects of the substance (eg, arguments with spouse about consequences of intoxication; physical fights)

Symptoms that have never met the criteria for substance dependence for this class of substances.[13]

Dependence is defined along more biologic terms to include concepts of tolerance and withdrawal as well as failed attempts to quit the substance. *DSM-IV* criteria define *dependence* as a maladaptive pattern of substance use, leading to clinically significant impairment or distress, as manifested by three or more of the following, occurring at any time in the same 12-month period:

1. Tolerance, as defined by either of the following:
   A need for markedly increased amounts of the substance to achieve intoxication or desired effect
   Markedly diminished effect with continued use of the same amount of substance
2. Withdrawal, as manifested by either of the following:
   The characteristic withdrawal syndrome for the substance
   Taking the same (or a closely related) substance to relieve or avoid withdrawal symptoms
3. Often taking the substance in larger amounts or over a longer period than was intended
4. Having a persistent desire or making unsuccessful efforts to cut down or control substance use
5. Spending a great deal of time in activities to obtain the substance, use the substance, or recover from its effects
6. Giving up or reducing important social, occupational, or recreational activities because of substance use
7. Continuing the substance use despite knowledge of having a persistent or recurrent physical or psychological problem that is likely to have been caused or exacerbated by the substance (eg, continued drinking despite recognition that an ulcer was made worse by alcohol consumption).[13]

ACUTE PHARMACOLOGIC EFFECTS OF DRUGS OF ABUSE
Amphetamines

At abused doses, amphetamine increases the concentration of dopamine in the synaptic cleft in four ways: (1) It binds to the presynaptic membrane of dopaminergic neurons and induces the release of dopamine from the nerve terminal; (2) it interacts with dopamine-containing synaptic vesicles, releasing free dopamine into the nerve terminal; (3) it effectively binds to monoamine oxidase in dopaminergic neurons to prevent the degradation of dopamine; and (4) it binds to the dopamine reuptake transporter, causing it to act in reverse and transport free dopamine out of the nerve terminal. High-dose amphetamine has a similar effect on noradrenergic neurons; it can induce the release of noradrenaline into the synaptic cleft and inhibit the noradrenaline reuptake transporter.[14–16] Methylphenidate has pharmacologic effects similar to those of amphetamine but perhaps with a somewhat lower abuse potential.[17] Both compounds are schedule II agents with the Drug Enforcement Administration. Chronic use can lead to dyskinesias as well as potential increased risk of cerebrovascular accidents.

Marijuana

The majority of research on marijuana focuses upon Δ^9-9 tetrahydrocannabinol (THC), which is the chemical responsible for marijuana's pharmacologic activity.[18,19] THC produces unique psychologic effects during acute intoxication, including feelings of euphoria, sedation, altered sensory inputs, distortion of time perception, and impaired cognitive function. In addition, it produces alveolar dilatation, tachycardia, vasodilation, and suppressed immune function.[20]

Cocaine

Cocaine is one of the most potent chemicals with respect to brain neurochemistry, and this results in a high addictive potential. Cocaine blocks the presynaptic reuptake of norepinephrine and dopamine, which produces sympathetic changes, such as vasoconstriction, tachycardia, and hypertension. Precise effects depend upon such factors as the purity of the drug, route of administration, chronicity of use, and use of other drugs simultaneously that usually adulterate commercially available cocaine. Additives include caffeine, lidocaine, amphetamines, phencyclidine (PCP), and heroin to provide additional central nervous system effects. Cocaine affects heavily the reward pathway centers of the brain as well as the "fight or flight" response to an impending threat. There is a shift of blood into the skeletal musculature away from the skin and viscera, and central nervous system neurotransmitters and hormones become depleted with chronic use. Cocaine has been noted to increase sexual excitation and even to produce spontaneous orgasms. It can cause seizures, with resultant complications, including anoxic brain injury. It neurochemically inactivates the feeding center in the lateral hypothalamus, so supersedes appetitive drive leading to loss of appetite and body weight. Chronically depleted dopamine as occurs with chronic use has been noted to lead to hyperprolactinemia along with its clinical manifestations of amenorrhea, sexual dysfunction, gynecomastia, and galactorrhea. Cocaine also appears to cause adrenocortical hypertrophy with dysregulation of the hypothalamic-pituitary-adrenal axis. With chronic use, users often develop depression, avolition, insomnia, paranoia, and extreme irritability.[21]

Alcohol

Alcohol (ethanol) produces multiple effects, including incoordination, anxiolysis, cognitive changes, and modulation of locomotor activity. Data support a clear role of the γ-aminobutyric acid system in modulating alcohol's effects—especially upon the anxiolytic, motor, amnestic, and hypnotic features produced with acute intoxication. However, pure benzodiazepine receptor antagonists (flumazenil) do not appear to counteract ethanol's actions. Other potential neurologic systems involved in producing ethanol's myriad of central nervous system actions include the serotonergic system, N-methyl-D-aspartate (NMDA) receptors with chronic use, and the dopaminergic system in reinforcing the pleasurable effects of alcohol.[22] With heavy chronic use, alcohol has been linked to multiple cognitive changes including Wernicke-Korsakoff syndrome, alcoholic dementia, polyneuropathy, and increased risk of both hemorrhagic and ischemic strokes.

Hallucinogens

Hallucinogens generally refer to a group of compounds that alter consciousness without delirium, sedation, excessive stimulation, or cognitive impairment. The prototypical agent in this group is lysergic acid diethylamide (LSD). True LSD hallucinations have been noted to be rare. Rather, the group produces perceptual distortions of actual stimuli and are, thus, illusionogenic. Agents within this class typically are either indoles (LSD or psilocybin) or substituted phenethylamines (mescaline, methylenedioxymethamphetamine [MDMA]). Indole compounds have a structure similar to that of serotonin, and may involve alterations in serotonergic transmission. Substituted phenylethylamines appear more closely linked to the catecholamine neurotransmitters (ie, norepinephrine), and MDMA appears structurally similar to amphetamines. Absorption of LSD occurs rapidly from the gastrointestinal system, and the onset of behavioral effects occurs approximately 60 minutes after initial ingestion with a peak occurrence in 2 to 4 hours. Dizziness, parathesias, altered visual and hearing senses, and changes in mood with emotional intensification and dissociative phenomena are common. Somatic symptoms occur initially, and are followed by the illusory symptoms. Synesthesia is commonly reported. Autonomically, pupillary dilation, hyperreflexia, hypertension, piloerection, tachycardia, and hyperthermia are commonly reported following ingestion of hallucinogenic compounds.[23]

Nicotine

Nicotine appears to increase acetylcholine (Ach) release from the parietal cortex. Nicotine can also stimulate norepinephrine secretion from peripheral adrenergic neurons. Repeated doses of nicotine results in the development of tolerance to its effects.[24] Autonomic effects include tachycardia, and continued chronic use of tobacco increases one's risk of stroke, cardiovascular disease, and peripheral vascular disease, in addition to a host of malignancies.

Opiates

Opiate receptors are found predominantly in the central nervous system, the gastrointestinal tract, and peripheral tissues. There are three classes of opiate receptors including mu, delta, and kappa, and the mu receptors are generally thought to be responsible for supraspinal analgesia. Opiates more commonly cause dysphoria than euphoria, and iatrogenic addiction in individuals without a preexisting addiction history is rare. Physiologic effects of opiate administration include dysphoria, somnolence, diminished respiratory rate, and, in overdose, death.[25] Intravenous use of heroin has been linked to infection and acute transverse myelopathy.

Phencyclidine

PCP produces a myriad of effects in the central nervous system by binding to high-affinity PCP receptors, which also bind sigma opiates and doxolanes. PCP is an extremely potent compound among drugs of abuse, and psychotic reactions have been observed at undetectably low serum concentrations. Low doses commonly induce attentional and perceptual changes similar to those seen in schizophrenia, and intoxication can result in coma, seizures, respiratory arrest, and death. Other manifestations include severe hyperthermia, hypertension, nystagmus, and rhabdomyolysis. Primate research has demonstrated that PCP is an extremely addicting drug of abuse.[26]

Solvents

Solvent abuse is growing in young adults. In the United Kingdom, it has been noted that up to 10% of young adults have experimented with solvent abuse. Potential aerosolized chemicals are numerous within this category and include carbon tetrachloride, chloroform, dichloromethane, n-hexane, trichloroethylene, and even halothane. The acute effects of volatile substance inhalation include a rapid onset of intoxication and rapid recovery with elements of euphoria and disinhibition followed by hallucinations, nausea, and vomiting. Death due to arrhythmia has been noted to happen in even first-time, nonhabituated users. Long-term exposure to n-hexanes and nitrous oxide is associated with peripheral neuropathy, while prolonged abuse (notably of toluene or chlorinated solvents) can cause permanent damage to the central nervous system (cerebellar damage), heart, liver, kidney, and lungs.[27]

SECOND MESSENGER SYSTEMS IN DRUG ABUSE

Knowledge about second messenger systems is crucial to the understanding of the biology of addiction as well as to efforts to develop potential treatments for addictive behaviors. A recent excellent review of this topic identified three neurobiological circuits associated with the development and maintenance of drug dependence.[28] The reader is referred to this review for a more in-depth assessment of these pathways.

The early stages of addictive behavior, which incorporate preoccupation and craving, appear to involve glutamatergic projections to the extended amygdala and nucleus accumbens from the prefrontal cortex and basolateral amygdala.[28,29] Compulsive drug-seeking behavior is thought to encourage ventral striatal–ventral pallidal-talamic-cortical loops that eventually involve dorsal striatal–dorsal pallidal-thalamic-cortical loops, which are then exaggerated by diminished activity in reward circuits. Finally, the mesocorticolimbic dopamine system has proven important in the positive reinforcing effects of drugs associated with the binge-intoxication stage of addiction.[28] In addition to the neuroanatomic circuitry involved, drugs of abuse lead to intracellular signal transduction changes leading to alterations in nuclear function and rates of genetic transcription. This has been noted to lead to altered neuronal activity and, ultimately, to changes in function of associated neural circuits.[28,30]

Glutamatergic systems are also believed to play a major role in the pathology of addiction, and alcohol has been noted to act as an NMDA antagonist as part of its reward mechanism pathway. Acute and protracted abstinence from alcohol appears to involve overactive glutamate systems, which may explain the efficacy of acamprosate in the treatment of alcohol dependence.[31] Repeated self-administration of stimulants appears to decrease basal release of glutamate, so may stimulate drug-seeking behavior. Similarly, glutamate appears to play a large role in behavioral sensitization to drugs of abuse. Koob[28] notes that previous studies have shown that NMDA receptor antagonists block the long-term potentiation and depression associated with repeated administration of these stimulant drugs. Similarly, topiramate appears to also decrease alcohol consumption via its NMDA receptor antagonism.[28] This has important implications for the future of treating psychostimulant addiction (cocaine and amphetamine) because few effective pharmacologic interventions are available now for this particular form of addiction. An adequate understanding of these different pathways is important to the development of future pharmacotherapy for addictive disorders, and it is important to realize that the craving pathways and the reinforcement pathways appear to be different. Koob and colleagues[28] rightly notes that optimal treatments will be those that treat both kinds of pathways.

NEUROPHARMACOLOGICAL TREATMENT OF ALCOHOL AND DRUG ABUSE
General Treatment Principles

Individuals with alcoholism and drug-abuse disorders are clinically heterogeneous. Undeniably, the goal of all treatment is abstinence. While this implies multimodal strategies in various settings for successful treatment, the neurobiology of the disease of addiction predominates and, thus, pharmacotherapy for various treatment parameters has become increasingly important.[32] Following harm-reduction principles, short of remission and abstinence, therapeutic targets should focus on assisting individuals in both reducing the frequency and number of substances used and the frequency and severity of relapse. Lastly, all treatment should provide individuals with optimal psychological functioning and improved quality of life. This section will not review current strategies for detoxification and withdrawal. Instead, we will focus predominantly on neuropharmacological strategies to treat abuse and dependence.

Alcoholism

In general, pharmacotherapy for alcoholism has largely been limited to the use of benzodiazepines for detoxification purposes. Until 1994, only one medication was approved in the United States for treating alcohol dependence. That was disulfuram (Antabuse).[33] Disulfuram inhibits aldehyde dehydrogenase, thus altering the metabolism of alcohol and the accumulation of acetaldehyde. Increased levels of acetaldehyde can cause a range of symptoms from merely general malaise and unpleasantness to death. While useful for some patients, most patients that drink while on disulfuram and get sick simply stop the disulfuram. Some even have learned to drink through the sickness and override its noxious effects.

In 1994, the Food and Drug Administration (FDA) approved naltrexone (ReVia, Depade) for the treatment of alcohol dependence. Naltrexone blocks central mu opioid receptors, which results in a reduction in both the craving and rewarding effects of alcohol.[34] Thus, the use of the medication in the first 12 weeks of abstinence is key in reducing craving and relapse. Naltrexone does not help people with withdrawal symptoms or detox from alcohol or help them stop drinking. Naltrexone is only helpful after one stops drinking to maintain abstinence and avoid relapse. Not all patients benefit from naltrexone. In part, this may be a compliance issue in that alcoholics need to be at least 80% compliant with daily administration for the drug to be effective. The problem of compliance with daily administration was eliminated in 2006 with the introduction of long-acting naltrexone (Vivitrol) in depot injection, which requires monthly administration.[35] Drinking while taking either form of naltrexone does not make one sick. The starting dose of oral naltrexone is 25–50 mg daily. Discontinuations with oral preparations are largely due to nausea and diffuse gastrointestinal complaints. Slow titration of oral naltrexone from 25 mg orally to 50 mg over 5 to 7 days increases both tolerability and compliance. The injectable depot naltrexone is 380 mg intramuscularly monthly.

The basis of craving and withdrawal during the early phases of abstinence may be aberrant glutamate function. Some experts think that NMDA antagonists are useful for stabilizing the aberrant glutamate function during early abstinence. In 2004, the FDA approved acamprosate (Campral) for the treatment of alcohol dependence, making that drug the third for this application.[36] The usual dose of 666 mg three times a day is well tolerated and assists with maintaining and sustaining total abstinence time. However, the results from controlled trials with acamprosate have not yielded consistent results. It may well be that the best use of acamprosate would be in combination chemotherapy.[37,38]

There has always been a keen interest in serotonin as it relates to appetitive drives, including drives associated with alcoholism. Serotonin agonists and reuptake inhibitors have all been reported as therapeutic options. However, the results have been inconsistent. Therefore, these agents are best used in conditions where anxiety and depression are comorbid.[37,39,40]

On the other hand, serotonin antagonists, specifically ondansetron (Zofran), either alone or in combination with naltrexone, can block the desire to drink.[41,42] The benefits may be limited to early-onset alcoholics as compared with late-onset alcoholics.

One of the most vexing problems in treating alcoholics is to get buy-in for abstinence. Many of the drug therapies are geared to assist with abstinence efforts, but none are effective in reducing drinking behavior in patients who are still drinking. Johnson and colleagues[43] have pioneered the use of topiramate (Topomax), 300-mg maximum daily dose, in a double-blind, randomized clinical trial of 150 alcoholics, many of whom were actively drinking. The results were nothing short of amazing with significant reductions in both craving and drinking, thus promoting abstinence.[43]

Opioids

Full agonist substitutive therapy with methadone has been the primary mode of therapy for addiction to opioids.[44] The primary goals of therapy are to prevent an abstinence syndrome, reduce narcotic cravings, and block the euphoric effects of illicit opioid use. There are two key phases to methadone treatment. In the first phase, patients are titrated to adequate steady-state dosing. Once stabilized on a satisfactory dosage, the second phase begins. This is maintenance, which is often used as a long-term therapy until the patient is ready for detoxification. Treatment with methadone is restricted to specially licensed clinics that provide treatment along with psychosocial rehabilitative services.

Since 2002, office-based opioid therapy was made possible with the use of buprenorphine alone (Buprenex, Subutex) or in combination with naltrexone (Suboxone) **(Table 2)**.[14]

Clinical trials comparing buprenorphine with methadone for opioid maintenance have shown that buprenorphine (<40 mg) is as effective as low-dose methadone (<40 mg).[45] However, a meta-analysis of five studies that compared the two therapies showed that 8 to 12 mg of buprenorphine is not as effective as 50 to 80 mg of methadone.[46] A 2004 Cochrane review[47] confirmed these findings. Therefore, patients requiring higher methadone doses may not be good candidates for buprenorphine.

As with methadone, buprenorphine is an effective agent in suppressing opioid withdrawal while blocking the effects of other opioids. Another strategy for suppressing withdrawal symptoms, but without the use of opiates, is to use clonidine (Catapres).[48] First described for suppressing withdrawal symptoms by Gold and colleagues,[49] clonidine is the only nonopioid demonstrating efficacy comparable to methadone and buprenorphine for withdrawal,[50] though the FDA has not yet approved clonidine for such use.

Cocaine

Pharmacologic management of cocaine craving and dependence has not been as successful as that of alcohol. Dopamine agonists, antidepressants, antipsychotics,

Table 2			
Available buprenorphine formulations			
Medication	**Indication**	**Description**	**Dose**
Buprenorphine tablet (Subutex)	Opioid maintenance and detoxification	White oval tablet	2 or 8 mg sublingual
Combination buprenorphine/ naloxone (Suboxone) in a 4:1 ratio	Opioid maintenance and detoxification	Orange hexagonal tablet	2/0.5 and 8/2 mg sublingual

and other agents inclusive of disulfuram have shown clear-cut efficacy.[51] Some studies have shown no short-term improvement superior to placebo with these multiple agents. Others have shown improvement, but that improvement has not held up over time. Grabowski and colleagues[52,53] have used both methylphenidate (Ritalin) and d-amphetamine (Dexedrine) as replacement therapies. Their results have been promising. Recently, modafinil (Provigil) has also shown promising results.[54] All these studies need replication and need to demonstrate long-term efficacy.

While therapies for cocaine abuse and dependence are studied, a new focus has been on the use of therapies to block the effects of cocaine. Disulfuram (Antabuse) does both. That is, it dampens the subjective effects of cocaine and reduces the use of the drug.[55] The development of a cocaine vaccine by Kosten[51] shows promising effects in forming an antibody response to reduce craving and cocaine use.

Psychostimulants

Like with other drugs of abuse, dopamine, serotonin, noradrenergic, γ-aminobutyric acid, endocannabinoids, glutamate, and opioid mechanisms of addiction to psychostimulants have been proposed.[56] However, in human trials, there are no effective therapeutic medical interventions for the treatment of psychostimulant addiction. Sustaining treatment and preventing relapse are enormously difficult, especially in cases involving methamphetamine. The main use of antidepressants is to control the depression that accompanies the withdrawal of psychostimulants. Bupropion (Wellbrutrin, Wellbutrin SR, Wellbutrin XL) has been found to be somewhat effective in nonheavy users.[56,57] Similarly, mirtazapine (Remeron) was able to reduce methamphetamine withdrawal symptoms independent of its effects on depression.[58] Aripiprazole (Abilify), a D2 partial agonist, has also been found to reduce methamphetamine withdrawal symptoms while simultaneously decreasing the effects of its use.[59,60] While all these are promising agents for detoxification from psychostimulants, specifically methamphetamine, continued research and surveillance will be required to improve outcomes.

SUMMARY

Trends related to use, abuse, social perception, and policies on addictions, like the neurobiology of psychoactive substance abuse, are constantly evolving. Addiction to substances of abuse is a psychiatric disorder with neurologic complications that affect many individuals in the general population. Different theories concerning the neurobiological aspects of addiction have been reviewed with special attention to dysregulation of the reward circuit and the inhibitory control system within the corticobasal ganglia-thalamocortical pathways. The behavioral neuroanatomy and behavioral neurochemistry of these pathways have direct implications for treatment. The most recent pharmacotherapy with various modes of action has been presented for some of the most common substances of abuse as part of a comprehensive treatment program.

REFERENCES

1. Sampson PD, Streissguth AP, Bookstein FL, et al. Incidence of fetal alcohol syndrome and prevalence of alcohol-related neurodevelopmental disorder. Teratology 1997;56(5):317–26.
2. Stratton KR, Howe CJ, Battaglia FC. Fetal alcohol syndrome: diagnosis, epidemiology, prevention, and treatment. Washington, DC: National Academy Press; 1996.
3. Sokol RJ, Delaney-Black V, Nordstrom B. Fetal alcohol spectrum disorder. JAMA 2003;290(22):2996–9.
4. Carlen PL, McAndrews MP, Weiss RT, et al. Alcohol-related dementia in the institutionalized elderly. Alcohol Clin Exp Res 1994;18(6):1330–4.
5. Torvik A. Wernicke's encephalopathy—prevalence and clinical spectrum. Alcohol Alcohol Suppl 1991;1:381–4.
6. Hingson RW, Zha W, Weitzman ER. Magnitude of and trends in alcohol-related mortality and morbidity among U.S. college students ages 18–24, 1998–2005. J Stud Alcohol Drugs Suppl 2009;(16):12–20.
7. Nida. Nida epidemiologic trends in drug abuse. In: proceedings of the Community Epidemiology Work Group: highlights and executive summary, U.S.D.o.-H.a.H. Service, editor. 2008. National Institutes of Health.
8. Kliegman RM, Madurra D, Kiwi R, et al. Relation of maternal cocaine use to the risks of prematurity and low birth weight. J Pediatr 1994;124(5 Pt 1):751–6.
9. Singer L, Arendt R, Song LY, et al. Direct and indirect interactions of cocaine with childbirth outcomes. Arch Pediatr Adolesc Med 1994;148(9):959–64.
10. Qureshi AI, Suri MF, Guterman LR, et al. Cocaine use and the likelihood of nonfatal myocardial infarction and stroke: data from the Third National Health and Nutrition Examination Survey. Circulation 2001;103(4):502–6.
11. Westover AN, McBride S, Haley RW. Stroke in young adults who abuse amphetamines or cocaine: a population-based study of hospitalized patients. Arch Gen Psychiatry 2007;64(4):495–502.
12. Nanda A, Vannemreddy P, Willis B, et al. Stroke in the young: relationship of active cocaine use with stroke mechanism and outcome. Acta Neurochir Suppl 2006;96:91–6.
13. Association AP. Diagnostic and statistical manual of mental disorders. 4th edition. Washington, DC: American Psychiatic Association; 2000.
14. Angrist B, Sathananthan G, Wilk S, et al. Amphetamine psychosis: behavioral and biochemical aspects. J Psychiatr Res 1974;11:13–23.
15. Fitzgerald JL, Reid JJ. Effects of methylenedioxymethamphetamine on the release of monoamines from rat brain slices. Eur J Pharmacol 1990;191(2):217–20.
16. Snyder SH. The dopamine hypothesis of schizophrenia: focus on the dopamine receptor. Am J Psychiatry 1976;133(2):197–202.
17. Kollins SH, MacDonald EK, Rush CR. Assessing the abuse potential of methylphenidate in nonhuman and human subjects: a review. Pharmacol Biochem Behav 2001;68(3):611–27.

18. Gaoni Y, Mechoulam R. Isolation, structure, and partial synthesis of an active constituent of hashish. J Am Chem Soc 2002;86(8):1646–7.
19. Martin BR, Wiley JL. Mechanism of action of cannabinoids: how it may lead to treatment of cachexia, emesis, and pain. J Support Oncol 2004;2(4):305–14 [discussion: 314–6].
20. Adams IB, Martin BR. Cannabis: pharmacology and toxicology in animals and humans. Addiction 1996;91(11):1585–614.
21. Gold MS, Miller NS, Jonas JM. Cocaine (and crack): neurobiology. In: Lowinson JH, Ruiz P, Millman RB, editors. Substance abuse: a comprehensive textbook. Baltimore (MD): Williams & Wilkins; 1992.
22. Tabakoff B, Hoffman PL. Alcohol: neurobiology. In: Lowinson JH, Ruiz P, Millman RB, editors. Substance abuse: a comprehensive textbook. Baltimore (MD): Williams & Wilkins; 1992.
23. Ungerleider TJ, Pechnick RN. Hallucinogens. In: Lowinson JH, Ruiz P, Millman RB, editors. Substance abuse: a comprehensive textbook. Baltimore (MD): Williams & Wilkins; 1992.
24. Balfour DJ. The effects of nicotine on brain neurotransmitter systems. Pharmacol Ther 1982;16(2):269–82.
25. Lipman AJ, Jackson KC. Opioid pharmacotherapy. In: Warfield C, Bajwa Z, editors. Principles and practice of pain medicine. New York: McGraw Hill Publishers; 2004. p. 583–600.
26. Zukin SR, Zukin RS. Phencyclidine. In: Lowinson LH, Ruiz P, Millman RB, editors. Substance abuse: a comprehensive textbook. Baltimore (MD): Williams & Wilkins; 1992.
27. Flanagan RJ, Ruprah M, Meredith TJ, et al. An introduction to the clinical toxicology of volatile substances. Drug Saf 1990;5(5):359–83.
28. Koob GF, Kenneth Lloyd G, Mason BJ. Development of pharmacotherapies for drug addiction: a Rosetta stone approach. Nat Rev Drug Discov 2009;8(6):500–15.
29. Kalivas PW, McFarland K. Brain circuitry and the reinstatement of cocaine-seeking behavior. Psychopharmacology (Berl) 2003;168(1–2):44–56.
30. Nestler EJ. Molecular neurobiology of addiction. Am J Addict 2001;10(3):201–17.
31. De Witte P, Littleton J, Parot P, et al. Neuroprotective and abstinence-promoting effects of acamprosate: elucidating the mechanism of action. CNS Drugs 2005;19(6):517–37.
32. Swift R. Emerging approaches to managing alcohol dependence. Am J Health Syst Pharm 2007;64(5 Suppl 3):S12–22.
33. Fuller RK, Branchey L, Brightwell DR, et al. Disulfiram treatment of alcoholism. A Veterans Administration cooperative study. JAMA 1986;256(11):1449–55.
34. Anton RF. Naltrexone for the management of alcohol dependence. N Engl J Med 2008;359(7):715–21.
35. Garbutt JC, Kranzler HR, O'Malley SS, et al. Efficacy and tolerability of long-acting injectable naltrexone for alcohol dependence: a randomized controlled trial. JAMA 2005;293(13):1617–25.
36. Mason BJ. Acamprosate for alcohol dependence: an update for the clinician. Focus 2006;4(4):505–11.
37. Anton RF, O'Malley SS, Ciraulo DA, et al. Combined pharmacotherapies and behavioral interventions for alcohol dependence: the COMBINE study: a randomized controlled trial. JAMA 2006;295(17):2003–17.
38. Besson J, Aeby F, Kasas A, et al. Combined efficacy of acamprosate and disulfiram in the treatment of alcoholism: a controlled study. Alcohol Clin Exp Res 1998;22(3):573–9.

39. George DT, Rawlings R, Eckardt MJ, et al. Buspirone treatment of alcoholism: age of onset, and cerebrospinal fluid 5-hydroxyindolacetic acid and homovanillic acid concentrations, but not medication treatment, predict return to drinking. Alcohol Clin Exp Res 1999;23(2):272–8.

40. Lejoyeux M. Use of serotonin (5-hydroxytryptamine) reuptake inhibitors in the treatment of alcoholism. Alcohol Alcohol Suppl 1996;1:69–75.

41. Johnson BA, Ait-Daoud N, Prihoda TJ. Combining ondansetron and naltrexone effectively treats biologically predisposed alcoholics: from hypotheses to preliminary clinical evidence. Alcohol Clin Exp Res 2000;24(5):737–42.

42. Sellers EM, Toneatto T, Romach MK, et al. Clinical efficacy of the 5-HT3 antagonist ondansetron in alcohol abuse and dependence. Alcohol Clin Exp Res 1994; 18(4):879–85.

43. Johnson BA, Rosenthal N, Capece JA, et al. Improvement of physical health and quality of life of alcohol-dependent individuals with topiramate treatment: US multisite randomized controlled trial. Arch Intern Med 2008;168(11):1188–99.

44. Heroin Abuse and Addiction. National Institute on Drug Abuse, U.S. Department of Health and Human Services. Rockville (MD): National Institutes of Health; 2000.

45. Kosten TR, Schottenfeld R, Ziedonis D, et al. Buprenorphine versus methadone maintenance for opioid dependence. J Nerv Ment Dis 1993;181(6):358–64.

46. Barnett PG, Rodgers JH, Bloch DA. A meta-analysis comparing buprenorphine to methadone for treatment of opiate dependence. Addiction 2001;96(5):683–90.

47. Mattick RP, Kimber J, Breen C, et al. Buprenorphine maintenance versus placebo or methadone maintenance for opioid dependence. Cochrane Database Syst Rev 2003;(2):CD002207.

48. Kleber HD, Riordan CE, Rounsaville B, et al. Clonidine in outpatient detoxification from methadone maintenance. Arch Gen Psychiatry 1985;42(4):391–4.

49. Gold MS, Redmond DE Jr, Kleber HD. Clonidine in opiate withdrawal. Lancet 1978;1(8070):929–30.

50. O'Connor PG, Carroll KM, Shi JM, et al. Three methods of opioid detoxification in a primary care setting. A randomized trial. Ann Intern Med 1997;127(7):526–30.

51. Kosten T. Pathophysiology and treatment of cocaine dependence, the fifth generation of progress. In: Davis KL, Charney DS, Coyle JT, et al, editors. Neuropsychopharmacology. Baltimore (MD): Lippincott, Williams & Wilkins; 2002. p. 1461–75.

52. Grabowski J, Rhoades H, Schmitz J, et al. Dextroamphetamine for cocaine-dependence treatment: a double-blind randomized clinical trial. J Clin Psychopharmacol 2001;21(5):522–6.

53. Grabowski J, Roache JD, Schmitz JM, et al. Replacement medication for cocaine dependence: methylphenidate. J Clin Psychopharmacol 1997;17(6):485–8.

54. Anderson AL, Reid MS, Li SH, et al. Modafinil for the treatment of cocaine dependence. Drug Alcohol Depend 2009;104(1–2):133–9.

55. Carroll KM, Fenton LR, Ball SA, et al. Efficacy of disulfiram and cognitive behavior therapy in cocaine-dependent outpatients: a randomized placebo-controlled trial. Arch Gen Psychiatry 2004;61(3):264–72.

56. Elkashef AM, Rawson RA, Anderson AL, et al. Bupropion for the treatment of methamphetamine dependence. Neuropsychopharmacology 2008;33(5): 1162–70.

57. Reichel CM, Murray JE, Grant KM, et al. Bupropion attenuates methamphetamine self-administration in adult male rats. Drug Alcohol Depend 2009;100(1–2): 54–62.

58. Kongsakon R, Papadopoulos KI, Saguansiritham R. Mirtazapine in amphetamine detoxification: a placebo-controlled pilot study. Int Clin Psychopharmacol 2005; 20(5):253–6.
59. Newton TF, Reid MS, De La Garza R, et al. Evaluation of subjective effects of aripiprazole and methamphetamine in methamphetamine-dependent volunteers. Int J Neuropsychopharmacol 2008;11(8):1037–45.
60. Bergman J. Medications for stimulant abuse: agonist-based strategies and preclinical evaluation of the mixed-action D-sub-2 partial agonist aripiprazole (Abilify). Exp Clin Psychopharmacol 2008;16(6):475–83.

Neurotoxicity of Radiation Therapy

Edward J. Dropcho, MD[a,b,]*

KEYWORDS

- Radiation adverse effects • Brain neoplasms • Myelopathy
- Brachial plexopathy • Lumbosacral plexopathy

Therapeutic irradiation can cause significant injury to any part of the central or peripheral nervous systems. This review will discuss the neurotoxicity of radiation therapy according to the affected anatomic site, including brain, cranial nerves, spinal cord, and nerve plexuses.

ACUTE ENCEPHALOPATHY

Brain injury by radiation therapy (RT) has traditionally been classified according to its time of onset into acute, early delayed, and late forms. The acute reaction to fractionated RT usually occurs during the first several days of treatment and consists of headache, nausea, fever, somnolence, and worsening of preexisting focal symptoms. Acute RT encephalopathy tends to occur more frequently and to be more severe among patients with increased intracranial pressure. Acute toxicity occurs in approximately 5% of patients within a few days following stereotactic radiosurgery for brain metastases or other tumors, consisting of headache, seizures, and/or temporary worsening of focal neurologic symptoms. Acute toxicity generally responds well to increased doses of dexamethasone.

EARLY DELAYED ENCEPHALOPATHY

"Early delayed" encephalopathy is a broad designation referring to reversible clinical and/or radiographic worsening occurring from a few weeks up to several months after brain irradiation. This includes a number of clinical scenarios, which may have differing pathophysiologies.

The "somnolence syndrome" occurs in about one-half of children given whole-brain RT for a primary tumor or leukemia prophylaxis. The syndrome is probably more frequent and more severe in children younger than 3 years. It occurs 3 to 8 weeks after

[a] Department of Neurology, Indiana University Medical Center, CL 292, Indianapolis, IN 46202, USA
[b] Neuro-Oncology Program, Indiana University Simon Cancer Center, Indianapolis, IN 46202, USA
* Department of Neurology, Indiana University Medical Center, CL 292, Indianapolis, IN 46202.
E-mail address: edropcho@iupui.edu

Neurol Clin 28 (2010) 217–234
doi:10.1016/j.ncl.2009.09.008
0733-8619/09/$ – see front matter © 2010 Elsevier Inc. All rights reserved.

completion of RT and consists of drowsiness, nausea, and irritability, and less commonly fever or transient papilledema. Symptoms resolve completely within 3 to 6 weeks. Corticosteroids hasten recovery and may also prevent the syndrome if given during the course of RT.

The syndrome of "pseudoprogression" occurs in up to 25% of patients with glioblastoma within the first 2 months after completion of standard 6000 cGy fractionated RT and concurrent daily temozolomide chemotherapy.[1] MRI scans show worsening contrast enhancement and/or "edema"; some patients have worsening neurologic symptoms. The clinical and radiographic changes generally improve over a few months; a minority of patients develop definite RT necrosis (see the following section). The pathophysiology of pseudoprogression is not clear, but it is likely a result of an interaction between RT and temozolomide, as the incidence of this syndrome seems considerably higher compared with patients who receive RT alone. The practical clinical difficulty is distinguishing pseudoprogression from true early tumor progression.

Within 3 to 9 months following stereotactic radiosurgery for primary or metastatic brain tumors, 5% to 25% of patients develop symptomatic or asymptomatic radiographic worsening (increased contrast enhancement and increased edema).[2] Patients with parasagittal meningioma seem to have a special predilection for developing this complication.[3] Most patients subsequently show clinical and radiographic improvement over the subsequent few months. Dexamethasone is generally effective in improving symptoms.

A relatively unusual sequel to RT for gliomas in adults is the development within 6 to 36 months of multifocal patchy or spotty enhancing MRI lesions, within the RT ports but often not immediately adjacent to the surgical cavity margins.[4] The lesions are either asymptomatic or associated with worsening focal deficits. They have a variable course, including spontaneous resolution over several months, stabilization, appearance of new lesions together with resolution of others, or (rarely) progression to focal necrosis.

Multifocal MRI lesions may also occur in children after RT for medulloblastoma or other tumors, especially when RT is combined with high-dose or intensified systemic chemotherapy.[5,6] The lesions generally appear 6 to 12 months after RT. Up to one-half of patients have accompanying neurologic symptoms. In most patients, the clinical and radiographic changes resolve over several months, although a few patients are left with significant permanent neurologic deficits.

FOCAL CEREBRAL NECROSIS

Focal cerebral radiation necrosis can occur after treatment of primary or metastatic brain tumors, or following incidental irradiation of the brain during treatment of extraneural tumors such as pituitary adenoma, nasopharyngeal carcinoma,[7] or skull base tumors.[8] Among patients with glioblastoma or anaplastic glioma who receive standard fractionated external beam RT (6000 cGy in daily fractions of 180–200 cGy), the actuarial incidence of focal necrosis is 10% to 15% in persons surviving at least 12 months after diagnosis.[9] The risk of RT necrosis increases with higher total RT doses, and with larger daily RT fractions.

Focal brain necrosis can also occur after "nonstandard" forms of RT, including hyperfractionated RT, proton beam or heavy-particle RT, interstitial brachytherapy, and stereotactic radiosurgery. Symptomatic focal brain necrosis occurs in 2% to 5% of patients treated with stereotactic radiosurgery ("gamma knife") for brain metastases.[10] Symptomatic cystic lesions or focal necrosis requiring surgery occur in 4% to 5% of patients following radiosurgery for an arteriovenous malformation.[11,12] The risk of necrosis increases with RT dose and target volume. There are anecdotal reports of focal necrosis following radiosurgical thalamotomy or pallidotomy for Parkinson disease.[13]

The histopathology of focal radiation necrosis features predominant involvement of white matter, with relative sparing of cerebral cortex and deep gray matter structures. In addition to confluent foci of coagulative necrosis, there is variable demyelination, loss of oligodendrocytes, axonal loss, focal calcifications, fibrillary gliosis, and scattered perivascular infiltrates of mononuclear cells. A nearly constant feature is extensive vascular injury, most commonly seen as fibrinoid necrosis of vessel walls, hyaline thickening of vessel walls, thrombotic occlusion of small vessels, and formation of telangiectasias.

The interval between completion of standard fractionated RT and the clinical onset of cerebral necrosis ranges from a few months to more than 5 years, with a peak onset around 12 to 15 months.[9] The clinical presentation of focal RT necrosis is that of a subacute space-occupying lesion, which is nonspecific and in brain tumor patients is indistinguishable from tumor recurrence or progression. Standard CT or MR scans show a mass lesion with a combination of edema and patchy or ring enhancement. Small series have attempted to identify imaging features that could reliably distinguish RT necrosis from tumor recurrence,[14,15] but these have not been validated in larger studies. Definitive diagnosis of RT necrosis requires pathologic confirmation, although the frequent intermingling of areas of tumor cells (glioma or brain metastasis) with areas of necrosis creates the possibility of sampling error from a stereotactic biopsy.[16,17]

Other neuroimaging techniques may be useful in diagnosing RT necrosis after fractionated RT or stereotactic radiosurgery for gliomas or brain metastases. On fluorodeoxyglucose positron-emission tomography (FDG-PET) scans, recurrent anaplastic glioma or brain metastasis is generally hypermetabolic, whereas focal necrosis is usually hypometabolic.[18,19] Methionine-PET scanning may have better specificity than FDG-PET, but it is not generally available. With MR spectroscopy, elevated choline:creatine ratios and choline: N-aspartyl acetate (NAA) ratios are more indicative of tumor than RT necrosis.[20–22] The diagnostic cutoff values for these ratios vary somewhat among the published studies. On diffusion-weighted MRI, recurrent tumor tends to have a lower apparent diffusion coefficient (ADC) than necrosis.[22] On perfusion MRI, tumor usually has a higher relative cerebral blood volume (rCBV) than necrosis.[17] Some published studies used more than one imaging modality to improve the overall diagnostic reliability. Each of these techniques has fairly good reliability, particularly in cases of "pure" RT necrosis or "pure" recurrent tumor, but each has false positives and false negatives. Their ability to distinguish recurrent tumor from RT necrosis is often limited by spatial resolution, partial volume effect, and/or the frequent intermingling of tumor cells (glioma or brain metastasis) and radiation-induced changes. There are also some inherent limitations, such as instances of proven RT necrosis being hypermetabolic on FDG-PET, or having elevated choline: creatine and choline: NAA ratios.

Dexamethasone usually produces clinical and sometimes radiographic improvement in patients with focal RT necrosis. In most cases this improvement is temporary or patients become steroid-dependent, but some patients maintain their improvement even after steroids are discontinued.[9] There are anecdotal reports of clinical and radiographic improvement in patients treated with warfarin, hyperbaric oxygen,[23] vitamin E, or pentoxifylline. There are recent reports of improvement, sometimes striking, in patients treated with bevacizumab, a monoclonal antibody against vascular endothelial growth factor (VEGF), which acts to decrease vascular permeability and normalize the blood-brain barrier.[24] Surgical debulking of necrotic brain tissue may help patients who do not show adequate response to conservative measures and who have a focal accessible mass lesion. Some patients with focal RT necrosis continue to deteriorate despite surgical debulking because of progressive necrosis adjacent to the original site.

DIFFUSE CEREBRAL INJURY IN ADULTS

The most frequent neurotoxic effect of cranial RT at any patient age is not focal necrosis but diffuse cerebral injury. For adults with glioblastoma or other malignant primary brain tumors, only a small minority survives long enough for delayed diffuse cerebral injury to become an issue. Among anaplastic glioma patients surviving longer than 18 to 24 months, serial CT or MR scans in the majority show diffuse cortical atrophy, ventricular dilatation, and signal abnormalities in the hemispheric white matter. These neuroimaging abnormalities may progressively worsen over time. The radiographic changes are more severe with higher RT doses, with larger volumes of brain irradiated, and with increasing patient age.

Some anaplastic glioma survivors with these radiographic abnormalities develop moderate to severe neurocognitive deficits not attributable to direct tumor effects. The most severely affected patients are disabled by progressive dementia and gait disturbance. Patients older than 50 years of age at diagnosis are more likely to develop severe neuroimaging changes and significant cognitive impairment than younger patients.

Radiation-induced diffuse cerebral injury is perhaps a more important issue for low-grade gliomas, because at the time of initial diagnosis most patients are young adults with a high level of neurologic function, and an anticipated survival of at least several years. Following RT for low-grade glioma, most patients develop some degree of cerebral atrophy and hemispheric white matter changes on serial MR scans.[25,26] The severity of radiographic changes correlates with the volume of brain irradiated and with the total radiation dose. Most patients with these radiographic changes do not have obvious clinical deficits. The few published studies of serial neuropsychologic testing of "long-term" low-grade glioma survivors show conflicting results as to whether radiation causes significant neurocognitive deficits.[25,27–30] The published studies are generally flawed by heterogeneity of RT, incomplete patient follow-up, and short periods of follow-up. There is a rough correlation between the severity of radiographic abnormalities and the severity of clinical neuropsychologic deficits.[26,30] The incidence and severity of neurocognitive deficits are probably worse in older patients, and in patients who receive a higher total radiation dose, a higher daily radiation dose fraction, or radiation to a large brain volume.

Delayed neurotoxicity is a serious consideration in the treatment of patients with primary CNS lymphoma. Current treatment generally includes whole-brain RT (usually 4,000 cGy) and chemotherapy including high-dose methotrexate. Up to 25% of 5-year survivors develop a disabling syndrome of progressive dementia, gait instability/apraxia, and urinary incontinence.[31] MRI scans show diffuse atrophy and white matter signal abnormalities. Patients with neurotoxicity often have a shortened survival despite no recurrence of the tumor. Autopsy shows prominent and diffuse myelin loss, pallor, and gliosis in the hemispheric white matter.[32] Some cases additionally have small vessel disease. Most but not all series show a correlation between increasing patient age and a higher risk of neurotoxicity. There is disagreement as to whether reducing or omitting whole-brain RT in patients who achieve a complete remission to initial high-dose methotrexate would reduce the risk of delayed neurotoxicity without compromising tumor outcome.

Whole-brain RT given for treatment or prophylaxis of brain metastases rarely causes focal necrosis but can cause diffuse brain injury. Up to one-half of patients with brain metastases who survive more than 1 year after 3000 to 4000 cGy develop changes on serial CT or MR scans including diffuse cerebral atrophy, ventricular enlargement, and signal abnormalities in the hemispheric white matter.[33] Most patients with these neuro-imaging changes do not develop gross neurologic deficits or cognitive impairment, although there are few studies of detailed serial neuropsychologic examinations. A small proportion of long-term survivors with brain metastases develop progressive dementia, psychomotor retardation, gait disturbance, and urinary incontinence appearing 6 to 18 months after whole-brain RT. The clinical similarity of this syndrome to normal pressure hydrocephalus has led some patients to undergo ventriculo-peritoneal cerebrospinal fluid (CSF) shunting, which can produce partial improvement in some patients. To date, there is no reliable way to predict which patients would benefit from a shunt.[34]

Prophylactic whole-brain RT significantly reduces the incidence of brain metastases in patients with small cell lung carcinoma who have a complete response to initial systemic treatment.[35] Recent studies have shown significant neuropsychologic impairment in some long-term survivors after prophylactic RT, but the overall incidence and severity of deficits do not exceed those in patients who never received RT.[35,36] Severe cognitive impairment is more likely to occur in patients who receive high daily dose RT fractions and/or concomitant systemic chemotherapy during prophylactic RT.[37]

Drugs including methylphenidate, modafinil, and donepezil have recently been used in an effort to improve patients' cognitive functioning after RT for anaplastic glioma or brain metastases. To date, most studies have been small and uncontrolled, with mixed results.[38]

DIFFUSE CEREBRAL INJURY IN CHILDREN

The developing brain is clearly more sensitive to irradiation than the adult brain. Prospective studies have consistently found mean full-scale IQ scores to be at least 10 points below normal among disease-free survivors of childhood medulloblastoma or other primary brain tumors who received whole-brain RT.[39,40] This is believed to be because of deficits in the "core functions" of memory, attention, and processing speed. IQ scores often continue to decline over several years, as children fall farther behind in the acquisition of cognitive skills. Survivors whose full-scale IQ still lies in the normal range commonly have neurobehavioral problems and learning disabilities, including maladaptive behavior, attention-deficit disorders, visual perceptual difficulties, impaired fine motor coordination, poor school performance, and the need for special education.[41]

Among children who receive whole-brain RT for medulloblastoma or other brain tumors, the two main factors that determine the severity of cognitive impairment are the RT dose and the age when RT is administered. Cognitive decline is more frequent and more severe in children given whole-brain RT at a younger age, especially before 3 years of age.[42,43] These children have average declines of 20 to 25 points in full-scale IQ and are much more likely to have IQ scores below 80 than are older children. Reduction in the dose of craniospinal axis RT and in the size of the posterior fossa "boost volume" probably reduces but does not eliminate significant long-term neurocognitive deficits.[44,45] Younger children remain at higher risk of neurotoxicity, even with reduced RT doses.

Standard diagnostic CT or MRI scans show diffuse cerebral atrophy and signal abnormalities in hemispheric white matter in up to one-half of children with primary brain tumors following 2500- to 4000-cGy whole-brain RT. A distinctive pattern called "mineralizing microangiopathy" also occurs in up to one-third of patients, consisting of calcifications in the basal ganglia, dentate nuclei, and cerebral gray-white matter junction. More recent neuroimaging techniques have provided further insight. Quantitative MR imaging demonstrates a dose-dependent reduction in the development of normal-appearing white matter in children after whole-brain RT.[46,47] These changes are more severe in children irradiated at a younger age. The reduction in normal-appearing white matter is correlated with decline in IQ scores.[46] Other quantitative MR studies of medulloblastoma survivors showed decreased volume of the corpus callosum, reduced thickness of the cerebral cortex, and reduction in hippocampal volume development. Diffusion tensor imaging shows diminished fractional anisotropy in normal-appearing white matter, reflecting microscopic damage. The frontal lobe white matter may be selectively more affected than parietal lobe.[48] Reduction in fractional anisotropy correlates with decline in full-scale IQ scores in medulloblastoma survivors.[49]

Significant cognitive impairment and learning disabilities are less common and less severe among children who receive RT to a limited brain target rather than to the whole brain. Impaired intellectual function may still occur after limited-field RT directed at the cerebral hemisphere, diencephalon, or posterior fossa.[43,50] There is increasing evidence of cognitive dysfunction in children after treatment of cerebellar tumors.[51]

Prophylactic whole-brain RT (1200–2400 cGy) and intrathecal methotrexate given to children with acute lymphoblastic leukemia (ALL) each carry a significant risk of producing diffuse cerebral injury. Modern treatment protocols for ALL generally omit whole-brain RT and rely on intrathecal and systemic chemotherapy for central nervous system (CNS) prophylaxis, except in the minority of children (<20%) who are at high risk for CNS relapse.[52] A very small number of ALL patients develop a devastating delayed leukoencephalopathy, most likely caused by a synergistic neurotoxic effect of RT and methotrexate. With that exception, ALL survivors generally have less severe radiographic and clinical signs of neurocognitive toxicity than children with primary brain tumors, presumably because of lower doses (or omission) of whole-brain RT.

The full-scale IQ scores of ALL survivors often remain in the average range, but are either less than the IQ of "controls" or show a decline on serial testing.[53,54] Children may have significant neuropsychologic dysfunction and learning disabilities despite IQ scores in the average range. There is a rough correlation between the whole-brain RT dose and the incidence and severity of neurocognitive toxicity, although significant toxicity has been reported in "chemotherapy-only" protocols. Early age at ALL diagnosis is generally associated with a higher risk of significant cognitive impairment. Several studies have also shown female gender to be an independent predictor of worse neurocognitive outcome.

Standard MRI scans show diffuse cerebral "atrophy" and/or white matter signal changes in a minority of ALL children following CNS prophylaxis.[55] In some patients the radiographic changes actually improve on subsequent scans. Presence of neuroimaging changes on standard MRI does not correlate very well with the results of neuropsychologic testing. In contrast, quantitative MRI in ALL survivors shows a correlation between reduced volume of normal-appearing white matter and worse deficits in IQ scores, attention, and academic performance.[56] These radiographic changes and neurocognitive outcomes are generally worse in children who received whole-brain RT than those who did not.

Methylphenidate has recently been shown to improve attention problems in survivors of childhood brain tumors or leukemia.[57] The impact this may have on children's academic achievement is not yet clear.

CEREBROVASCULAR DISEASE

Stenosis or occlusion of the extracranial or intracranial cerebral arteries can occur after RT given for tumors of the neck, head, or brain.[58,59] Transient ischemic attacks or cerebral infarcts usually occur at least 5 to 10 years after RT, but shorter latent periods are possible. Angiography shows stenosis or occlusion, often multifocal, of one or more major arteries lying within the RT ports. The pathology of RT-induced large-vessel disease resembles "ordinary" atherosclerosis. Many of the reported patients had hyperlipidemia. Endothelium is believed to be the primary site of injury, with a possible additional factor of injury to the vasa vasorum. Carotid endarterectomy is often made difficult by a lengthy span of diseased artery, and scarring of periarterial tissues, but the reported morbidity is fairly low.[60] Carotid angioplasty and stenting may be a reasonable alternative to endarterectomy.[61] There are no reliable data addressing the relative long-term merits of surgery, stenting, antiplatelet agents, statins, or anticoagulation for these patients.

RT-induced vasculopathy often takes the form of moyamoya syndrome following irradiation of the circle of Willis during early childhood, usually for optic pathway or hypothalamic glioma, craniopharyngioma, or other suprasellar tumor.[58,62] Children with type 1 neurofibromatosis treated for optic pathway glioma are at especially high risk for developing this complication.[63,64] The latent period from RT to diagnosis of moyamoya syndrome is usually 5 years or less. Clinical manifestations include multiple strokes, recurrent transient ischemic attacks, headache, seizures, and progressive cognitive impairment. The vascular pathology resembles that of idiopathic or "primary" moyamoya syndrome and features intimal fibrosis and marked proliferation of endothelial and myointimal cells, without inflammation or much atheroma. Patients may benefit from a surgical revascularization procedure.[58,62,64]

The development of one or more intracranial cavernous angiomas is an increasingly recognized sequel to cranial RT during childhood. The cumulative incidence is at least 5% within 10 years after RT.[65,66] Symptomatic intracranial hemorrhage is uncommon, but the lesions may slowly expand and become symptomatic over time.

Other unusual cerebrovascular disorders may occur as late effects of cranial RT. Multiple lacunar lesions may occur within 5 years after RT in children, especially if RT is given before 5 years of age.[67] The lesions are usually clinically silent and not correlated with strokelike events or cognitive decline. Focal intratumoral hemorrhage may occur after stereotactic radiosurgery for brain metastases, especially with melanoma.[68] A syndrome resembling complicated migraine, with unilateral headache and reversible focal deficits, may occur 1 to 20 years after cranial RT in children or adults.[69,70]

RADIATION-INDUCED CENTRAL NERVOUS SYSTEM TUMORS

Radiation-induced intracranial tumors most commonly occur in survivors of childhood medulloblastoma, other brain tumors, or leukemia.[71] Among 14,000 survivors of childhood cancer who received brain RT, the relative risk of developing subsequent meningioma was increased by nearly 10-fold, and the risk of glioma by nearly 7-fold.[72] Most gliomas occurred within 5 years after the initial RT, whereas the latency time for meningiomas was at least 15 years in two-thirds of cases. There was a significant relationship between the dose of cranial RT and the incidence of subsequent glioma or meningioma. In another study of 2000 survivors of childhood ALL, the cumulative incidence of subsequent glioma or meningioma was 5% at 30 years.[73] Glioma and meningioma are the most common nonhematologic tumors occurring as second neoplasms in survivors of childhood ALL. The incidence of secondary brain tumors in leukemia survivors is expected to decline as fewer patients receive whole-brain RT for CNS prophylaxis.[74]

Long-term follow-up series of patients who received fractionated RT for pituitary adenoma show a cumulative incidence of RT-induced tumor of 2% to 3% at 15 to 20 years.[75,76] Gliomas and meningiomas are roughly equally represented.

There are reports of glioma (mainly glioblastoma) occurring within the field of stereo-tactic radiosurgery given for meningioma, vestibular schwannoma, arteriovenous malformation, or other lesions.[77,78]

RT-induced meningiomas do not show any unusual distribution of histologic subtypes, but they are more likely to be multiple, to show histologic anaplasia, and to recur after surgery compared with "sporadic" meningiomas.[79,80] Approximately 50% of RT-induced gliomas are glioblastoma and another 25% are anaplastic astrocytoma. Up to 10% of the gliomas are multifocal.[81] There are no distinctive histologic features of RT-induced gliomas, and no striking differences in clinical behavior as compared with malignant gliomas in general.

Sarcoma of the skull base, calvarium, or dura is a rare complication of RT for primary brain tumors, pituitary tumors, or leukemia prophylaxis.[82] Tumors include osteosarcoma, fibrosarcoma, or malignant fibrous histiocytoma. Clinical outcome is poor.

CRANIAL NERVE INJURY

Radiation injury to the optic nerve and chiasm most often occurs in patients treated for tumors of the orbit, paranasal sinus, nasopharynx, pituitary adenoma, or craniopharyngioma,[83] or less commonly following whole-brain RT for primary or metastatic brain tumors. In most reported patients, the optic nerve exposure after fractionated RT was 5000 cGy or more.[84] Optic neuropathy may also occur after stereotactic radiosurgery for treatment of pituitary adenoma or meningioma.[85] Radiation-induced optic neuropathy generally presents within 12 to 18 months of RT as subacute painless monocular or binocular loss of acuity and/or visual field deficits.[83,84] MRI scanning shows patchy enhancement of one or both optic nerves and occasionally of the optic chiasm.[86] The optic nerves may also be slightly enlarged. Most patients with radiation optic neuropathy deteriorate rapidly over several weeks and are left with irreversible, severe vision loss and optic atrophy. Partial spontaneous improvement occurs in a small minority. There are anecdotal reports of partial improvement with corticosteroids, warfarin, or hyperbaric oxygen, although most patients do not respond to any treatment.[86]

Second to optic neuropathy, hypoglossal palsy is the most frequent RT-induced cranial neuropathy, occurring 2 to 10 years after treatment of primary head and neck tumors.[87] The probable mechanism is entrapment of the nerve by fibrosis. Less common is unilateral palsy of the vagus nerve, spinal accessory nerve, or multiple lower cranial nerve palsies. Some patients with "RT-induced bulbar palsy" have myokymia or complex repetitive electromyogram (EMG) discharges in multiple muscles innervated by the lower cranial nerves.[88,89] Cranial nerves III-VII are relatively resistant to damage by fractionated photon RT, but may be injured by stereotactic radiosurgery or proton beam RT for vestibular schwannoma, skull base meningioma, or pituitary adenoma.[90] Hearing loss is a common complication of cranial RT but is generally due to a conductive loss or to cochlear damage rather than injury to the auditory nerve itself.

MYELOPATHY

Radiation-induced spinal cord injury most often occurs after "incidental" irradiation of the spinal cord as part of treatment for an extraneural primary tumor, and less often among patients in whom the spinal cord itself is targeted in treatment of a glioma or as part of craniospinal axis RT for medulloblastoma. The most common form of radiation myelopathy is a transient syndrome usually occurring within 4 to 6 months after treatment. This syndrome consists solely of paresthesias or "electric shock" sensations radiating down the spine (L'hermitte's phenomenon) and frequently extending down the limbs as well. These symptoms are often precipitated or worsened by neck flexion or physical exertion. MR scans are unrevealing. Transient radiation myelopathy is believed to be caused by demyelination of the posterior columns, but there is no neuropathologic proof of this. The syndrome resolves gradually over several months.

Delayed severe radiation myelopathy generally occurs 1 to 2 years after RT. Exceptional patients have latent intervals as short as 3 months or as long as 10 years. Delayed radiation myelopathy usually presents with numbness or dysesthesias in the legs, followed by weakness and sphincter dysfunction, with an upper level of cord dysfunction ascending to lie within the irradiated area. Pain is not a prominent complaint. In most patients the neurologic deficit progresses over weeks to months in a steady or (less commonly) stepwise fashion, leading to paraplegia or quadriplegia in at least 50% of patients. A few patients show partial spontaneous recovery, but it is rare for ambulation to be regained once it is lost.

MR scans in delayed radiation myelopathy usually show widening of the affected cord and abnormal signal intensity on T2-weighted images.[91] Most patients have abnormal intramedullary contrast enhancement, either in a streaky or less commonly a ring-enhancing pattern. The MR abnormalities often extend beyond the radiation ports and generally persist for several months, followed by spinal cord atrophy in long-term survivors.

Evidence from autopsied patients and from animal studies indicates that severe, delayed radiation myelopathy results from a combination of damage to small blood vessels and direct injury to glia and myelin; in individual patients, one or the other mechanism may predominate.[92] Coalescing foci of demyelination and axonal degeneration are accompanied by wallerian degeneration above and below the necrotic zones. There is a spectrum of severity of changes in small blood vessels, including fibrinoid necrosis of the vessel walls, hyaline thickening, and obliteration of lumens.

The incidence of delayed radiation myelopathy is less than 0.5% after a total dose of 4500 to 5000 cGy, and 5% after total doses of 5700 to 6100 cGy, when "standard" RT is given in once-daily fractions of 180 to 200 cGy.[93] The risk increases with higher total RT doses and/or larger daily RT fractions. There is no clear evidence indicating differential susceptibility of one region of the spinal cord versus another, nor is there a clear relationship between the length of spinal cord irradiated and the risk of delayed radiation myelopathy.[93] There are recent reports of radiation myelopathy occurring after stereotactic radiosurgery for primary or metastatic spinal tumors.[94,95] Delayed myelopathy has occurred after "safe" radiation doses in combination with high-dose or intensive chemotherapy regimens.[96,97]

Treatment options for patients with severe radiation myelopathy are very limited. Some patients show stabilization or partial improvement on corticosteroids. There are reports of partial improvement or stabilization following warfarin[98] or hyperbaric oxygen.[99,100]

BRACHIAL PLEXOPATHY

Breast carcinoma is the tumor most often associated with radiation brachial plexopathy, accounting for 40% to 75% of reported patients, followed by lung carcinoma and then by lymphoma.[101,102] Radiation-induced brachial plexopathy may rarely occur as a relatively mild reversible syndrome, or much more commonly as a delayed and progressive syndrome. Delayed radiation brachial plexopathy occurs after a latent interval varying from a few months up to more than 10 years, with peak onset of neurologic symptoms occurring 2 to 4 years after RT.[101] There is a rough correlation between the risk of delayed brachial plexopathy and the total dose of RT administered to the plexus. The tolerance dose or "safety threshold" for the brachial plexus is estimated to be 5600 cGy given in daily 200-cGy fractions.[103] The risk of delayed brachial plexopathy may be increased when large RT fields are used, when patients receive two separate courses of "subthreshold" RT, and possibly when patients receive concomitant chemotherapy plus RT.[103]

The exact pathophysiology of delayed RT injury to the brachial (or lumbosacral) plexus remains unclear. Extensive fibrosis within and surrounding nerve trunks of the plexus, with demyelination and loss of axons, are consistently present at surgery or autopsy. Most experimental animal studies implicate microvascular injury as the key event, although peripheral axons and myelin sheaths are also clearly susceptible to direct damage by irradiation.

Delayed RT brachial plexopathy generally presents with numbness and paresthesias of the hand and fingers, with weakness tending to develop later in the course.[101,102] The clinical presentation of radiation brachial plexopathy cannot be absolutely distinguished from that of brachial plexus metastasis, although the presence of Horner's syndrome and/or early and severe pain are strongly suggestive of brachial plexus metastasis.[101,102,104]

Needle EMG testing may be useful in diagnosing radiation brachial plexopathy, in that myokymia is present in one or more muscles in 50% to 70% of affected patients.[102,104] The number of myokymic discharges may vary considerably among muscles innervated by the same trunks and cords of the plexus. Myokymia is rarely if ever present in patients with brachial plexus metastases.

CT or MR scanning is often but not always useful in distinguishing between RT brachial plexopathy and plexus metastases.[104] Patients with RT plexopathy may have low or high signal intensities in the plexus on T2-weighted images, and some patients show gadolinium enhancement.[105] Some patients have no obvious tumor mass on MR scans and have changes read as "consistent with radiation injury," but later turn out to have plexus metastases. FDG-PET scanning may be useful in identifying metastatic breast cancer in or near the brachial plexus not clearly imaged by CT or MR scanning.[106]

In approximately two-thirds of patients with radiation brachial plexopathy, the motor and sensory deficits gradually worsen over several years to a level of severe neurologic disability, whereas other patients have a spontaneous cessation of progression after 1 to 3 years. Spontaneous recovery of neurologic function is highly unusual. In some patients the dysesthesias and pain diminish concurrently with worsening weakness, whereas other patients suffer from persistent or even increasing pain with progressive motor and sensory loss.

Treatment options for patients with RT brachial plexopathy are not very satisfactory. There are numerous anecdotal reports or small uncontrolled studies of surgical neurolysis, ie, opening the epineural sheath and resecting scar tissue, with or without placement of an omental flap to "revascularize" the plexus. Some patients had significant pain relief following surgery,[107] but there is very little information on patients' long-term course. Neurolysis rarely relieves motor or sensory deficits, and it is not clear whether it can halt the progression of deficits.[108] Surgery causes a significant deterioration in sensory or motor function in 20% to 50% of patients.[107] There are reports of long-lasting pain relief in patients with RT brachial plexopathy following dorsal root entry zone lesions[109] or chemical sympathectomy.[110] Warfarin was associated with neurologic improvement in a few patients.[111] A randomized trial of hyperbaric oxygen failed to show neurologic benefit.[112]

LUMBOSACRAL PLEXOPATHY AND POLYRADICULOPATHY

RT injury to the lumbosacral plexus or cauda equina most commonly occurs after treatment of pelvic tumors, testicular tumors, or tumors involving para-aortic lymph nodes.[113–115] Injury may occur after external beam photon therapy, interstitial or intracavitary radiation implants, or combined photon and proton beam RT.[115,116] Relatively mild, reversible lumbosacral plexopathy may rarely occur within a few months after RT.[117] Delayed, severe plexopathy occurs after a median latent interval of approximately 5 years.

Delayed RT-induced lumbosacral plexopathy usually presents as asymmetric bilateral leg weakness.[114] Weakness may involve any muscles innervated by L2 through S1 but often has an L5-S1 predominance. Atrophy, fasciculations, and loss of muscle stretch reflexes accompany the weakness. Pain eventually occurs in approximately one-half of patients, but is usually not early or severe. One-third of patients have early and prominent numbness and paresthesias. Bladder or bowel symptoms are unusual, and if present are often attributable to RT-induced proctitis or bladder fibrosis.

Delayed RT injury to the cauda equina can mimic lumbosacral plexopathy. Patients develop asymmetric bilateral leg weakness, and less often pain or sensory loss, more than 10 years after RT.[116,118,119] Radiation injury to the cauda equina overlaps with what was previously described as a selective lower motor neuron syndrome.[120]

Needle EMG in RT lumbosacral plexopathy shows scattered myokymic discharges in approximately 60% of patients.[114] In the limited published literature, CT or MRI scanning is mainly useful in detecting lumbosacral plexus metastases, showing lymphadenopathy, tumor masses, thickening of the plexus, and/or bone erosion.[121] Whether there is a distinctive MRI appearance of RT plexopathy is not clear. In patients who develop delayed lumbosacral polyradiculopathy, MRI scans may show patchy or multinodular enhancement along the conus medullaris and cauda equina.[118,119]

The most frequent course of RT lumosacral plexopathy is one of slow progression over months to years. A few patients have a more rapid tempo of progression, and a few show stabilization of neurologic deficits after a period of progression.[115] Exceptional patients have significant spontaneous resolution of weakness and sensory symptoms.[122] There are anecdotal responses to warfarin. In patients with a cauda equina syndrome the neurologic deficits eventually stabilize, or may continue to worsen slowly over years.[118,119]

SUMMARY

Clinicians need to be aware of the many ways in which radiation-induced neurotoxicity can manifest itself, so that they carry out the appropriate steps in differential diagnosis and management. Future efforts will hopefully refine the uses and techniques of therapeutic irradiation further, leading to improved efficacy and reduced toxicity.

REFERENCES

1. Brandsma D, Stalpers L, Taal W, et al. Clinical features, mechanisms, and management of pseudoprogression in malignant gliomas. Lancet Oncol 2008; 9:453–61.

2. Chang JH, Chang JW, Choi JY, et al. Complications after gamma knife radiosurgery for benign meningioma. J Neurol Neurosurg Psychiatr 2003;74: 226–30.

3. Patil CG, Hoang S, Borchers DJ, et al. Predictors of peritumoral edema after stereotactic radiosurgery of supratentorial meningiomas. Neurosurgery 2008; 63:435–42.

4. Peterson K, Clark B, Hall WA, et al. Multifocal enhancing magnetic resonance imaging lesions following cranial irradiation. Ann Neurol 1995;38:237–44.

5. Helton KJ, Edwards M, Steen RG, et al. Neuroimaging-detected late transient treatment-induced lesions in pediatric patients with brain tumors. J Neurosurg 2005;102(Suppl 2):179–86.

6. Spreafico F, Gandola L, Marchiano A, et al. Brain magnetic resonance imaging after high-dose chemotherapy and radiotherapy for childhood brain tumors. Int J Radiat Oncol Biol Phys 2008;70:1011–9.

7. Lee AW, Foo W, Chappel R, et al. Effect of time, dose, and fractionation on temporal lobe necrosis following radiotherapy for nasopharyngeal carcinoma. Int J Radiat Oncol Biol Phys 1998;40:35–42.

8. Santoni R, Liebsch N, Finkelstein DM, et al. Temporal lobe damage following surgery and high-dose photon and proton irradiation in patients affected by chordomas and chondrosarcomas of the base of the skull. Int J Radiat Oncol Biol Phys 1998;41:59–68.

9. Ruben JD, Dally M, Bailey M, et al. Cerebral radiation necrosis: incidence, outcomes, and risk factors with emphasis on radiation parameters and chemotherapy. Int J Radiat Oncol Biol Phys 2006;65:499–508.

10. Swinson BM, Friedman WA. Linear accelerator stereotactic radiosurgery for metastatic brain tumors. Neurosurgery 2008;62:1018–32.

11. Pollock BE, Gorman DA, Coffey RJ. Patient outcomes after arteriovenous malformation radiosurgical management: results based on a 5–14 year follow up study. Neurosurgery 2003;52:1291–7.

12. Massengale JL, Levy RP, Marcellus M, et al. Outcomes of surgery for resection of regions of symptomatic radiation injury after stereotactic radiosurgery for arteriovenous malformations. Neurosurgery 2006;59:553–60.

13. Okun MS, Stover NP, Subramanian T, et al. Complications of gamma knife surgery for Parkinson disease. Arch Neurol 2001;58:1995–2002.

14. Mullins ME, Barest GD, Schaefer PW, et al. Radiation necrosis versus glioma recurrence: conventional MR imaging clues to diagnosis. AJNR Am J Neuroradiol 2005;26:1967–72.

15. Dequesada IM, Quisling RG, Yachnis A, et al. Can standard magnetic resonance imaging reliably distinguish between recurrent tumor from radiation necrosis after radiosurgery for brain metastases? Neurosurgery 2008;63: 898–904.

16. McGirt MJ, Bulsara KR, Cummings TJ, et al. Prognostic value of magnetic resonance imaging-guided stereotactic biopsy in the evaluation of recurrent malignant astrocytoma compared with a lesion due to radiation effect. J Neurosurg 2003;98:14–20.

17. Truong MT, St. Clair EG, Donahue BR, et al. Results of surgical resection for progression of brain metastases previously treated by gamma knife radiosurgery. Neurosurgery 2006;59:86–97.

18. Chao ST, Suh JH, Raja S, et al. The sensitivity and specificity of FDG PET in distinguishing recurrent brain tumor from radionecrosis in patients treated with stereotactic radiosurgery. Int J Cancer 2001;96:191–7.

19. Ross DA, Sandler HM, Balter JM, et al. Imaging changes after stereotactic radiosurgery of primary and secondary malignant brain tumors. J Neurooncol 2002; 56:175–81.
20. Schlemmer HP, Bachert P, Herfarth KK, et al. Proton MR spectroscopic evaluation of suspicious brain lesions after stereotactic radiotherapy. AJNR Am J Neuroradiol 2001;22:1316–24.
21. Weybright P, Sundgren PC, Maly P, et al. Differentiation between brain tumor recurrence and radiation injury using MR spectroscopy. AJR Am J Roentgenol 2005;185:1471–6.
22. Zeng QS, Li C, Liu H, et al. Distinction between recurrent glioma and radiation injury using magnetic resonance spectroscopy in combination with diffusion-weighted imaging. Int J Radiat Oncol Biol Phys 2007;68:151–8.
23. Chuba PJ, Aronin P, Bhambhani K, et al. Hyperbaric oxygen therapy for radiation-induced brain injury in children. Cancer 1997;80:2005–12.
24. Gonzalez J, Kumar AJ, Conrad CA, et al. Effect of bevacizumab on radiation necrosis of the brain. Int J Radiat Oncol Biol Phys 2007;67:323–6.
25. Armstrong CL, Hunter JV, Ledakis GE, et al. Late cognitive and radiographic changes related to radiotherapy: initial prospective findings. Neurology 2002; 59:40–8.
26. Postma TJ, Klein M, Verstappen CC, et al. Radiotherapy-induced cerebral abnormalities in patients with low-grade glioma. Neurology 2002;59:121–3.
27. Surma-aho O, Niemela M, Vilkki J, et al. Adverse long-term effects of brain radiotherapy in adult low-grade glioma patients. Neurology 2001;56:1285–90.
28. Klein M, Heimans JJ, Aaronson NK, et al. Effect of radiotherapy and other treatment-related factors on mid-term to long-term cognitive sequelae in low-grade gliomas: a comparative study. Lancet 2002;360:1361–8.
29. Laack NN, Brown PD, Ivnik RJ, et al. Cognitive function after radiotherapy for supratentorial low-grade glioma: a North Central Cancer Treatment Group prospective study. Int J Radiat Oncol Biol Phys 2005;63:1175–83.
30. Correa DD, DeAngelis LM, Shi W, et al. Cognitive functions in low-grade gliomas: disease and treatment effects. J Neurooncol 2007;81:175–84.
31. Omuro AM, Ben-Porat L, Panageas KS, et al. Delayed neurotoxicity in primary central nervous system lymphoma. Arch Neurol 2005;62:1595–600.
32. Lai R, Abrey LE, Rosenblum MK, et al. Treatment-induced leukoencephalopathy in primary CNS lymphoma: a clinical and autopsy study. Neurology 2004;62: 451–6.
33. Shibamoto Y, Baba F, Oda K, et al. Incidence of brain atrophy and decline in mini-mental state examination score after whole-brain radiotherapy in patients with brain metastases: a prospective study. Int J Radiat Oncol Biol Phys 2008; 72:1168–73.
34. Thiessen B, DeAngelis LM. Hydrocephalus in radiation leukoencephalopathy: results of ventriculoperitoneal shunting. Arch Neurol 1998;55:705–10.
35. Vines EF, Le Pechoux C, Arriagada R. Prophylactic cranial irradiation in small cell lung Cancer. Semin Oncol 2003;30(1):38–46.
36. Grosshans DR, Meyers CA, Allen PK, et al. Neurocognitive function in patients with small cell lung cancer: effect of prophylactic cranial irradiation. Cancer 2008;112:589–95.
37. Fonseca R, O'Neill BP, Foote RL, et al. Cerebral toxicity in patients treated for small cell carcinoma of the lung. Mayo Clin Proc 1999;74:461–5.
38. Gehring K, Sitskoom MM, Aaronson NK, et al. Interventions for cognitive deficits in adults with brain tumours. Not Found In Database 2008;7:548–60.

39. Mulhern RK, Merchant TE, Gajjar A, et al. Late neurocognitive sequelae in survivors of brain tumours in childhood. Lancet Oncol 2004;5:399–408.
40. Palmer SL, Reddick WE, Gajjar A. Understanding the cognitive impact on children who are treated for medulloblastoma. J Pediatr Psychol 2007;32: 1040–9.
41. Maddrey AM, Bergeron JA, Lombardo ER, et al. Neuropsychological performance and quality of life of 10 year survivors of childhood medulloblastoma. J Neurooncol 2005;72:245–53.
42. Walter AW, Mulhern RK, Gajjar A, et al. Survival and neurodevelopmental outcome of young children with medulloblastoma at St. Jude Children's Research Hospital. J Clin Oncol 1999;17:3720–8.
43. Fouladi M, Gilger E, Kocak M, et al. Intellectual and functional outcome in children 3 years old or younger who have CNS malignancies. J Clin Oncol 2005;23:7152–60.
44. Ris MD, Packer R, Goldwein J, et al. Intellectual outcome after reduced-dose radiation therapy plus adjuvant chemotherapy for medulloblastoma: a Children's Cancer Group study. J Clin Oncol 2001;19:3470–6.
45. Mulhern RK, Palmer SL, Merchant TE, et al. Neurocognitive consequences of risk-adapted therapy for childhood medulloblastoma. J Clin Oncol 2005;23: 5511–9.
46. Mulhern RK, Palmer SL, Reddick WE, et al. Risks of young age for selected neurocognitive deficits in medulloblastoma are associated with white matter loss. J Clin Oncol 2001;19:472–9.
47. Reddick WE, Glass JO, Palmer SL, et al. Atypical white matter volume development in children following craniospinal irradiation. Neuro Oncol 2005;7: 12–9.
48. Qiu D, Kwong DL, Chan GC, et al. Diffusion tensor magnetic resonance imaging finding of discrepant fractional anisotropy between the frontal and parietal lobes after whole-brain irradiation in childhood medulloblastoma survivors. Int J Radiat Oncol Biol Phys 2007;69:846–51.
49. Mabbott DJ, Noseworthy MD, Bouffet E, et al. Diffusion tensor imaging of white matter after cranial radiation in children for medulloblastoma: correlation with IQ. Neuro Oncol 2006;8:244–52.
50. Kiehna EN, Mulhern RE, Li C, et al. Changes in attentional performance of children and young adults with localized primary brain tumors after conformal radiation therapy. J Clin Oncol 2006;24:5283–90.
51. Cantelmi D, Schweizer TA, Cusimano MD. Role of the cerebellum in the neurocognitive sequelae of treatment of tumours of the posterior fossa: an update. Lancet Oncol 2008;9:569–76.
52. Pui CH, Howard SC. Current management and challenges of malignant disease in the CNS in paediatric leukaemia. Lancet Oncol 2008;9:257–68.
53. Spiegler BJ, Kennedy K, Maze R, et al. Comparison of long-term neurocognitive outcomes in young children with acute lymphoblastic leukemia treated with cranial radiation or intravenous methotrexate. J Clin Oncol 2006;24:3858–64.
54. Waber DP, Turek J, Catania L, et al. Neuropsychological outcomes from a randomized trial of triple intrathecal chemotherapy compared with 18 Gy cranial radiation as CNS treatment in acute lymphoblastic leukemia. J Clin Oncol 2007;25:4914–21.
55. Paakko E, Harila-Saari A, Vainionpaa L, et al. White matter changes on MRI during treatment in children with acute lymphoblastic leukemia: correlation with neuropsychological findings. Med Pediatr Oncol 2000;35:456–61.

56. Reddick WE, Shan ZY, Glass JO, et al. Smaller white matter volumes are associated with larger deficits in attention and learning among long-term survivors of acute lymphoblastic leukemia. Cancer 2006;106:941–9.
57. Thompson SJ, Leigh L, Christensen R, et al. Immediate neurocognitive effects of methylphenidate on learning-impaired survivors of childhood cancer. J Clin Oncol 2001;19:1802–8.
58. Omura M, Aida N, Sekido K, et al. Large intracranial vessel occlusive vasculopathy after radiation therapy in children: clinical features and usefulness of magnetic resonance imaging. Int J Radiat Oncol Biol Phys 1997; 38:241–9.
59. Dorresteijn LD, Kappelle AC, Boogerd W, et al. Increased risk of ischemic stroke after radiotherapy on the neck in patients younger than 60 years. J Clin Oncol 2001;20:282–8.
60. Lesche G, Castier Y, Chataigner O, et al. Carotid artery revascularization through a radiated field. J Vasc Surg 2003;38:244–50.
61. Harrod-Kim P, Kadkhodayan Y, Derdeyn CP, et al. Outcomes of carotid angioplasty and stenting for radiation-associated stenosis. AJNR Am J Neuroradiol 2005;26:1781–8.
62. Grill J, Couanet D, Cappelli C, et al. Radiation-induced cerebral vasculopathy in children with neurofibromatosis and optic pathway glioma. Ann Neurol 1999;45: 393–6.
63. Desai SS, Paulino AC, Mai WY, et al. Radiation-induced moyamoya syndrome. Int J Radiat Oncol Biol Phys 2006;65:1222–7.
64. Ullrich NJ, Robertson R, Kinnamon DD, et al. Moyamoya following cranial irradiation for primary brain tumors in children. Neurology 2007;68:932–8.
65. Lew SM, Morgan JN, Psaty E, et al. Cumulative incidence of radiation-induced cavernomas in long-term survivors of medulloblastoma. J Neurosurg 2006; 104(Suppl 2):103–7.
66. Strenger V, Sovinz P, Lackner H, et al. Intracerebral cavernous hemangioma after cranial irradiation in childhood: incidence and risk factors. Strahlenther Onkol 2008;184:276–80.
67. Fouladi M, Langston J, Mulhern R, et al. Silent lacunar lesions detected by magnetic resonance imaging of children with brain tumors: a late sequela of therapy. J Clin Oncol 2000;18:824–31.
68. Suzuki H, Toyoda S, Muramatsu M, et al. Spontaneous haemorrhage into metastatic brain tumours after stereotactic radiosurgery using a linear accelerator. J Neurol Neurosurg Psychiatr 2003;74:908–12.
69. Partap S, Walker M, Longstreth WT, et al. Prolonged but reversible migraine-like episodes long after cranial irradiation. Neurology 2006;66:1105–7.
70. Pruitt A, Dalmau J, Detre J, et al. Episodic neurologic dysfunction with migraine and reversible imaging findings after radiation. Neurology 2006;67: 676–8.
71. Pettorini BL, Park YS, Caldarelli M, et al. Radiation-induced brain tumours after central nervous system irradiation in childhood: a review. Childs Nerv Syst 2008; 24:793–805.
72. Neglia JP, Robison LL, Stovall M, et al. New primary neoplasms of the central nervous system in survivors of childhood cancer: a report from the Childhood Cancer Survivor Study. J Natl Cancer Inst 2006;98:1528–37.
73. Hijiya N, Hudson MM, Lensing S, et al. Cumulative incidence of secondary neoplasms as a first event after childhood acute lymphoblastic leukemia. J Am Med Assoc 2007;297:1207–15.

74. Bhatia S, Sather HN, Pabustan OB, et al. Low incidence of second neoplasms among children diagnosed with acute lymphoblastic leukemia after 1983. Blood 2002;99:4257–64.
75. Tsang RW, Laperriere NJ, Simpson WJ, et al. Glioma arising after radiation therapy for pituitary adenoma. Cancer 1993;72:2227–33.
76. Minniti G, Traish D, Ashley S, et al. Risk of second brain tumor after conservative surgery and radiotherapy for pituitary adenoma: update after an additional 10 years. J Clin Endocrinol Metab 2005;90:800–4.
77. Balasubramanian A, Shannon P, Hodaie M, et al. Glioblastoma after stereotactic radiotherapy for acoustic neuroma. Neuro Oncol 2007;9:447–53.
78. Berman EL, Eade TN, Brown D, et al. Radiation-induced tumor after stereotactic radiosurgery for an arteriovenous malformation. Neurosurgery 2007;61: 1099.
79. Sadetzki S, Flint-Richter P, Ben-Tal T, et al. Radiation-induced meningioma: a descriptive study of 253 cases. J Neurosurg 2002;97:1078–82.
80. Al-Mefty O, Topsakal C, Pravdenkova S, et al. Radiation-induced meningiomas: clinical, pathological, cytokinetic, and cytogenetic characteristics. J Neurosurg 2004;100:1002–13.
81. Salvati M, D'Elia A, Melone GA, et al. Radio-induced gliomas: 20-year experience and critical review of the pathology. J Neurooncol 2008;89: 169–77.
82. Chang SM, Barker FG, Larson DA, et al. Sarcomas subsequent to cranial irradiation. Neurosurgery 1995;36:685–90.
83. Kline LB, Kim JY, Ceballos R. Radiation optic neuropathy. Ophthalmology 1985; 92:1118–26.
84. Parsons JT, Bova FJ, Fitzgerald CR, et al. Radiation optic neuropathy after megavoltage external-beam irradiation: analysis of time-dose factors. Int J Radiat Oncol Biol Phys 1994;30:755–63.
85. Girkin CA, Comey CH, Lunsford LD, et al. Radiation optic neuropathy after stereotactic radiosurgery. Ophthalmology 1997;104:1634–43.
86. Roden D, Bosley TM, Fowble B, et al. Delayed radiation injury to the retrobulbar optic nerves and chiasm. Ophthalmology 1990;97:346–51.
87. Lin YS, Jen YM, Lin JC. Radiation-related cranial nerve palsy in patients with nasopharyngeal carcinoma. Cancer 2002;95:404–9.
88. Shapiro BE, Rordorf G, Schwamm L, et al. Delayed radiation-induced bulbar palsy. Neurology 1996;46:1604–6.
89. Chew NK, Sim BF, Tan CT, et al. Delayed post-irradiation bulbar palsy in nasopharyngeal carcinoma. Neurology 2001;57:529–31.
90. Morita A, Coffey RJ, Foote RL, et al. Risk of injury to cranial nerves after gamma knife radiosurgery for skull base meningiomas: experience in 88 patients. J Neurosurg 1999;90:42–9.
91. Melki PS, Halimi P, Wibault P, et al. MRI in chronic progressive radiation myelopathy. J Comput Assist Tomogr 1994;18:1–6.
92. Schultheiss TE, Stephens LC, Maor MH. Analysis of the histopathology of radiation myelopathy. Int J Radiat Oncol Biol Phys 1988;14:27–32.
93. Schultheiss TE, Kun LE, Ang KK, et al. Radiation response of the central nervous system. Int J Radiat Oncol Biol Phys 1995;31:1093–112.
94. Dodd RL, Ryu M, Gibbs IC, et al. CyberKnife radiosurgery for benign intradural extramedullary spinal tumors. Neurosurgery 2006;58:674–85.
95. Gibbs IC, Ryu M, Dodd R, et al. Image-guided robotic radiosurgery for spinal metastases. Radiother Oncol 2007;82:185–90.

96. Seddon BM, Cassoni AM, Galloway MJ, et al. Fatal radiation myelopathy after high-dose busulfan and melphalan chemotherapy and radiotherapy for Ewing's sarcoma. Not Found In Database 2005;17:385–90.
97. Gatcombe H, Lawson J, Phuphanich S, et al. Treatment related myelitis in Hodgkin's lymphoma following stem cell transplant, chemotherapy and radiation. J Neurooncol 2006;79:293–8.
98. Koehler PJ, Verbiest H, Jager J, et al. Delayed radiation myelopahy: serial MR-imaging and pathology. Clin Neurol Neurosurg 1996;98:197–201.
99. Angibaud G, Ducasse JL, Baille G, et al. Potential value of hyperbaric oxygenation in the treatment of post-radiation myelopathies. Rev Neurol 1995;151:661–6.
100. Calabro F, Jinkins JR. MRI of radiation myelitis: a report of a case treated with hyperbaric oxygen. Eur Radiol 2000;10:1079–84.
101. Kori SH, Foley KM, Posner JB. Brachial plexus lesions in patients with cancer: 100 cases. Neurology 1981;31:45–50.
102. Harper CM, Thomas JE, Cascino TL, et al. Distinction between neoplastic and radiation-induced brachial plexopathy, with emphasis on the role of EMG. Neurology 1989;39:502–6.
103. Olsen NK, Pfeiffer P, Johannsen L, et al. Radiation-induced brachial plexopathy: neurological follow-up in 161 recurrence-free breast cancer patients. Int J Radiat Oncol Biol Phys 1993;26:43–9.
104. Thyagarajan D, Cascino T, Harms G. Magnetic resonance imaging in brachial plexopathy of cancer. Neurology 1995;45:421–7.
105. Qayyum A, MacVicar AD, Padhani AR, et al. Symptomatic brachial plexopathy following treatment for breast cancer: utility of MR imaging with surface-coil techniques. Radiology 2000;214:837–42.
106. Ahmad A, Barrington S, Maisey M, et al. Use of positron emission tomography in evaluation of brachial plexopathy in breast cancer patients. Br J Cancer 1999;79:478–82.
107. Dubuisson AS, Kline DG, Weinshel SS. Posterior subscapular approach to the brachial plexus: report of 102 patients. J Neurosurg 1993;79:319–30.
108. Lusk MD, Kline DG, Garcia CA. Tumors of the brachial plexus. Neurosurgery 1987;21:439–53.
109. Teixeira MJ, Fonoff ET, Montenegro MC. Dorsal root entry zone lesions for treatment of pain related to radiation-induced plexopathy. Spine 2007;32:E316–9.
110. Fathers E, Thrush D, Huson SM, et al. Radiation-induced brachial plexopathy in women treated for carcinoma of the breast. Clin Rehabil 2002;16:160–5.
111. Soto O. Radiation-induced conduction block: resolution following anticoagulant therapy. Muscle Nerve 2005;31:642–5.
112. Pritchard J, Anand P, Broome J, et al. Double-blind randomized phase II study of hyperbaric oxygen in patients with radiation-induced brachial plexopathy. Radiother Oncol 2001;58:279–86.
113. Pettigrew LC, Glass JP, Maor M, et al. Diagnosis and treatment of lumbosacral plexopathies in patients with cancer. Arch Neurol 1984;41:1282–5.
114. Thomas JE, Cascino TL, Earle JD. Differential diagnosis between radiation and tumor plexopathy of the pelvis. Neurology 1985;35:1–7.
115. Georgiou A, Grigsby PW, Perez CA. Radiation induced lumbosacral plexopathy in gynecologic tumors: clinical findings and dosimetric analysis. Int J Radiat Oncol Biol Phys 1993;26:479–82.
116. Pieters RS, Niemierko A, Fullerton BC, et al. Cauda equina tolerance to high-dose fractionated irradiation. Int J Radiat Oncol Biol Phys 2006;64:251–7.

117. Brydoy M, Storstein A, Dahl O. Transient neurological adverse effects following low dose radiation therapy for early stage testicular seminoma. Radiother Oncol 2007;82:137–44.
118. Hsia AW, Peterson K. Post-irradiation polyradiculopathy mimics leptomeningeal tumor on MRI. Neurology 2003;60:1694–6.
119. Ducray F, Guillevin R, Psimaras D, et al. Postradiation lumbosacral radiculopathy with spinal root cavernomas mimicking carcinomatous meningitis. Neuro Oncol 2008;10:1035–9.
120. Bowen J, Gregory R, Squier M, et al. The post-irradiation lower motor neuron syndrome: neuronopathy or radiculopathy? Brain 1996;119:1429–39.
121. Taylor BV, Kimmel DW, Krecke KN, et al. Magnetic resonance imaging in cancer-related lumbosacral plexopathy. Mayo Clin Proc 1997;72:823–9.
122. Dahele M, Davey P, Reingold S, et al. Radiation-induced lumbosacral plexopathy: an important enigma. Clin Oncol 2006;18:427–8.

Neurologic Manifestations of Transplant Complications

Saša A. Živković, MD, PhD[a,b,*], Hoda Abdel-Hamid, MD[c]

KEYWORDS

- Posttransplant recovery • Neurotoxicity
- Opportunistic infections • Transplant complications

Transplantation medicine has rapidly advanced over the last two decades and is becoming part of daily clinical practice of many physicians with increasing numbers of transplant recipients and improved survival. Annually, there are more than 27,000 solid-organ transplants performed in the United States alone (**Table 1**),[1] in addition to more than 18,000 hematopoietic stem cell transplantations ([HCST]; bone marrow or peripheral blood stem cells).[2] Although transplant recipients are similar to other patients who are immunosupressed, complexities of associated metabolic and toxic disturbances distinguish this group of patients and offer unique challenges in diagnosis and management of various clinical problems. Despite tremendous advances, posttransplant clinical course is still marred by a wide spectrum of complications affecting survival and quality of life of transplant recipients.

Neurologic complications are a significant source of morbidity after organ transplantation and affect more than 20% of transplant recipients (**Table 2**).[3–12] Underlying etiology is usually related to surgical procedure of transplantation, primary disorders causing failure of transplanted organ, opportunistic infections, and neurotoxicity of

This work was supported in part by Health Resources and Services Administration contract 231-00-0115. The content is the responsibility of the authors alone and does not necessarily reflect the views or policies of the Department of Health and Human Services, nor does mention of trade names, commercial products, or organizations imply endorsement by the US Government.

[a] Neurology Service, VA Pittsburgh Healthcare System, University Drive C, Pittsburgh, PA 15240, USA
[b] Department of Neurology, University of Pittsburgh School of Medicine, PUH F878, 200 Lothrop Street, Pittsburgh, PA 15213, USA
[c] Division of Pediatric Neurology, Children's Hospital Pittsburgh, University of Pittsburgh School of Medicine, CHP 2nd floor, 45th Street and Penn Avenue, Pittsburgh, PA 15201, USA
* Corresponding author. Department of Neurology, University of Pittsburgh School of Medicine, Pittsburgh, PA.
E-mail address: zivkovics@upmc.edu (S.A. Živković).

Neurol Clin 28 (2010) 235–251
doi:10.1016/j.ncl.2009.09.011
0733-8619/09/$ – see front matter. Published by Elsevier Inc.

Table 1		
Number of solid-organ transplantations in the United States in 1998 and 2008		
	1998	2008
Kidney	12,452	16,517
Liver	4516	6318
Pancreas	244	436
Kidney/pancreas	972	837
Heart	2348	2163
Lung	869	1478
Heart/lung	47	27
Intestine	70	185

Data from Health Resources and Services Administration, Healthcare Systems Bureau, Division of Transplantation, US Department of Health and Human Services. 2008 Annual Report of the US Organ Procurement and Transplantation Network and the Scientific Registry of Transplant Recipients: Transplant Data 1998–2007. Rockville (MD); United Network for Organ Sharing, Richmond (VA); University Renal Research and Education Association, Ann Arbor (MI). 2009.

immunosuppressive medications.[13,14] Immunosuppressive regimen may be changed in more than 10% of transplant recipients because of neurologic complications.[15] Although similar clinical spectrum of neurologic complications is found in adult and pediatric transplant recipients, neurologic complications seem to be less common and more severe in pediatric patients.[6,16]

Clinical spectrum of posttransplant neurologic complications spans widely from alterations of consciousness and behavior, involuntary movements, cerebrovascular complications, to opportunistic central nervous system (CNS) infections, neuromuscular complications and epileptic seizures.

ALTERED CONSCIOUSNESS AND ENCEPHALOPATHY

Alterations of consciousness and encephalopathy are common after transplantation ranging from confusion and delirium to stupor and coma. Frequently, the presence of multiple concurrent potential causes of altered responsiveness complicates identification of a single underlying cause.[17] Severe medical illness, advanced age, and pre-existing cognitive difficulties increase the risk for posttransplant delirium. Spectrum of causes of altered consciousness in transplant recipients changes depending on the time elapsed since the transplantation procedure. Immediately after transplantation, anoxic brain injury associated with intraoperative cardiac arrest may be quite severe, and the presence of myoclonic status is indicative of a poor prognosis.. Subsequently, in the subacute postoperative period, various toxic and metabolic disturbances and opportunistic infections prevail.[17] Common metabolic disturbances include hyperammonemia, uremia, and glucose abnormalities (hypo- or hyperglycemia). Graft failure may also precipitate alteration of consciousness, especially with worsening ammonemia and uremia. Liver allograft recipients who have prior history of alcohol abuse are at higher risk for posttransplant delirium.[18] Central pontine myelinolysis is specific for liver allograft recipients and manifests with pseudobulbar palsy and stupor occurring usually within weeks from liver transplantation (**Table 3**).[19] Wernicke encephalopathy, with a triad of altered mental status, ophthalmoplegia, and ataxia, has been described in HSCT recipients who have severe refractory acidosis at 4 weeks after transplantation.[20] Neurotoxicity of calcineurin inhibitors ([CNI]; tacrolimus, cyclosporin)

Table 2
Neurologic complications after organ transplantation

		Ad/P	n	Total (%)	Seizure (%)	CNS Infection (%)	Encephalopathy (%)	Stroke (%)	Neuromuscular (%)
Bronster et al[4]	Liver	Ad	463	20	8.2	1.2	11.8	2.1	nd
Lewis and Howdle[7]	Liver	Ad	657	27	6.0	1.1	11.0	4.0	4.0
Erol et al[10]	Liver	P	40	35	15.0	nd	12.0	nd	nd
Denier et al[9]	Bone marrow	Ad	361	16	5.0	4.2	2.8	1.7	3.3
Faraci et al[5]	Bone marrow	P	272	14	7.0	2.6	6.3	1.1	1.8
Zivkovic et al[8]	Intestine	Ad	54	85	17.0	7.0	43.0	4.0	7.0
Zierer et al[11]	Heart	Ad	200	23	7.0	1.5	nd	9.0	1.0
Mayer et al[6]	Heart	Ad	107	30	5.6	3.7	2.8	8.4	13.1
Mayer et al[6]	Heart	P	77	23	9.1	1.3	1.3	6.5	3.9
Zivkovic et al[12]	Lung	Ad	132	68	8.0	1.0	25.0	7.0	21.0
Wong et al[3]	Lung	P	132	45	27.0	1.5	6.7	3.7	nd

Abbreviations: Ad, adult; nd, no data; P, pediatric.
Data from Refs. [1,3-12]

Table 3
Allograft-specific neurologic complications

Allograft	Syndrome	Manifestations
Liver	Central pontine myelinolysis	Stupor, quadriparesis
Heart	Cardioembolic stroke	Focal weakness, numbness, aphasia
Kidney	Diabetic neuropathy	Weakness, numbness, neuropathic pain
Lung	Phrenic nerve palsy	Dyspnea
Bone marrow	Graft-versus-host disease	Weakness, myalgia (polymyositis)

manifesting with altered consciousness, seizures, and cortical blindness is more common with higher intravenous dosing in the early postoperative period.[21–24] Impaired renal function may precipitate neurotoxicity of renally metabolized medications including acyclovir or cephalosporins, and benzodiazepines may accumulate with hepatic insufficiency. Combined use of antibiotic linezolid and serotonin reuptake-inhibiting antidepressants may precipitate serotonin syndrome.[25]

PSYCHIATRIC COMPLICATIONS

Patients who have a transplant may exhibit a variety of behavioral abnormalities and psychiatric disorders ranging from depressed mood to mania and psychosis.[26–28] Precipitating factors include use of various medications, such as corticosteroids and tacrolimus; complex drug-drug interactions and metabolic disturbances; and posttraumatic stress related to transplantation or exacerbation of preexisting psychiatric conditions.[26,28–31] Psychiatric complications may also stem from the original cause of organ failure (eg, Wilson's disease).[32] Transplant recipients and their family members may also suffer from posttransplant posttraumatic stress disorder, which affects medical compliance, morbidity, and quality of life.[31]

MOVEMENT DISORDERS

New onset of abnormal involuntary movements after transplantation is usually drug induced. The most common is tremor related to the use of CNI. Severity of CNI-related tremor varies widely, but only rarely does it limit patient's activity or require medication adjustment.[21,33] Parkinsonian symptoms related to pre-transplant hepatocerebral degeneration with liver failure may improve after successful liver transplantation, similarly as movement disorder associated with Wilson's disease.[32,34] Use of neuroleptics can trigger drug-induced parkinsonism or tardive movement disorders.[35] Non-epileptic myoclonus in transplant recipients is usually drug-induced, particularly with opiates and antidepressants, and this is usually self-limited and stops shortly after offending medication is discontinued.

CEREBROVASCULAR COMPLICATIONS

Cerebrovascular complications are most frequent after heart transplantation; ischemic stroke or transient ischemic attacks were reported in 9% of cardiac allograft recipients, and up to 4% and 7% of liver and kidney transplant recipients, respectively (see **Table 2**).[7,11,36] Increased risk of stroke was observed in patients who had cardiac transplants and a history of use of intra-aortic balloon pumps.[11] Although cerebrovascular complications are common after kidney transplantation, the risk decreases after successful transplantation when compared with similar patients on transplant waiting lists.[36] Opportunistic infections also increase risk of stroke.[37,38] Bacterial septic endocarditis may precipitate hemorrhagic cardioembolic stroke, whereas vasoinvasive fungal infections (aspergillosis) may cause thrombosis. Cardioembolic stroke may be also associated with nonbacterial thrombotic endocarditis or atrial fibrillation.[38] Systemic bacterial and fungal infections without direct CNS involvement, thrombocytopenia and coagulopathy, are associated with an increased risk for intracerebral hemorrhage.[37,39,40] Posttransplant thrombocytopenia increases risk for intracranial hemorrhage in HSCT recipients, especially in patients who have platelet counts of 20,000 or lower.[41] History of polycystic kidney disease in renal transplant recipients is also associated with a tenfold increase of the risk for intracerebral hemorrhage.[39] Rarely, transplant recipients may develop thrombotic microangiopathy, similar to thrombotic thrombocytopenic purpura.[42] Increased incidence of hypercoagulable state related to protein S deficiency was reported after bone marrow transplantation.[43]

SEIZURES

Seizures are common in transplant recipients, occurring in 7% to 27% of solid-organ recipients and 5% to 7% of patients who have HSCT (see **Table 2**). New onset of posttransplant seizures is not automatically indicative of poor prognosis because most patients do well, and do not require long-term therapy with antiepileptic medications.[44,45] However, postanoxic myoclonus status after cardiac arrest is an indicator of poor prognosis, and seizures may precede other manifestations of severe neurologic conditions. Most commonly, seizures present as generalized tonic-clonic events with primary or secondary generalization. Simple or complex partial seizures are suggestive of a localized process (eg, abscess, stroke) that may be reflected by focal electroencephalogram (EEG) findings. Nonconvulsive seizures are difficult to distinguish from toxic-metabolic encephalopathy without EEG. Frequent causes of posttransplant seizures include CNI neurotoxicity, transient metabolic disturbances, and CNS infections.[44,45] Seizures related to CNI neurotoxicity frequently originate from occipital regions.[46] Cardioembolic stroke is frequently followed by seizures.[11] Less commonly, antibiotics or chemotherapy medications may cause seizures (imipenem, cephalosporins, busulfan).

MYELOPATHIES

Spinal cord disorders are rare in transplant recipients. However, gradual onset of weakness and sensory loss accompanied with sphincter incontinence may be caused by myelopathy. Potential causes after transplantation include epidural abscess and hematoma, whereas chronic use of corticosteroids may lead to epidural lipomatosis.[47] Opportunistic viral infections caused by human T-lymphotropic virus 1 (HTLV-1), human herpesvirus 6 and 7 (HHV-6, HHV-7), varicella zoster virus (VZV), Epstein–Barr virus (EBV), or cytomegalovirus (CMV) may lead to myelopathy or polyradiculopathy.[48,49] Stem-cell transplantation and chemotherapy may increase risk for radiation myelitis with lower doses of radiation resulting in severe weakness and disability.[50]

NEUROMUSCULAR COMPLICATIONS

Various postoperative entrapment neuropathies related to traction and stretch injury are specific for different types of transplanted organs; lower trunk brachial plexopathy is seen after thoracic and liver transplantations, whereas femoral neuropathy is more common after kidney transplantation. Peroneal neuropathy usually occurs later and is associated with local compression at the fibular head in patients who are obtunded and cachectic. The exposure to corticosteroids (especially intravenous) and neuro-muscular junction blocking agents, multiple organ failure and sepsis increase risk for critical illness myopathy (CIM) and critical illness polyneuropathy (CIP).[51] In liver transplant recipients, severe quadriparesis attributable to CIM was reported in 7% of subjects within 2 weeks of transplantation.[52] Onset of weakness related to CIM can be quite sudden and dramatic (acute quadriplegic myopathy), but prognosis seems to be somewhat better than with CIP.[53] Worsening of weakness in patients who have diabetic neuropathy after pancreatic transplantation was also attributed to superimposed CIM/CIP.[54] CIM/CIP frequently affects respiratory function and delays ventilator weaning[55] and many patients experience prolonged recovery.[53] Thoracic organ transplantation may lead to phrenic nerve injury caused by cold-induced injury (ice packing) or mechanical damage and up to 3.2% of lung-transplant recipients may suffer from phrenic palsy.[56] Guillain-Barré syndrome has been rarely reported in transplant recipients, and it may be difficult to distinguish from CIM/CIP without electrodiagnostic testing and cerebrospinal fluid analysis. After HCST, chronic graft-versus-host-disease (GVHD) may be associated with inflammatory myopathy or neuropathy or even myasthenia gravis.[57] Posttransplant toxic neuropathy usually follows subacute clinical course and is mostly related to antibiotics (linezolid) or chemotherapy agents (bortezomib, thalidomide). Concurrent therapy with statins or colchicine and cyclosporine may cause myopathy leading to rhabdomyolysis. Rarely, peripheral nerve disorders were reported in patients treated with tacrolimus, including multifocal demyelinating polyneuropathy resembling chronic inflammatory demyelin-ating polyneuropathy.[58]

HEADACHE AND PAIN

Headaches are frequently overshadowed by other systemic or neurologic complaints and symptoms in transplant recipients. However, new onset of severe headache may be an early manifestation of an opportunistic infection or CNI neurotoxicity, and CNIs may aggravate preexisting migraine disorder.[59] Headaches related to fungal sinusitis are worrisome because direct spread of infection to the CNS may follow. Within a week of transplantation, some cardiac-transplant recipients may develop symptoms of vascular headaches associated with nausea, flushed faces, and bounding pulses that may be responsive to treatment with β-blockers.[60] Herpes zoster has been re-ported in up to 8.6% of solid organ transplant recipients and almost half may later develop postherpetic neuralgia.[61]

Toxic neuropathies may be associated with severe neuropathic discomfort. More recently, complex regional pain syndrome was described in patients treated with CNI, sirolimus, and everolimus.[62,63]

VISUAL DISTURBANCES

Visual disturbances after organ transplantation are frequently related to cortical blind-ness associated with posterior reversible encephalopathy syndrome (PRES) and neurotoxicity of CNI.[24] Patients may experience homonymous sectional visual loss that usually improves after resolution of PRES. Additionally, transient visual loss and visual hallucinations caused by occipital lobe seizures may be the only clinical mani-festations of PRES.[46] Ocular infections following systemic opportunistic fungal and viral infections requires prompt evaluation and treatment to avoid more significant complications.[64] Less commonly, transplant recipients may suffer from optic neurop-athy caused by tacrolimus.[65]

OPPORTUNISTIC CENTRAL NERVOUS SYSTEM INFECTIONS

Chronic immunosuppression required to control allograft rejection maintains long-term risk for opportunistic infections. Most patients are maintained on prophylactic antimicrobial regimens, but details of practice vary between different transplant centers. HSCT recipients (bone marrow or peripheral blood stem cells) are at highest risk for infection immediately after transplantation when the immune system has still not reconstituted. In solid-organ allograft recipients, the risk for infection is between the second and sixth month after transplantation, and then generally decreases as immunosuppressive therapy is tapered. Highest risk was reported with intestinal and multivisceral transplants (7%), followed by bone marrow transplantation (4%), and heart (3%) and liver allografts (1%).[4,7–9,66] The risk for infection is determined by the intensity of epidemiologic exposure to pathogens and the characteristics of the immunosuppression regimen.[67] Additionally, chronic immunosuppression may lead to reactivation of ubiquitous latent viral infections (eg, VZV, JC virus).

Various environmental and geographic endemic factors may increase the risk for particular infectious agents (eg, coccidioidomycosis in the Southwestern United States) (**Box 1**).[68] As opposed to individuals who are nonimmunosuppressed, posttransplant meningitis is usually caused by fungi, and bacterial infections are more commonly caused by Listeria or Nocardia species rather than typical bacterial pathogens. Most patients who have fungal meningitis first develop systemic infection that later spreads to the CNS, typically septicemia, sinusitis, or pneumonia. Posttransplant fungal CNS infections carry a high mortality of 90% or higher.[69]

Box 1
Risk factors for exposure to opportunistic infectious agents

Nocardia

    Unwashed vegetables

Listeria

    Unpasteurized dairy

LCMV (lymphocytic choriomeningitis virus)

    Hamsters

HTLV

    Intravenous drug abuse, Japan, Caribbean

Coccidioides immitis

    Southwestern United States (desert regions)

Histoplasma

    Ohio, Indiana, Mississippi valley

Trypanosoma cruzi

    South America

Toxoplasma

    Cats

Ameba

    Freshwater swimming

Patients usually present with altered level of consciousness and systemic signs of infection, although initially immunosuppression may blunt early systemic signs of infection. Focal neurologic symptoms in the context of an underlying septicemia suggest a possible brain abscess that is also usually fungal in patients who have had a transplant, and neuroimaging studies (preferably MRI) demonstrate multiple contrast-enhancing lesions. In the absence of direct CNS involvement, systemic opportunistic infections may also lead to septic encephalopathy.[70]

Posttransplant viral CNS infections are associated with reactivation of a latent infection (eg, JC virus) or with new exposure (eg, West Nile virus). Most common causes of viral posttransplant encephalitis include HSV, VZV, EBV and CMV viruses. More recently, HHV6 was described as a cause of limbic encephalitis in HSCT recipients.[71] Slowly progressive multifocal leukoencephalopathy related to JC virus carries a poor prognosis and is fortunately uncommon.[72] Less commonly, environmental exposure to rabies virus or West Nile virus may precipitate CNS infection in transplant recipients.[73] Toxoplasmosis is the most common parasitic infection in transplant recipients and is related to activation of latent infection (more common with HSCT) or transmission by way of an infected organ from seropositive donors (most common with heart transplantation).[74] Chronic immunosuppression can also activate latent Strongyloides infection. Acquired amebic encephalitis is fortunately rare and when present carries a high mortality.[75] Continuous emergence of new infectious agents in transplant recipients requires constant adjustment of diagnostic and treatment strategies.

In addition to direct effects of systemic and CNS infections, frequent use of antibiotics and antivirals may precipitate neurotoxic effects involving central end peripheral nervous system including seizures (imipenem, cephalosporins), encephalopathy (acyclovir), or toxic neuropathy (linezolid).

NEUROTOXICITY OF IMMUNOSUPPRESSIVE MEDICATIONS

Neurotoxicity of immunosuppressive medications is most commonly seen after treatment with CNI and corticosteroids, which both form the backbone of most antirejection protocols (**Table 4**). Typical adverse effects of CNI include tremor, headaches, and PRES manifesting with cortical blindness, altered consciousness, and seizures.[21–24,33] Neuroimaging studies commonly show typical findings of PRES with bilateral T2 and fluid-attenuated inversion recovery hyperintensities on MRI in posterior brain regions, and drug levels are frequently elevated although normal levels are also not uncommon.[24] Neurotoxicity of CNI is more frequent early when higher intravenous dosing is used to prevent rejection.[21,23] Corticosteroids may be associated with dysthymia, tremor, steroid myopathy, steroid psychosis, CIM/CIP, or epidural lipomatosis.[30,47] However, neurologic complications are also seen with other

Table 4 Neurotoxic effects of immunosuppressive medications		
	Common	Uncommon
Corticosteroids	Tremor (*mild*), dysthymia	Epidural lipomatosis, psychosis
Tacrolimus, cyclosporine	Tremor, headache, confusion, PRES	Ataxia, polyneuropathy, CRPS
Sirolimus	Tremor, headache	PRES, CRPS
Mycophenolate	Headache	
Muromonab	Aseptic meningitis	

Abbreviation: CRPS, complex regional pain syndrome.

immunosuppressive medications including antilymphocyte antibodies muromonab (OKT3) and antithymocyte globulin antibodies (aseptic meningitis), mycophenolate (headache), and sirolimus (PRES, very rare).[76,77]

POSTTRANSPLANT MALIGNANCIES

Recurrence of hematologic malignancies after HCST affects CNS in 3% of patients who have leukemia and is associated with a high mortality.[78] Relapse is more common with autologous HSCT, and occurs at 3 months or later after transplantation. Additionally, newly developed posttransplant lymphoproliferative disorder (PTLD) affects approximately 2% of solid-organ and HSCT recipients and is frequently associated with an EBV infection. Its occurrence is highest after heart, heart-lung, and intestinal transplantation. CNS involvement is found in approximately 15% of affected patients and is associated with poor prognosis.[79] Higher incidence of solid-brain tumors was reported in solid-organ transplant recipients, but this association remains somewhat controversial.[80] Risk of solid-brain tumors is higher in allogeneic HSCT recipients who were previously treated with total-body irradiation.

ADULT VERSUS PEDIATRIC TRANSPLANTATION

Pediatric transplant recipients offer unique challenges in diagnosis and treatment of neurologic and other posttransplant complications as we have to simultaneously maintain allograft function and normal child development. Development is affected by primary organ failure and associated metabolic disturbances, chronic immunosuppression, and posttransplant complications. Longitudinal studies showed mixed impact of successful transplantation in childhood on long-term linear growth and bone mineralization.[81] Delay in linear growth may also be attributable to a medication effect, such as steroid exposure following transplantation.[82]

Some of the specificities of pediatric transplantation include higher prevalence of hereditary conditions causing primary organ failure. Another problem after pediatric transplantation is noncompliance with immunosuppressive medications that may trigger rejection and allograft dysfunction. Following transplantation, children may be at a higher risk for developing primary infection with various organisms, which may be caused by their lack of exposure to certain organisms and the lack of acquired immunity to common diseases, if they lack immunizations. Lack of acquired immunity related to previous exposure to infectious agents and frequently incomplete immunizations place children at higher risk for opportunistic infections than found in adult patients who have received a transplant.[83]

There are few studies directly comparing posttransplant neurologic complications in pediatric and adult recipients.[6,16] Overall, neurologic complications seem to be less common and more severe in the pediatric population compared with adults.[6,16] However, recovery of pediatric transplant recipients may be quite remarkable compared with adults because of the plasticity of the brain, and most pediatric recipients do well after successful transplantation without significant long-term neurologic disability.[84]

EFFECTS OF TRANSPLANTATION ON NEUROLOGIC DISORDERS

Organ transplantation has variable effects on different neurologic disorders associated with the primary cause of organ failure, but is usually not curative. However, many transplant recipients will stabilize or improve, including patients who have Wilson's disease (liver transplantation) and familial amyloidosis (liver and heart transplantation).[32,85] Diabetic neuropathy usually improves after transplantation, and posttransplant worsening in kidney and pancreas allograft recipients has been attributed to CIP/CIM.[54] Successful renal transplantation leads to more significant and uniform improvement of uremic neuropathy, although the extent of improvement depends on the severity of pretransplantation nerve damage.[86] Hepatic encephalopathy and myelopathy usually improve after successful liver transplantation.

PHARMACOKINETICS AND DRUG-DRUG INTERACTIONS

Complex pharmacokinetics of immunosuppressive and other medications in organ transplant recipients is influenced by liver and kidney drug clearance and complex drug-drug interactions. In patients who have liver and kidney transplants, delayed graft function may significantly alter drug levels. Free fractions of medications with significant protein binding (eg, phenytoin) are also affected by hypoalbuminemia, displacement of protein-bound medication and inactivation of appropriate P450 enzymes.[87] Herbal preparations may also affect pharmacokinetics of immunosuppressants and their effects may be difficult to predict. Our understanding of the role of transporter proteins (P-glycoprotein, multidrug resistance protein-2) continues to evolve, and genetic variability may explain susceptibility of individual patients to toxicity of particular drugs.[88]

RECOMMENDED EVALUATION OF NEUROLOGIC COMPLICATIONS FOLLOWING TRANSPLANTATION

Detailed and systematic evaluation facilitates early diagnosis and timely treatment of posttransplant neurologic complications starting with a thorough review of the history of present illness, consideration of type and timing of transplantation, and cause of primary organ failure. Additionally, we have to consider a possible occurrence of an opportunistic infection or neurotoxicity of immunosuppressive medications. Less commonly, allograft rejection may be associated with neurologic manifestations (eg, hepatic encephalopathy with liver allograft dysfunction). Opportunistic CNS infections usually present in the context of systemic infection, and timely identification of etiology allows appropriate treatment. We have to consider potential exposures to common and endemic infectious agents (see **Box 1**).

As clinical features may be quite complex, extensive batteries of laboratory tests, neuroimaging, and neurophysiologic studies may be needed to establish the underlying cause (**Table 5**). Neuroimaging studies play a significant role in the evaluation of neurologic complications after transplantation because they may provide clues to the underlying etiology and suggest appropriate work-up and management.[89] If readily available, MRI of the brain or spine is usually preferred to CT, but CT may be easier to obtain and is frequently the initial study.

If CNS infection is suspected, cerebrospinal-fluid analysis is needed to establish the diagnosis, but this should not delay the treatment. Viral polymerase chain reactions (PCR) are preferred to serology because they are much more sensitive, but there is still a role for microbial cultures and serology.[90] Innovative diagnostic methods may be needed to diagnose an infection caused by new emerging infectious agents.[91] EEG is helpful in evaluation of suspected seizures and altered consciousness. Careful interpretation of EEG is essential for accurate diagnosis of nonconvulsive seizures in patients who are critically ill because subtle epileptiform changes may be missed. Presence of triphasic waves is strongly suggestive of a toxic-metabolic encephalopathy, especially with renal or hepatic failure.[92] Nerve conduction studies and needle

Table 5
Recommended testing for evaluation of posttransplant neurologic complications

1 Laboratory testing	Basic tests: blood counts, electrolytes, glucose, magnesium, hepatic and renal function tests Toxicology: serum levels of immunosuppressive and other medications Metabolic: B12/folate, methylmalonic acid, pyridoxine, thiamine, vitamin E levels Serology: cryptococcal and other fungal antigens, viral PCR and antibodies Microbiology: acid-fast, bacterial ,and fungal cultures CSF analysis: cell count and differential, protein, glucose, acid-fast/bacterial/fungal culture, cryptococcal and other fungal antigens, viral/mycobacterial/toxoplasma PCR and antibody titers Consider cytology and flow cytometry
2 Imaging studies	MRI of brain: MR angiogram (aneurysm); MR venogram (cerebral sinus thrombosis) MRI of spine CT of sinuses: evaluation of fungal sinusitis CT of head and spine: used mostly if MRI is not feasible MRI of brachial and lumbosacral plexus
3 Electrodiagnostic studies	EMG/NCS: evaluation of nerve entrapment, polyneuropathy or myopathy EEG: helpful in evaluation of seizure tendency or metabolic encephalopathy SSEP: rarely used, may be helpful for localization of pathology
4 Other tests	Echocardiogram: investigation of possible embolic source and endocarditis Brain biopsy: investigation of PTLD, glioma, or brain abscess Muscle and nerve biopsy: investigation of vasculitis or polymyositis

Abbreviation: SSEP, somatosensory evoked potentials.

electromyography are helpful in investigations of subacute onset of weakness and sensory loss. A special technique for direct muscle stimulation is helpful in evaluation of suspected CIM, but a muscle biopsy is needed to confirm the diagnosis.[93] Muscle biopsy may also prove diagnosis of polymyositis in patients who have GVHD. Nerve biopsy is performed infrequently, except if lymphomatous infiltration is suspected. Brain biopsy is rarely pursued, but it may be necessary to identify PTLD, glioma, or brain abscess.

TREATMENT OF POSTTRANSPLANT NEUROLOGIC COMPLICATIONS
Toxic/Metabolic Encephalopathy and Psychiatric Disorders

Guidelines of treatment of posttransplant metabolic encephalopathy and psychiatric disorders related to allograft insufficiency do not differ from patients who have not had a transplant. However, it is important to consider complexities of pharmacokinetics and drug-drug interactions because these patients are frequently treated with a large number of medications and may have renal or hepatic impairment.

If encephalopathy is related to allograft rejection (eg, hepatic encephalopathy), unless function of allograft is reestablished, other treatment modalities usually have limited efficacy.

Hyperammonemia related to hepatic glutamine synthase or urea cycle enzyme defect may respond to a combination of plasma exchange and alternate waste nitrogen agents.[94] In patients who have drug-related toxic encephalopathy, it is most important to identify the offending agent and discontinue its use.

Cerebrovascular Complications

Cerebrovascular complications remain frequent with cardiac transplantation, especially in patients who have prolonged coronary bypass and cross-clamp times during surgery. Careful titration of blood pressure is needed because postoperative hypotensive and hypertensive episodes may precipitate ischemic stroke or cerebral hemorrhage.[11] Increased rate of posttransplant atrial fibrillation has been reported in lung and heart transplant recipients, but its clinical significance remains uncertain.[11] Additionally, use of CNI may lead to hypertension and hyperlipidemia, requiring increased attention in long-term follow-up of patients who received a transplant. Patients who receive intestinal and multivisceral transplants and who have hypercoagulable conditions may require lifelong anticoagulation.[95]

Seizures

Approach to treatment of convulsive status epilepticus is unchanged in transplant recipients because the immediate intent is to break the epileptic status and stabilize patients. Most patients do not require long-term preventive treatment, and phenytoin was safely discontinued after 3 months in a small series of subjects who received liver-transplants.[45] Long-term phenytoin use may affect immunosuppressant levels and interfere with metabolism of cyclosporine and tacrolimus. Therefore, use of levetiracetam has been advocated because this medication does not affect metabolism of CNI and is not significantly affected by liver failure after liver transplantation.[96] Levetiracetam may have unwanted behavioral side effects and its clearance is affected by kidney function. Other options include gabapentin, pregabalin, and topiramate, but valproic acid is used only in non-liver allograft recipients because of its potential hepatotoxicity.

Critical Illness Myopathy/Critical Illness Polyneuropathy

There is currently no treatment of CIM/CIP and management is based mostly on the avoidance of risk factors and the reduction of the use of intravenous corticosteroids and neuromuscular blocking drugs in patients who are critically ill. Recent studies showed decreased incidence of CIM/CIP with intensive insulin treatment of hyperglycemia.[55] These patients may require intense physical therapy and recovery may be incomplete.[53]

Opportunistic Infections

Accurate diagnosis and prompt treatment are necessary for effective treatment of CNS and systemic infections in patients who are immunosuppressed. Cerebrospinal fluid analysis is essential for accurate diagnosis of CNS infection, but empiric broad spectrum treatment guided by infectious disease service recommendations should not be delayed before a specific infectious agent is identified. While determining the most likely cause of infection we have to consider elapsed time since transplantation, possible endemic exposure, and onset of infection resistant to medications used in prophylactic regimen.[97]

Neurotoxicity of Immunosuppressive Medications

Severe neurotoxicity may warrant adjustment of immunosuppression and switching between different CNI (eg, tacrolimus to cyclosporine) may be helpful in individual cases.[15,23,33,90] Although neurotoxicity of CNI frequently occurs with normal serum levels, decrease of the dosing or substitution with alternate CNI commonly leads to spontaneous improvement.[22-24] We should also correct hypomagnesemia if present. Patients who have CNI-induced seizures should be treated with appropriate antiepileptic medications. Treatment of neurotoxic effects of other immunosuppressants (eg, OKT3) is mostly based on removal of offending agent and supportive measures.

REFERENCES

1. Health Resources and Services Administration, Healthcare Systems Bureau, Division of Transplantation, US Department of Health and Human Services. 2008 Annual Report of the US Organ Procurement and Transplantation Network and the Scientific Registry of Transplant Recipients: Transplant Data 1998–2007. Rockville, MD; United Network for Organ Sharing, Richmond, VA; University Renal Research and Education Association, Ann Arbor (MI), 2009.
2. Pasquini MC, Wang Z, Schneider L. Current use and outcome of hematopoietic stem cell transplantation. CIBMTR Newsletter 2007;13(2):5–8.
3. Wong M, Mallory GB Jr, Goldstein J, et al. Neurologic complications of pediatric lung transplantation. Neurology 1999;53(7):1542–9.
4. Bronster DJ, Emre S, Boccagni P, et al. Central nervous system complications in liver transplant recipients–incidence, timing, and long-term follow-up. Clin Transplant 2000;14(1):1–7.
5. Faraci M, Lanino E, Dini G, et al. Severe neurologic complications after hematopoietic stem cell transplantation in children. Neurology 2002;59(12):1895–904.
6. Mayer TO, Biller J, O'Donnell J, et al. Contrasting the neurologic complications of cardiac transplantation in adults and children. J Child Neurol 2002;17(3):195–9.
7. Lewis MB, Howdle PD. Neurologic complications of liver transplantation in adults. Neurology 2003;61(9):1174–8.
8. Zivkovic S, Abu-Elmagd K, Bond G, et al. Long-term follow-up of neurologic complications of multivisceral and intestinal transplantation. Neurology 2005; 64(Suppl 1):A123.
9. Denier C, Bourhis JH, Lacroix C, et al. Spectrum and prognosis of neurologic complications after hematopoietic transplantation. Neurology 2006;67(11): 1990–7.
10. Erol I, Alehan F, Ozcay F, et al. Neurological complications of liver transplantation in pediatric patients: a single center experience. Pediatr Transplant 2007;11(2): 152–9.
11. Zierer A, Melby SJ, Voeller RK, et al. Significance of neurologic complications in the modern era of cardiac transplantation. Ann Thorac Surg 2007;83(5):1684–90.
12. Zivkovic SA, Jumaa M, Barisic N, et al. Neurologic complications following lung transplantation. J Neurol Sci 2009;280(1–2):90–3.
13. Patchell RA. Neurological complications of organ transplantation. Ann Neurol 1994;36(5):688–703.
14. Pless M, Zivkovic SA. Neurologic complications of transplantation. Neurologist 2002;8(2):107–20.
15. DiMartini A, Fontes P, Dew MA, et al. Age, model for end-stage liver disease score, and organ functioning predict posttransplant tacrolimus neurotoxicity. Liver Transpl 2008;14(6):815–22.
16. Menegaux F, Keeffe EB, Andrews BT, et al. Neurological complications of liver transplantation in adult versus pediatric patients. Transplantation 1994;58(4): 447–50.

17. Wijdicks EF. Impaired consciousness after liver transplantation. Liver Transpl Surg 1995;1(5):329–34.
18. Buis CI, Wiesner RH, Krom RA, et al. Acute confusional state following liver transplantation for alcoholic liver disease. Neurology 2002;59(4):601–5.
19. Estol CJ, Faris AA, Martinez AJ, et al. Central pontine myelinolysis after liver transplantation. Neurology 1989;39(4):493–8.
20. Bleggi-Torres LF, de Medeiros BC, Ogasawara VS, et al. Iatrogenic Wernicke's encephalopathy in allogeneic bone marrow transplantation: a study of eight cases. Bone Marrow Transplant 1997;20(5):391–5.
21. Eidelman BH, Abu-Elmagd K, Wilson J, et al. Neurologic complications of FK 506. Transplant Proc 1991;23(6):3175–8.
22. Wijdicks EF, Wiesner RH, Dahlke LJ, et al. FK506-induced neurotoxicity in liver transplantation. Ann Neurol 1994;35(4):498–501.
23. Wijdicks EF, Wiesner RH, Krom RA. Neurotoxicity in liver transplant recipients with cyclosporine immunosuppression. Neurology 1995;45(11):1962–4.
24. Small SL, Fukui MB, Bramblett GT, et al. Immunosuppression-induced leukoencephalopathy from tacrolimus (FK506). Ann Neurol 1996;40(4):575–80.
25. DeBellis RJ, Schaefer OP, Liquori M, et al. Linezolid-associated serotonin syndrome after concomitant treatment with citalopram and mirtazepine in a critically ill bone marrow transplant recipient. J Intensive Care Med 2005;20(6):351–3.
26. Abbott KC, Agodoa LY, O'Malley PG. Hospitalized psychoses after renal transplantation in the United States: incidence, risk factors, and prognosis. J Am Soc Nephrol 2003;14(6):1628–35.
27. Dew MA, DiMartini AF. Psychological disorders and distress after adult cardiothoracic transplantation. J Cardiovasc Nurs 2005;20(Suppl 5):S51–66.
28. Krahn LE, DiMartini A. Psychiatric and psychosocial aspects of liver transplantation. Liver Transpl 2005;11(10):1157–68.
29. Corruble E, Buhl C, Esposito D, et al. Psychosis associated with elevated trough tacrolimus blood concentrations after combined kidney-pancreas transplant. Int J Neuropsychopharmacol 2006;9(4):493–4.
30. Warrington TP, Bostwick JM. Psychiatric adverse effects of corticosteroids. Mayo Clin Proc 2006;81(10):1361–7.
31. DiMartini A, Dew MA, Kormos R, et al. Posttraumatic stress disorder caused by hallucinations and delusions experienced in delirium. Psychosomatics 2007;48(5):436–9.
32. Medici V, Mirante VG, Fassati LR, et al. Liver transplantation for Wilson's disease: the burden of neurological and psychiatric disorders. Liver Transpl 2005;11(9):1056–63.
33. Wijdicks EF. Neurotoxicity of immunosuppressive drugs. Liver Transpl 2001;7(11):937–42.
34. Stracciari A, Guarino M, Pazzaglia P, et al. Acquired hepatocerebral degeneration: full recovery after liver transplantation. J Neurol Neurosurg Psychiatr 2001;70(1):136–7.
35. Pavletic ZS, Bishop MR, Markopoulou K, et al. Drug-induced parkinsonism after allogeneic bone marrow transplantation. Bone Marrow Transplant 1996;17(6):1185–7.
36. Lentine KL, Rocca Rey LA, Kolli S, et al. Variations in the risk for cerebrovascular events after kidney transplant compared with experience on the waiting list and after graft failure. Clin J Am Soc Nephrol 2008;3(4):1090–101.
37. Estol CJ, Pessin MS, Martinez AJ. Cerebrovascular complications after orthotopic liver transplantation: a clinicopathologic study. Neurology 1991;41(6):815–9.

38. Coplin WM, Cochran MS, Levine SR, et al. Stroke after bone marrow transplantation: frequency, aetiology and outcome. Brain 2001;124(Pt 5):1043–51.
39. Wijdicks EF, Torres VE, Schievink WI, et al. Cerebral hemorrhage in recipients of renal transplantation. Mayo Clin Proc 1999;74(11):1111–2.
40. Wijdicks EF, de Groen PC, Wiesner RH, et al. Intracerebral hemorrhage in liver transplant recipients. Mayo Clin Proc 1995;70(5):443–6.
41. Pomeranz S, Naparstek E, Ashkenazi E, et al. Intracranial haematomas following bone marrow transplantation. J Neurol 1994;241(4):252–6.
42. Trimarchi HM, Truong LD, Brennan S, et al. FK506-associated thrombotic microangiopathy: report of two cases and review of the literature. Transplantation 1999;67(4):539–44.
43. Gordon BG, Haire WD, Patton DF, et al. Thrombotic complications of BMT: association with protein C deficiency. Bone Marrow Transplant 1993;11(1):61–5.
44. Estol CJ, Lopez O, Brenner RP, et al. Seizures after liver transplantation: a clinicopathologic study. Neurology 1989;39(10):1297–301.
45. Wijdicks EF, Plevak DJ, Wiesner RH, et al. Causes and outcome of seizures in liver transplant recipients. Neurology 1996;47(6):1523–5.
46. Steg RE, Kessinger A, Wszolek ZK. Cortical blindness and seizures in a patient receiving FK506 after bone marrow transplantation. Bone Marrow Transplant 1999;23(9):959–62.
47. Zampella EJ, Duvall ER, Sekar BC, et al. Symptomatic spinal epidural lipomatosis as a complication of steroid immunosuppression in cardiac transplant patients. Report of two cases. J Neurosurg 1987;67(5):760–4.
48. Gruhn B, Meerbach A, Egerer R, et al. Successful treatment of Epstein-Barr virus-induced transverse myelitis with ganciclovir and cytomegalovirus hyperimmune globulin following unrelated bone marrow transplantation. Bone Marrow Transplant 1999;24(12):1355–8.
49. Zarranz JJ, Rouco I, Gomez-Esteban JC, et al. Human T lymphotropic virus type I (HTLV-1) associated myelopathy acquired through a liver transplant. J Neurol Neurosurg Psychiatr 2001;71(6):818.
50. Schwartz DL, Schechter GP, Seltzer S, et al. Radiation myelitis following allogeneic stem cell transplantation and consolidation radiotherapy for non-Hodgkin's lymphoma. Bone Marrow Transplant 2000;26(12):1355–9.
51. Hermans G, De Jonghe B, Bruyninckx F, et al. Clinical review: critical illness polyneuropathy and myopathy. Crit Care 2008;12(6):238.
52. Campellone JV, Lacomis D, Kramer DJ, et al. Acute myopathy after liver transplantation. Neurology 1998;50(1):46–53.
53. Guarneri B, Bertolini G, Latronico N. Long-term outcome in patients with critical illness myopathy or neuropathy: the Italian multicentre CRIMYNE study. J Neurol Neurosurg Psychiatr 2008;79(7):838–41.
54. Dyck PJ, Velosa JA, Pach JM, et al. Increased weakness after pancreas and kidney transplantation. Transplantation 2001;72(8):1403–8.
55. Hermans G, Wilmer A, Meersseman W, et al. Impact of intensive insulin therapy on neuromuscular complications and ventilator dependency in the medical intensive care unit. Am J Respir Crit Care Med 2007;175(5):480–9.
56. Maziak DE, Maurer JR, Kesten S. Diaphragmatic paralysis: a complication of lung transplantation. Ann Thorac Surg 1996;61(1):170–3.
57. Stevens AM, Sullivan KM, Nelson JL. Polymyositis as a manifestation of chronic graft-versus-host disease. Rheumatology (Oxford) 2003;42(1):34–9.
58. Wilson JR, Conwit RA, Eidelman BH, et al. Sensorimotor neuropathy resembling CIDP in patients receiving FK506. Muscle Nerve 1994;17(5):528–32.

59. Steiger MJ, Farrah T, Rolles K, et al. Cyclosporin associated headache. J Neurol Neurosurg Psychiatr 1994;57(10):1258–9.
60. Sila CA. Spectrum of neurologic events following cardiac transplantation. Stroke 1989;20(11):1586–9.
61. Gourishankar S, McDermid JC, Jhangri GS, et al. Herpes zoster infection following solid organ transplantation: incidence, risk factors and outcomes in the current immunosuppressive era. Am J Transplant 2004;4(1):108–15.
62. Grotz WH, Breitenfeldt MK, Braune SW, et al. Calcineurin-inhibitor induced pain syndrome (CIPS): a severe disabling complication after organ transplantation. Transpl Int 2001;14(1):16–23.
63. Collini A, De Bartolomeis C, Barni R, et al. Calcineurin-inhibitor induced pain syndrome after organ transplantation. Kidney Int 2006;70(7):1367–70.
64. Papanicolaou GA, Meyers BR, Fuchs WS, et al. Infectious ocular complications in orthotopic liver transplant patients. Clin Infect Dis 1997;24(6):1172–7.
65. Brazis PW, Spivey JR, Bolling JP, et al. A case of bilateral optic neuropathy in a patient on tacrolimus (FK506) therapy after liver transplantation. Am J Ophthalmol 2000;129(4):536–8.
66. van de Beek D, Patel R, Daly RC, et al. Central nervous system infections in heart transplant recipients. Arch Neurol 2007;64(12):1715–20.
67. Fishman JA. Infection in solid-organ transplant recipients. N Engl J Med 2007; 357(25):2601–14.
68. Martin-Davila P, Fortun J, Lopez-Velez R, et al. Transmission of tropical and geographically restricted infections during solid-organ transplantation. Clin Microbiol Rev 2008;21(1):60–96.
69. Singh N, Husain S. Infections of the central nervous system in transplant recipients. Transpl Infect Dis 2000;2(3):101–11.
70. Finelli PF, Uphoff DF. Magnetic resonance imaging abnormalities with septic encephalopathy. J Neurol Neurosurg Psychiatr 2004;75(8):1189–91.
71. Seeley WW, Marty FM, Holmes TM, et al. Post-transplant acute limbic encephalitis: clinical features and relationship to HHV6. Neurology 2007; 69(2):156–65.
72. Shitrit D, Lev N, Bar-Gil-Shitrit A, et al. Progressive multifocal leukoencephalopathy in transplant recipients. Transpl Int 2005;17(11):658–65.
73. DeSalvo D, Roy-Chaudhury P, Peddi R, et al. West Nile virus encephalitis in organ transplant recipients: another high-risk group for meningoencephalitis and death. Transplantation 2004;77(3):466–9.
74. Derouin F, Pelloux H. Prevention of toxoplasmosis in transplant patients. Clin Microbiol Infect 2008;14(12):1089–101.
75. Mendez O, Kanal E, Abu-Elmagd KM, et al. Granulomatous amebic encephalitis in a multivisceral transplant recipient. Eur J Neurol 2006;13(3):292–5.
76. Pittock SJ, Rabinstein AA, Edwards BS, et al. OKT3 neurotoxicity presenting as akinetic mutism. Transplantation 2003;75(7):1058–60.
77. Bodkin CL, Eidelman BH. Sirolimus-induced posterior reversible encephalopathy. Neurology 2007;68(23):2039–40.
78. Singhal S, Powles R, Treleaven J, et al. Central nervous system relapse after bone marrow transplantation for acute leukemia in first remission. Bone Marrow Transplant 1996;17(4):637–41.
79. Buell JF, Gross TG, Hanaway MJ, et al. Posttransplant lymphoproliferative disorder: significance of central nervous system involvement. Transplant Proc 2005;37(2):954–5.

80. Schiff D. Gliomas following organ transplantation: analysis of the contents of a tumor registry. J Neurosurg 2004;101(6):932–4.
81. Shemesh E, Shneider BL, Savitzky JK, et al. Medication adherence in pediatric and adolescent liver transplant recipients. Pediatrics 2004;113(4):825–32.
82. Alonso EM. Growth and developmental considerations in pediatric liver transplantation. Liver Transpl 2008;14(5):585–91.
83. Fonseca-Aten M, Michaels MG. Infections in pediatric solid organ transplant recipients. Semin Pediatr Surg 2006;15(3):153–61.
84. Martin AB, Bricker JT, Fishman M, et al. Neurologic complications of heart transplantation in children. J Heart Lung Transplant 1992;11(5):933–42.
85. Adams D, Samuel D, Goulon-Goeau C, et al. The course and prognostic factors of familial amyloid polyneuropathy after liver transplantation. Brain 2000;123(Pt 7):1495–504.
86. Bolton CF. Electrophysiologic changes in uremic neuropathy after successful renal transplantation. Neurology 1976;26(2):152–61.
87. Fredericks S, Holt DW, MacPhee IA. The pharmacogenetics of immunosuppression for organ transplantation: a route to individualization of drug administration. Am J Pharmacogenomics 2003;3(5):291–301.
88. Mourad M, Wallemacq P, De Meyer M, et al. Biotransformation enzymes and drug transporters pharmacogenetics in relation to immunosuppressive drugs: impact on pharmacokinetics and clinical outcome. Transplantation 2008;85(Suppl 7):S19–24.
89. Zivkovic S. Neuroimaging and neurologic complications after organ transplantation. J Neuroimaging 2007;17(2):110–23.
90. Guarino M, Benito-Leon J, Decruyenaere J, et al. EFNS guidelines on management of neurological problems in liver transplantation. Eur J Neurol 2006;13(1):2–9.
91. Palacios G, Druce J, Du L, et al. A new arenavirus in a cluster of fatal transplant-associated diseases. N Engl J Med 2008;358(10):991–8.
92. Brenner RP. The interpretation of the EEG in stupor and coma. Neurologist 2005;11(5):271–84.
93. Rich MM, Bird SJ, Raps EC, et al. Direct muscle stimulation in acute quadriplegic myopathy. Muscle Nerve 1997;20(6):665–73.
94. Berry GT, Bridges ND, Nathanson KL, et al. Successful use of alternate waste nitrogen agents and hemodialysis in a patient with hyperammonemic coma after heart-lung transplantation. Arch Neurol 1999;56(4):481–4.
95. Giraldo M, Martin D, Colangelo J, et al. Intestinal transplantation for patients with short gut syndrome and hypercoagulable states. Transplant Proc 2000;32(6):1223–4.
96. Chabolla DR, Wszolek ZK. Pharmacologic management of seizures in organ transplant. Neurology 2006;67(12 Suppl 4):S34–8.
97. Roos KL. Central nervous system infections in solid organ, bone marrow, or stem cell transplant recipients. Continuum 2004;10(2):61–73.

Neurologic Presentations of AIDS

Elyse J. Singer, MD[a,b,]*, Miguel Valdes-Sueiras, MD[a],
Deborah Commins, MD, PhD[c], Andrew Levine, PhD[a]

KEYWORDS

• AIDS • HIV • Brain • Opportunistic infection

The human immunodeficiency virus (HIV), the cause of acquired immunodeficiency syndrome (AIDS), has infected an estimated 33 million individuals worldwide.[1] HIV is a member of the lentivirus genus, part of the Retroviridae (retrovirus) family.[2] HIV is associated with immunodeficiency, neoplasia, and neurologic disease.

The development of an identifiable neurologic syndrome in an HIV-infected person is the culmination of a chain of events, determined by properties of HIV itself, genetic characteristics of the host, and interactions with the environment (including treatment). HIV-associated neurologic syndromes can be classified as primary HIV neurologic disease (in which HIV is both necessary and sufficient to cause the illness), secondary or opportunistic neurologic disease (in which HIV interacts with other pathogens, resulting in opportunistic infections [OI] and tumors), and treatment-related neurologic disease (such as immune reconstitution inflammatory syndrome [IRIS]).

HIV is neuroinvasive (can enter the central nervous system [CNS]), neurotrophic (can live in neural tissues), and neurovirulent (causes disease of the nervous system).[2] Presumed mechanisms of CNS invasion include the "Trojan horse" mechanism in which HIV-infected monocytes are admitted by the blood-brain barrier and mature into long-lived, persistently infected perivascular macrophages; infection of the choroid plexus; and direct infection of capillary endothelial cells, among others. HIV-infected cells include capillary endothelium, microglia, monocytes, macrophages, astrocytes, and choroid plexus.[3] Neurons and oligodendrocytes are rarely, if ever, infected (although this is still under discussion), and "indirect" mechanisms are postulated to account for most damage.[4] There is a burst of viral replication in primary

This work was supported by Grants NS38841, U01MH083500, and R03DA026099, from the National Institutes of Health.
[a] Department of Neurology, David Geffen School of Medicine at UCLA, 11645 Wilshire Boulevard, Suite 770, Los Angeles, CA 90025, USA
[b] National Neurological AIDS Bank, 11645 Wilshire Boulevard, Suite 770, Los Angeles, CA 90025, USA
[c] Department of Pathology, University of Southern California Keck School of Medicine, 2011 Zonal Avenue, Los Angeles, CA 90089, USA
* Corresponding author. Department of Neurology, David Geffen School of Medicine at UCLA, 11645 Wilshire Boulevard, Suite 770, Los Angeles, CA 90025.
E-mail address: esinger@ucla.edu (E.J. Singer).

Neurol Clin 28 (2010) 253–275
doi:10.1016/j.ncl.2009.09.018
0733-8619/09/$ – see front matter © 2010 Elsevier Inc. All rights reserved.

infection, followed by an aggressive immune response that declines over time, and by a long period of subclinical infection, followed by recrudescence of disease, and death.[2] Persistent infection and inflammation results in blood-brain barrier breakdown, neuronal and axonal injury, neurotoxicity, and clinical symptoms; damage to the immune system, particularly cell-mediated immunity, results in vulnerability to OI.

In addition to its importance as a cause of neurologic problems, HIV infection of the CNS constitutes a serious barrier to management and eradication of the virus. The CNS is incompletely permeable to antiretroviral drugs, resulting in subtherapeutic levels of many antiretrovirals[5]; it is part of a protected reservoir[6] (along with the gut and several other organs), where HIV can evade the immune system; and it provides an environment where HIV can replicate, mutate, and reinfect the circulation. HIV stimulates a persistent inflammatory response that may activate pathways leading to other neurodegenerative diseases.[7]

HIV-1–ASSOCIATED SYNDROMES IN PRIMARY INFECTION

Acute HIV infection is the period from initial infection to complete seroconversion. During this time 40% to 90% of individuals describe physical symptoms, similar to influenza, or mononucleosis. The most common features include a short period of fever, lymphadenopathy, night sweats, headache, or rash.[8,9] Early CNS infection is usually asymptomatic, but cerebrospinal fluid (CSF)[10] and imaging studies[11] can detect abnormalities even during the "asymptomatic" period that presage later neurologic events.

A minority of seroconverters will experience a neurologic event that brings them to medical attention, such as aseptic meningitis, Bell's palsy,[12,13] or inflammatory neuropathy. Individuals with symptomatic neurologic disease tend to have higher CSF HIV levels than those without neurologic symptoms. Neurologic symptoms may occur before an HIV diagnosis is suspected, for example, before there are sufficient HIV antibodies to produce a positive HIV enzyme-linked immunosorbent antibody (ELISA, also called an HIV enzyme immunoassay). In such cases, a polymerase chain reaction (PCR) test for HIV may lead to the diagnosis. Early diagnosis of acute HIV infection is important, as these individuals are at high risk of transmitting the virus.

The most common neurologic syndrome associated with primary HIV infection is an acute aseptic (viral) meningitis or meningoencephalitis. The symptoms are similar to other viral meningitides, with fever, headache, stiff neck, and photophobia. CSF shows a mild lymphocytic pleocytosis, normal or slightly elevated total protein, and normal glucose.[14] HIV may be detectable by p24 antigen or PCR testing.[15] Most individuals will recover with supportive care. A few will have recurrent bouts of septic meningitis.

Information on the management of HIV aseptic meningitis is limited to case reports. Initiating treatment with cART, or changing and intensifying the regimen to include more CNS-penetrating drugs, may suppress the symptoms.[16] Others have recurrent meningitis when they stop combined antiretroviral therapy (cART), for example, during structured treatment interruptions.[17]

HIV-associated Neurocognitive Disorder

The most common CNS manifestation of HIV is a chronic neurodegenerative condition characterized by cognitive, central motor, and behavioral abnormalities. A variety of names (eg, AIDS dementia complex, HIV-associated dementia, HIV-associated cognitive motor complex) have been applied to this syndrome. HIV-associated neurocognitive disorder (HAND)[18] has recently become a widely accepted nosology for classifying individuals with varying levels of HIV-associated neurocognitive deficits.

HAND is stratified into (1) asymptomatic neurocognitive impairment (ANI), (2) minor neurocognitive disorder (MND), and (3) HIV-associated dementia (HAD). ANI is characterized a subclinical decline in cognition. MND is characterized as mild decline in cognition in addition to mild everyday functioning impairment that affects the more difficult activities of daily living. HAD is characterized by significant decline in cognition along with a significant degree of functional impairment that affects routine activities.[19] There is no diagnostic marker or combination of markers for HAND. The diagnosis is made in HIV-positive (HIV+) patients with cognitive impairment, after ruling out confounding conditions (CNS OI, neurosyphilis, substance abuse, delirium, toxic-metabolic disorders, psychiatric disease, age-related dementias).

Although HAND can affect any neuropsychological domain, the most commonly reported deficits are in attention/concentration, psychomotor speed, memory and learning, information processing, and executive function, whereas language and visuospatial abilities are relatively unaffected.[20] HAND has been characterized as a "subcortical dementia,"[21] in which deficits in working memory (eg, "short-term" memory, the ability to remember information over a brief period of time) and executive function (eg, planning, cognitive flexibility, abstract thinking, rule acquisition, initiating appropriate actions, and inhibiting inappropriate actions) tend to occur early on. Deficits in delayed recall are more typical of "cortical" dementias such as Alzheimer disease. Like other subcortical dementias, the pattern of episodic memory impairment in HAND is consistent with a mixed encoding and retrieval profile,[22] whereas that of Alzheimer disease consists of rapid forgetting due to inability to encode novel information.[23]

HIV can have profound effects on the pyramidal and extrapyramidal motor systems. Milder manifestations of CNS motor impairment include ataxia, motor slowing, incoordination, and tremor; this may progress to disabling weakness, spasticity, extrapyramidal movement disorders, and paraparesis.[24,25] Behavioral effects of HAND include apathy, irritability, and psychomotor retardation,[26–28] which can be mistaken for depression. This presentation is difficult to disentangle because of the high rate of major depression and dysthymia in the HIV population,[29] and because many symptoms queried in depression screening instruments, such as loss of appetite, can be due to HIV. Some AIDS patients develop "manic" symptoms.[30] Again, this must be disentangled from a preexisting bipolar disorder, or a reaction to drugs. So-called secondary or AIDS mania tends to occur in patients with poorly controlled disease, concurrent cognitive deficits, irritability, aggression, and talkativeness, and who have hallucinations and paranoia.[31]

The onset of HAND historically was associated with low CD4+ counts,[32] other AIDS symptoms,[33] elevated CSF viral load,[34] and elevated CSF markers of immune activation (eg, β2-microglobulin and neopterin).[35] Much of this dates back to the 1980s when no effective treatment was available and only the most demented patients came to medical attention.[36,37] At that time, a diagnosis of HAD was considered to be a precursor of death.[32] These aggressive forms of HAND remain prevalent in developing countries and among individuals with late diagnosis, or who have refused or failed cART. However, such presentations are uncommon in cART-treated individuals, who manifest a milder, more slowly progressing and less lethal "attenuated" form of HAND.[38,39] These mild presentations typically occur in persons with partial immune reconstitution, higher CD4+ counts, and suppressed viral loads, and are less strongly associated with markers of immune activation.[40–43] Due to increased awareness of HAND it is also possible that it is identified at an earlier stage.

The traditional neuroimaging approach (in which a diagnosis is made through qualitative image examination) is useful in excluding structural or inflammatory processes, such as abscess, or tumor, that may mimic HAND, but is limited as a diagnostic marker. The HAND brain may appear grossly normal until advanced disease, when atrophy may be noted. White matter changes may appear, typically in the periventricular region. These diseases must be differentiated from others that affect myelin such as progressive multifocal leukoencephalopathy (PML), and unrelated processes such as leukoariosis. At present, there are few ways to distinguish among these white matter abnormalities except for the pattern and distribution of the lesions, which are not definitive. Advanced, investigative neuroimaging techniques show promise as biomarkers of HAND.[44] Brain mapping indicates that there may be a unique pattern of atrophy in HAND that distinguishes it from other dementias. There are reports of ventricular enlargement, atrophy of the caudate, putamen, nucleus accumbens, and other subcortical regions that may characterize HAND.[45–47] Another technique that may identify HAND and measure its progression or improvement is magnetic resonance spectroscopy (MRS).[44,45] MRS is sensitive to the earliest signs of CNS infection. Lentz and colleagues[48] reported on subjects followed from early seroconversion and reported an initial decline in N-acetylaspartate (NAA), a marker of neuronal viability, in the frontocortical gray matter. NAA levels were found to be decreased in the centrum semiovale white matter of chronically HIV-infected subjects, but not in early infection. This study is still ongoing, so further follow-up will be needed to map changes over time. Paul and colleagues[49] reported that impaired neuropsychological performance in HIV is associated with reduced NAA and increased myoinositol (MI; a marker of gliosis) in the basal ganglia and frontal white matter, but not with markers in the parietal region (**Fig. 1**). Fluorodeoxyglucose (FDG) positron emission tomography (PET) studies in HIV are few, but show early hypermetabolism in the basal ganglia,[50] followed by hypometabolism in late HAND.[51] This pattern is unlike Alzheimer disease and other dementias.

Neurologic and neuropsychologic improvement of HAND after treatment with antiretrovirals was established with studies of zidovudine monotherapy in randomized placebo-controlled trials that demonstrated improved neuropsychological test scores versus placebo.[52,53] Current treatment of HIV is based on the use of cART, which includes 2 or more antiretroviral agents to suppress HIV and increase CD4+ counts. The most common initial cART regimens consist of 2 nucleoside or nucleotide reverse transcriptase inhibitors (NRTIs) combined with either a non-nucleoside reverse transcriptase inhibitor (NNRTI) or a "boosted" protease inhibitor (PI). Ritonavir (in small doses) is a PI most commonly used as a booster; it enhances other PIs so they can

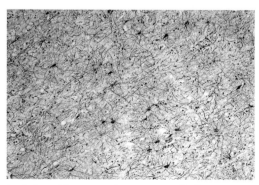

Fig. 1. Marked gliosis of the white matter is a common finding in HIV+ patients at autopsy and may underlie changes seen premortem by magnetic resonance spectroscopy. Immunoperoxidase stain (*brown*) for the astrocytic marker, glial fibrillary acidic protein (original magnification ×200).

be given in lower doses. No placebo-controlled trials of cART for HAND have been performed, because it would be unethical to refuse treatment to a symptomatic patient. Based on well-conducted (albeit not randomized, double blinded, or controlled) studies,[54] it seems that cART improves neuropsychological performance.[55] It also seems that cART has reduced the incidence of new cases of severe HAND (HAD), while apparently increasing the number and life span of individuals living with milder forms of HAND.[38,56]

The CNS penetration of the various components of a cART regimen may vary widely, and there is ongoing discussion regarding the importance of the CNS penetrability of a cART regimen. Letendre and colleagues[5] have proposed a CNS-Penetration Effectiveness (CPE) Rank, in which cART regimens are ranked by summing up various criteria associated with CNS effectiveness. In a large study, subjects whose regimens scored low on the CPE ranking had higher CSF viral loads.[5] In a related study, Marra and colleagues[57] confirmed the association of low CPE scores with higher probability of detectable CSF viral load, and poorer neuropsychological performance. An independent group[58] confirmed that higher CPE scores were associated with greater improvements in neuropsychological performance.

In addition to cART, there have been attempts to identify non-antiretroviral neuroprotective drugs to avert HAND. A review of clinical studies[59] have been performed on memantine (an N-methyl-D-aspartate antagonist drug), selegiline (a monoamine oxidase-B inhibitor), nimodipine (a calcium channel blocker), and nonapproved drugs Peptide T, CPI-1189, and others. None of the drugs studied was effective. Studies of valproic acid (an anticonvulsant) and minocycline (an antibiotic) are in progress.

There are a few studies of psychostimulant drugs to palliate neuropsychiatric symptoms frequently seen in HAND. These studies included a randomized, placebo-controlled trial of methylphenidate for severe HIV-associated fatigue,[60] and a single-blind, placebo-controlled, crossover-design study of methylphenidate for HIV-associated cognitive slowing.[61] Both showed significantly more improvement with methylphenidate than placebo.

HIV-Associated Vacuolar Myelopathy

Vacuolar myelopathy (VM) is the most common spinal cord disease in AIDS, found in up to 30% of autopsies in the pre-cART era.[62] VM is underdiagnosed,[63] and must be differentiated from other causes of myelopathy such as infection with human T-cell lymphotropic virus (HTLV) I or II, herpes simplex 1 or 2, varicella zoster, cytomegalovirus, enteroviruses, syphilis and tuberculosis, tumors, and nutritional deficiencies such as B12.[64] In the past, HIV VM was more common in patients with opportunistic conditions,[63] but this association has not been reviewed in the cART era.

The clinical presentation of HIV VM is slowly progressive leg weakness, which may be asymmetric at first, spasticity, dorsal column (vibration, position) sensory loss, ataxic gait, and urinary frequency and urgency.[65] Erectile dysfunction is an early sign in men. Paresthesias in the legs are common but neuropathic pain rarely rises to the level seen with peripheral neuropathy. There is prominent hyperreflexia, and extensor plantar responses. In advanced cases, patients may become wheelchair-bound and doubly incontinent.[65] The diagnosis should be questioned if symptoms present in an acute fashion, the arms are affected, there is a sensory level, or if there is back pain.

The most important test is a spinal magnetic resonance image (MRI), to rule out abscess or tumor. In many HIV VM cases, the MRI is normal. Some will have high signal hyperintense areas on T2-weighted imaging, primarily in the thoracic region and affecting the posterior columns, that do not enhance with contrast; these areas correlate to vacuolation on histopathology.[66] Cord atrophy has also been reported.[67] A lumbar puncture is important to exclude treatable infections or carcinomatous meningitis. Somatosensory evoked potentials are useful to disentangle cases in which both HIV VM and sensory neuropathy are present.[68]

The precise pathophysiology of HIV VM is unknown. The distribution of pathology, involving the posterior columns and pyramidal tracts, resembles B12 deficiency.[69] The relationship to productive HIV infection within the cord remains controversial.[70–73] Suspected mechanisms include defective methylation due to a deficiency of S-adenosylmethionine,[74] triggered by inflammatory products secreted by activated macrophages and microglia.[75,76]

There is no specific treatment for HIV VM. A pilot, open-label study of L-methionine to address the suspected abnormality of transmethylation mechanisms in HIV VM did not show benefit.[77] There are case reports of improvement with cART.[78–80] However, axonal degeneration is a late feature of HIV VM,[81] and would not be expected to resolve. Patients with HIV VM benefit from physical and occupational therapy, baclofen, tizanidine, dantrolene, and intramuscular botulinum toxin to manage spasticity, pain management, and anticholinergic drugs to improve bladder function.[65]

HIV-Associated Peripheral Neuropathies

Many peripheral neuropathic syndromes have been reported in the context of HIV infection. Here the discussion is confined to HIV-associated distal sensory neuropathy, neurotoxic nucleoside neuropathy, and inflammatory demyelinating neuropathy.

HIV-associated distal peripheral sensory neuropathy (DSPN) (also called predominantly sensory neuropathy, or distal symmetric peripheral neuropathy), is the most common neurologic problem in AIDS,[82] with incidences ranging from 19% to 66%, depending on the age, disease stage, and treatment history of the cohort.[83] The risk factors for HIV DSPN are older age, history of alcohol abuse, and advanced HIV disease (eg, a low nadir CD4+ count and high plasma HIV viral load),[84,85] prior use of a neurotoxic antiretroviral drug (eg, didanosine, stavudine, zalcitabine), and diabetes.

The most universally reported symptoms are paresthesias,[86] that virtually always begin in the feet, as this is a length-dependent neuropathy. Patients complain of burning, numbness, hot or cold sensations, and episodic electric-shock like sensations. Some complain of a sensation that they are walking on sand or glass. Many cannot bear to wear shoes. The symptoms ascend over time, as far as the thighs, and will also involve the hands in a glovelike fashion. Cramps and fasciculations may develop in the extremities. Most patients do not develop any motor weakness or muscle wasting until late in their course, and this is limited to the distal extremities.[87] The most common physical findings are decreased or absent ankle jerks, diminished vibratory sensation in the legs, and increased threshold to temperature and pinprick (alternatively, some patients develop hyperesthesia).[87] Some patients will have all the physical findings of neuropathy but do not report pain; they usually have an asymptomatic neuropathy. Others will have hyperreflexia proximally and hyporeflexia distally, in which case a mixed myelopathy and neuropathy should be suspected.

The pathogenesis of HIV DSPN is unknown. Related viruses such as feline immunodeficiency virus (FIV) also cause neuropathy in cats.[88] FIV (and HIV-1) infects and activates macrophages[88] and CD8+ lymphocytes[89] in the dorsal root ganglion, and these cells can release substances, such as tumor necrosis factor,[88] that are toxic to neurons and oligodendrocytes. The HIV protein gp120 is also neurotoxic, causing hyperesthesia, allodynia, and spinal gliosis.[90] The major neuropathologic features in HIV DSPN include a loss of unmyelinated axons in the distal regions of sensory nerves, followed by Wallerian degeneration of the distal myelinated fibers. Some degree of demyelination and remyelination has also been reported.[91]

In most cases, an electromyogram (EMG) and nerve conduction studies (NCS) are not necessary to diagnose HIV DSPN.[92] If an electrodiagnostic study is performed, it will demonstrate findings similar to other degenerative, predominantly axonal neuropathies, such as reduced or absent action potentials. A few patients have apparently normal studies. These patients most likely have a small-fiber neuropathy, and quantitative sensory testing may be helpful if there is a reason to document the clinical diagnosis. It is important to search for processes that can mimic or exacerbate HIV DSPN, including syphilis, diabetes, B12 or folate deficiency, thyroid disease, hepatitis C virus, and any neurotoxic medication.

Treatment of DSPN itself is generally frustrating. Studies of nerve growth factor[93] and the experimental drug prosaptide[94] were unproductive. Randomized, controlled clinical trials of drugs to control neuropathic pain showed positive results for lamotrigine,[95] for an experimental high-concentration capsaicin dermal patch,[96] cannabinoids,[97,98] and gabapentin.[99] Treatments that were ineffective included amitriptyline,[100,101] mexilitene,[100] memantine,[102] Peptide T,[103] and acupuncture.[101]

Nucleoside neuropathy in HIV+ patients (also called antiretroviral toxic neuropathy, or neurotoxic neuropathy), has classically been associated with 3 NRTI drugs: didanosine (ddI), zalcitabine (ddC), and stavudine (d4T). These drugs were used extensively early in the epidemic, and they are still used in resource-limited settings. Other risk factors include another, prior neuropathy, diabetes, alcoholism, poor nutrition, using higher doses of the offending nucleoside, and use of more than one potentially neurotoxic nucleoside.[86,104] The clinical and electrophysiological features of neurotoxic neuropathy are very similar to HIV DSPN,[105] but usually begin within 6 months of starting the offending drug, with a peak around 3 months.[106] It has been proposed that mitochondrial toxicity,[107] competitive inhibition of human mitochondrial DNA polymerase-γ,[108] downregulation of gene expression for brain-derived neurotrophic factor in the dorsal root ganglion,[109] and specific host genetic polymorphisms[110] may predispose to nucleoside neuropathy. The only specific treatment is to remove the offending drug; if this is impossible, it should be maintained at the lowest dose. Many patients take up to 3 weeks after the drug is discontinued to see any improvement[111]; reduction in symptoms usually occurs by 6 weeks, but some may take up to 6 months and a few never resolve.

Inflammatory Demyelinating Polyneuropathies

The true prevalence of this complication is unknown, but it seems to be relatively rare. There are 2 major types of HIV inflammatory demyelinating polyneuropathies (IDP). Acute IDP is similar to Guillain-Barré syndrome, and often occurs during or near primary infection.[112] Patients develop the rapid onset of ascending weakness, areflexia, autonomic instability, and some (usually minor) sensory symptoms,[113] but bowel and bladder function is spared. The disease can progress to involve the muscles of respiration. Unlike non-HIV Guillain-Barré, there is usually a mild lymphocytic pleocytosis. Since the advent of cART, a few cases have occurred during immune reconstitution.[114] Electrophysiological studies show patchy distribution of abnormalities, including slow or absent nerve conduction, and abnormal F waves.[115] Treatment consists of supportive care, intravenous γ-globulin, plasma exchange, and possibly cART,[116–118] and is based on case reports and extrapolation from the non-HIV literature.[119]

A chronic IDP (CIDP) may occur in late infection and is often associated with a CD4+ count of less than 50 cells/mm^3.[120] Unlike acute HIV IDP, this syndrome progresses slowly and may have a relapsing and remitting nature. CIDP must be differentiated from neuropathies caused by cytomegalovirus (CMV) and related viruses. Treatment of HIV CIDP is similar to that of non-HIV related CIDP, with the exception for the need to control HIV infection, and is based on case reports on HIV patients and the non-HIV literature.

Progressive Multifocal Leukoencephalopathy

PML is a demyelinating disease of the CNS.[121] PML is caused by the John Cunningham virus (JCV), a polyoma virus found worldwide, with a seroprevalence of 70% to 90%.[122,123] Previously a rare disease, PML became a frequent (up to 5%) complication of AIDS in the 1980s,[124] although the incidence has declined with cART.[125] PML has been recently reported to occur in association with the treatments for multiple sclerosis and rheumatologic disorders.[126]

Most cases of AIDS PML occur during severe immunosuppression (less than 100 CD4+ cells/mm^3), although exceptions occur in about 11% of cases.[124] Most present with the subacute onset of altered mental status, accompanied by focal symptoms referable to the location of the one or more PML lesions, such as hemiparesis, hemianopsia, ataxia, vertigo, speech disorders, and seizures.[125] Patients usually do not have headaches, fevers, nausea, vomiting, or papilledema.

A definitive diagnosis is established by biopsy or autopsy. However, a diagnosis of probable PML can be made with a supportive clinical history along with correlative radiological and laboratory findings. The most common neuroimaging findings[127] are one or more space-occupying white matter lesions that are nonenhancing, hyperintense on T2 and hypointense on T1, and sparse cortical U-fibers. However, some cases do enhance, a feature associated with a better prognosis.[128] There is no definitive MRI marker of PML. CSF examination is invaluable in ruling out other infections but otherwise is nonspecific, with mild pleocytosis, elevated total protein, and normal glucose. A positive JCV PCR is considered diagnostic in a case with typical clinical and imaging features; however, the sensitivity and specificity of this test is under discussion, as JCV has been detected in the CSF of immune suppressed persons without PML,[129] and may not be detected in cART-treated patients with tissue-diagnosed PML or those with low JCV viral loads.[130] In a severe case such as shown in **Fig. 2**, gross examination at autopsy may show multifocal areas of tan-gray discoloration and softening. The gray-white junction is a favored site. The larger lesions may

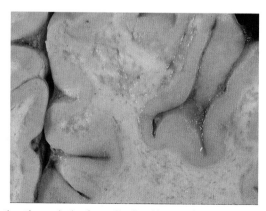

Fig. 2. Coronal section through the formalin-fixed brain of an HIV+ person who succumbed to progressive multifocal leukoencephalopathy shows the characteristic multifocal areas of white matter discoloration.

be necrotizing at the center with loss of both myelin and axons and replacement by confluent lipid-laden macrophages. At the periphery there are scattered virally infected oligodendroglial cells with enlarged nuclei that contain deep amphophilic (purple) viral inclusions. PML lesions also contain grossly enlarged, pleomorphic "pseudoneoplastic" astrocytes. If necessary, the diagnosis can be confirmed with immunohistochemistry or in situ hybridization for JCV.

There is no specific treatment for PML with or without AIDS. Multiple agents have been tried without success, including topotecan,[131] cytarabine,[132,133] and cidofovir.[134] However, cART has improved the course of AIDS PML, decreasing the mortality rate, improving the neuroimaging features, improving survival, and decreasing CSF JCV viral load.[125,135,136] Patients who survive AIDS PML are likely to have serious residual neurocognitive deficits. Levine and colleagues[137] reported that 8 patients with past PML differed as a group from AIDS patients without history of CNS OI regarding information processing and motor functioning. Further, although the PML group was less severely impaired overall than those with history of AIDS and toxoplasmosis, their deficits in information processing and motor functioning were the most severe of all groups examined.

Cytomegalovirus

CMV, a member of the Herpesvirus family, can infect the brain, spinal cord, meninges, retina, the dorsal root ganglion of peripheral nerves, and many visceral organs.[138] Approximately 60% of the population show evidence of exposure to CMV[139] but the prevalence is higher in homosexual men.[140] CMV establishes a lifelong, latent infection without clinical disease in immunocompetent individuals after initial infection, and may remain latent for years, or reactivate under conditions such as HIV or other immunodeficient states. CMV and HIV are known to transactivate each other in vitro.[141]

CMV of the nervous system typically presents in individuals with CD4+ counts of less than 50 cells/mm^3, CMV viremia, and one or more systemic site(s) of infection.[138] Neurologic CMV disease can present as encephalitis, ventriculitis, myelitis, radiculoganglionitis, and peripheral polyneuropathy, or various combinations thereof.[138,142] Presenting signs and symptoms are extremely variable depending on the area affected; CMV encephalitis and ventriculitis may present with fever, lethargy, confusion, or coma, seizures, and cranial nerve palsies, ataxia, and hemiparesis, or even coma; some patients present with dementia, which may or may not be due to a concurrent HIV encephalitis.[143,144] CMV infection of the spinal cord may cause either a transverse myelitis or a myeloradiculitis characterized by flaccid paraparesis associated with back pain, incontinence, areflexia, paresthesias and sensory loss, and ascending weakness.[145,146]

The CSF CMV PCR is considered the gold standard for identifying and quantifying CNS CMV and for following the response to therapy.[147] The literature also refers to a CSF profile that may consist of a polymorphonuclear pleocytosis,[148] but this is not a consistent finding.[145]

Unlike HIV, CMV can directly infect astrocytes, neurons, oligodendroglia, endothelial, ependyma, and meningeal cells,[149,150] and can directly kill neural cells, for example, by inducing apoptosis.[151,152] The most common pathologic finding is a microglial nodule encephalitis, but other findings include ventriculoencephalitis (a focal or diffuse destruction of the ependymal lining and necrosis of periventricular tissue), focal necrosis, and isolated cytomegalic cells (**Fig. 3**).[153]

Randomized, placebo-controlled trial data regarding treatment of CNS CMV are lacking. Based on data extrapolated from case reports and clinical trials of other organ

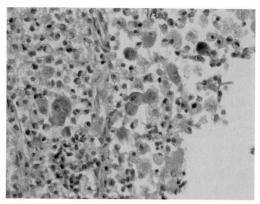

Fig. 3. Cytomegalovirus (CMV) infection of cells may result in the morphologic changes shown here, namely cytomegaly and both intranuclear and intracytoplasmic viral inclusions. Immunohistochemistry for CMV (not shown) may detect additional infected cells that appear normal. Hematoxylin and eosin stain (original magnification ×200).

systems, it is recommended that treatment be initiated immediately with intravenous ganciclovir, at an induction dose of 5 mg/kg twice daily.[54] Intravenous foscarnet 90 mg/kg twice a day can be used in lieu of ganciclovir,[54] but has greater renal toxicity. Cidofovir can be used if these regimens fail.[54] Based on information extrapolated from other CMV infections, patients should continue chronic suppressive therapy until CD4+ cell counts increase to more than 100 cells/mm³.[154] Patients who have not started cART should do so, and those with suboptimal cART should have that adjusted.[155]

Cryptococcal Meningitis

Cryptococcus neoformans is an encapsulated yeast found throughout the world. *C. neoformans* is spread through inhalation of spores, which can be found in dust and bird droppings. The initial infection is usually a self-limited pneumonitis. In most individuals the immune system clears the disease, but some of the organism remains in a latent state within granulomas,[156] from which it can disseminate to multiple organs, particularly in immunosuppressed patients. In AIDS, the most common presentation is a subacute meningoencephalitis, usually in a patient with less than 100 CD4+ cells/mm³. Cryptococcus has an affinity for the CNS, possibly related to its consumption of catecholamines.[157]

Common presenting symptoms of cryptococcal meningitis (CM) include malaise, headache, and fever. As the disease progresses, patients may develop seizures and signs of increased intracranial pressure (nausea, vomiting, visual loss, diplopia, coma).[156] A diagnosis of CM can be made by visualizing the yeast in CSF using India ink; or by detecting cryptococcal antigen in the CSF using the latex agglutination test.[54] If lumbar puncture is contraindicated, a presumptive diagnosis can be made with a serum antigen test. AIDS patients may not have a CSF cellular pleocytosis, abnormal protein, or low CSF glucose.[158] Neuroimaging may be normal, but abnormalities such as masses (cryptococcomas), dilated perivascular spaces, or pseudocysts are associated with higher blood and CSF antigen titers.[159]

Immediate treatment is essential to prevent loss of brain and loss of life, as this is a lethal disease, and even with optimal treatment the mortality rate is still 15%.[160] The recommended initial standard treatment is amphotericin B, at a dose of

0.7–1.0 mg daily, combined with flucytosine, at a dose of 100 mg/kg daily in 4 divided doses, for at least 2 weeks for those with normal renal function.[155] Primary treatment with fluconazole has failed.[161] In addition to antifungal therapy and cART, it is important to manage increased intracranial pressure, as this may lead to permanent neurologic deficits, blindness, and death.[162] The CSF can be removed by repeated lumbar puncture, or a lumbar drain or shunt may be necessary.[54] After at least a 2-week period of successful induction therapy, defined as significant clinical improvement and a negative repeat CSF culture, amphotericin B and flucytosine may be discontinued and follow-up therapy initiated with fluconazole 400 mg daily.[155] This regimen should continue for at least 8 weeks. Discontinuation of secondary prophylaxis can be considered in patients with sterile CSF, clinical improvement, and an increase in CD4+ cell count to at least 200 cells/mm^3.

With treatment, most HIV+ individuals will survive CM. Long-term outcomes in neurocognitive functioning have only recently been examined. In an exploratory study, Levine and colleagues examined neurocognitive functioning in a cohort of 15 individuals with a history of AIDS and CM, compared with 61 individuals with AIDS but without history of CNS disease. Those with a history of CM continued to demonstrate deficits in verbal fluency and motor functioning relative to HIV-infected controls without CM.

Toxoplasmosis Encephalitis

Toxoplasma gondii is a ubiquitous intracellular protozoan pathogen of both humans and animals. From 15% to 85% of the world's adult human population is infected with *T. gondii* depending on geographic location. The definitive host is the cat, but the parasite can be carried by all mammals. Infection can be acquired transplacentally, or by ingesting contaminated water, undercooked meat, soil, or cat feces. Once in the gut, the parasite disseminates to the brain, muscles, and eyes, and invades cells, where it forms intracellular cysts. Most primary infections are asymptomatic or there may be flulike symptoms. The parasite may remain latent for years; cases of AIDS-associated toxoplasmosis encephalitis (TE) almost always result from reactivation, usually when the CD4+ count has declined to less than 200 cells/mm^3; higher risk is present when the CD4+ count is less than 50 cells/mm^3.[155,163]

Fever, headache, focal neurologic deficit, cognitive dysfunction, seizures, and altered mental status are the most common presenting symptoms of TE.[164,165] Because these are highly inflammatory and necrotic lesions with mass effect, elevated intracranial pressure is often a serious problem. The typical neuroimaging presentation includes multiple (in 70% of cases), contrast-enhancing lesions, frequently surrounded by edema.[166] Most lesions are supratentorial, and located at the gray-white matter junction or in the basal ganglia. MRI typically shows several T2-weighted hyperintense lesions with enhancement on postcontrast T1 images.[166] Some lesions are hemmorhagic.[167] The most important differential diagnosis in AIDS patients is primary CNS lymphoma (PCNSL). Some investigators advocate the use of thallium-201 brain single-photon emission computed tomography (CT)[168] or positron emission tomography[169] (PET) to differentiate between PCNSL (which has a high rate of uptake) and TE (which does not). However, most physicians still require a tissue diagnosis before treating a patient for PCNSL because of the lack of specificity of these techniques. CSF frequently is not sampled in TE, because the mass lesions may make lumbar puncture unsafe; it is useful in excluding other pathogens. Almost all AIDS patients with TE are have toxoplasma immunoglobulin G (IgG) antibodies in blood. Although a definitive diagnosis requires brain biopsy, a response to empiric toxoplasmosis treatment is also considered to be diagnostic[54]; failure to respond is an indication for biopsy.[155] The response to antiparasitic therapy may be confounded, however, if corticosteroids are required to reduce brain inflammation, control intracranial pressure, and prevent herniation.

The treatment of choice for TE is a combination of pyrimethamine (200 mg oral loading dose followed by 50–75 mg by mouth per day), plus sulfadiazine 1000–1500 mg by mouth, 4 times a day (to treat the parasite) and leucovorin (folinic acid) 10–25 mg by mouth per day, to reduce toxicity caused by pyrimethamine.[54,155] An alternative regimen is pyrimethamine 200 mg by mouth loading dose followed by 50 mg by mouth per day, plus clindamycin 600 mg by mouth every 6 hours, plus pyrimethamine 25–50 mg PO daily plus leucovorin 10–25 mg PO daily. Acute therapy should be continued for at least 6 weeks, provided that the patient is improving, and longer in cases with extensive disease. Secondary prophylaxis should be continued until the lesions are resolved, symptoms have improved, cART has raised the CD4+ cell count to at least 200 cells/mm^3, and viral load is suppressed.[170]

Persistent neuropsychological deficits are evident in many survivors of TE. Examining the long-term neurocognitive outcomes of individuals who survived AIDS CNS OIs, Levine and colleagues[137] found that those with past TE performed worse on all but one neuropsychological domain than those with history of other AIDS CNS OI, including PML and CM.

Primary CNS Lymphoma in AIDS

PCNSL arises in, and is confined to, the CNS. PCNSL is the second most common mass lesion in AIDS. The major risk factor is a CD4+ count of less than 100 cells/mm^3. These tumors are promoted by immunosuppression, chronic antigenic stimulation, and cytokine overproduction. In the setting of immunosuppression, PCNSL is almost always associated with Epstein-Barr Virus (EBV),[171] a ubiquitous herpesvirus with a seroprevalence of 90%. Most EBV infections are asymptomatic, or present as acute mononucleosis. EBV can remain latent in B cells, and can immortalize the cell. In AIDS, immune surveillance fails and the immortalized EBV-infected B cells are no longer held in check.[172] Thus the risk of PCNSL is greatly increased. Prior to cART, PCNSL occurred in 5% of those AIDS patients with neurologic symptoms.[173,174] The use of cART has resulted in a lower incidence of PCNSL and improved survival.[175,176]

The presenting symptoms of PCNSL include lethargy, confusion, impaired memory, headache, seizures, or focal weakness. Many patients develop cranial neuropathies or ocular involvement. Increased intracranial pressure and herniation can result in papilledema, and coma if untreated.

The usual neuroimaging findings on CT or MRI are one or sometimes multiple, contrast-enhancing lesions surrounded by edema, with mass effect. On MRI, they are hyperintense on T1 imaging and often show a periventricular distribution. These lesions typically have a high uptake of radioactive tracers on thallium-201 single-photon emission CT[168] or fluorodeoxyglucose PET[169] as opposed to TE. If it is safe to perform a lumbar puncture, the CSF may be helpful. EBV can be detected and quantified by PCR in the CSF[177] and plasma[178] of these patients, and may be a biomarker of PCNSL. However, diagnosis ultimately depends on tissue examination.

AIDS PCNSLs are almost always high-grade, diffuse B-cell lymphomas, often of immunoblastic subtype. Compared with similar tumors seen in immunocompetent individuals, they are more likely to be multifocal and necrotic. Biopsy can be problematic,[179] especially a needle biopsy, because of the small sample, the possibility of extensive necrosis of the tumor, and the angiocentric nature. Administration of corticosteroids to reduce cerebral edema before biopsy can result in lysis of most neoplastic lymphocytes, resulting in a nondiagnostic biopsy.[179]

The tumor is treated with cranial irradiation (usual adult dose is fractionated 4000–5000 cGy), and by instituting or optimizing cART. Chemotherapy, if used, typically includes methotrexate, and there are also some positive results using antiviral therapies (eg, ganciclovir) that decrease EBV viral load,[180] but there are no large controlled trials that establish optimal therapy.

Unfortunately, many treatments for AIDS PCNSL can result in residual cognitive impairment, particularly when both whole brain radiation and methotrexate-based chemotherapy are used.[181] The literature on this topic almost exclusively involves non-HIV cases. Harder and colleagues[182] reported on the neurocognitive status and quality of life among 19 non-HIV patients treated for PCNSL. All patients were in remission after combined whole brain radiation and methotrexate-based chemotherapy. Neurocognitive and quality of life scores were compared with demographically matched controls who had systemic malignancies and had undergone chemotherapy or nonbrain radiotherapy. The investigators found neurocognitive impairment in 12 patients with PCNSL, with 4 showing severe cognitive deficits. Only 2 control subjects were cognitively impaired according to their criteria. Only 42% of the PCNSL patients returned to work, compared with 81% of controls.

Immune Reconstitution Inflammatory Syndrome

The immune reconstitution inflammatory syndromes (IRIS) is a serious problem complicating the treatment of AIDS.[183] IRIS refers to a group of syndromes characterized by paradoxic clinical worsening that usually occurs within the first 4 to 8 weeks after starting cART.[155] The reconstituted immune system generates an inflammatory response, resulting in either a worsening of a known, underlying infection, or the unmasking of a subclinical, indolent infection. This exaggerated "dysregulated" inflammatory response is characterized by massive infiltration of CD8+ cells. Neuroimaging features include development of, or increase in, contrast enhancement, and unusual patterns of contrast enhancement.[184] Intracranial pressure may increase,[185] requiring the use of corticosteroids. Among the most common CNS infections reported to be involved in IRIS are HIV encephalitis,[186–188] TE,[187,189] CM,[185] and PML.[155,184] Risk factors for IRIS include taking cART for the first time, active or subclinical OI, CD4+ counts of less than 50 cells/mm^3, high CD8+ cells, anemia, and a rapid decline in HIV viral load.[190,191] There are relatively few biopsy or autopsy studies of IRIS, in part because most patients survive the syndrome. Some studies have reported both active lesions containing the pathogen (HIV-associated multinucleated giant cells, JCV, *Toxoplasma* parasites, and so forth), and "sterile" lesions with inflammatory infiltrates. The treatment of CNS IRIS with corticosteroids has been advocated and remains controversial, as there are no formal studies, but should be considered if increased intracranial pressure is present.

The continuing evolution of the HIV epidemic has spurred an intense interest in a hitherto neglected area of medicine, neuroinfectious diseases and their consequences. This work has broad applications for the study of CNS tumors, dementias, neuropathies, and CNS disease in other immunosuppressed individuals.

REFERENCES

1. UNAIDS. Report on the global AIDS epidemic 2008. Geneva: UNAIDS; 2007.
2. Patrick MK, Johnston JB, Power C. Lentiviral neuropathogenesis: comparative neuroinvasion, neurotropism, neurovirulence, and host neurosusceptibility. J Virol 2002;76:7923–31.

3. Wiley CA, Schrier RD, Nelson JA, et al. Cellular localization of human immunodeficiency virus infection within the brains of acquired immune deficiency syndrome patients. Proc Natl Acad Sci U S A 1986;83:7089–93.

4. Kaul M, Lipton SA. Mechanisms of neuronal injury and death in HIV-1 associated dementia. Curr HIV Res 2006;4:307–18.

5. Letendre S, Marquie-Beck J, Capparelli E, et al. Validation of the CNS penetration-effectiveness rank for quantifying antiretroviral penetration into the central nervous system. Arch Neurol 2008;65:65–70.

6. Clements JE, Li M, Gama L, et al. The central nervous system is a viral reservoir in simian immunodeficiency virus-infected macaques on combined antiretroviral therapy: a model for human immunodeficiency virus patients on highly active antiretroviral therapy. J Neurovirol 2005;11:180–9.

7. Brew BJ, Crowe SM, Landay A, et al. Neurodegeneration and ageing in the HAART era. J Neuroimmune Pharmacol 2009;4:163–74.

8. Huang ST, Lee HC, Liu KH, et al. Acute human immunodeficiency virus infection. J Microbiol Immunol Infect 2005;38:65–8.

9. Fox R, Eldred LJ, Fuchs EJ, et al. Clinical manifestations of acute infection with human immunodeficiency virus in a cohort of gay men. AIDS 1987;1:35–8.

10. Resnick L, Berger JR, Shapshak P, et al. Early penetration of the blood-brain-barrier by HIV. Neurology 1988;38:9–14.

11. Tarasow E, Wiercinska-Drapalo A, Kubas B, et al. Cerebral MR spectroscopy in neurologically asymptomatic HIV-infected patients. Acta Radiol 2003;44:206–12.

12. Krasner CG, Cohen SH. Bilateral Bell's palsy and aseptic meningitis in a patient with acute human immunodeficiency virus seroconversion. West J Med 1993;159:604–5.

13. Serrano P, Hernandez N, Arroyo JA, et al. Bilateral Bell palsy and acute HIV type 1 infection: report of 2 cases and review. Clin Infect Dis 2007;44:e57–61.

14. Hollander H, Stringari S. Human immunodeficiency virus-associated meningitis. Clinical course and correlations. Am J Med 1987;83:813–6.

15. Hollander H, Levy JA. Neurologic abnormalities and recovery of human immunodeficiency virus from cerebrospinal fluid. Ann Intern Med 1987;106:692–5.

16. Wendel KA, McArthur JC. Acute meningoencephalitis in chronic human immunodeficiency virus (HIV) infection: putative central nervous system escape of HIV replication. Clin Infect Dis 2003;37:1107–11.

17. Worthington MG, Ross JJ. Aseptic meningitis and acute HIV syndrome after interruption of antiretroviral therapy: implications for structured treatment interruptions. AIDS 2003;17:2145–6.

18. Antinori A, Arendt G, Becker JT, et al. Updated research nosology for HIV-associated neurocognitive disorders. Neurology 2007;69:1789–99.

19. Woods SP, Moore DJ, Weber E, et al. Cognitive neuropsychology of HIV-associated neurocognitive disorders. Neuropsychol Rev 2009;19:152–68.

20. Reger M, Welsh R, Razani J, et al. A meta-analysis of the neuropsychological sequelae of HIV infection. J Int Neuropsychol Soc 2002;8:410–24.

21. Tross S, Price RW, Navia B, et al. Neuropsychological characterization of the AIDS dementia complex: a preliminary report. AIDS 1988;2:81–8.

22. Delis DC, Peavy G, Heaton R, et al. Do patients with HIV-associated minor cognitive/motor disorder exhibit a 'subcortical' memory profile? Evidence using the California verbal learning test. Assessment 1995;2:151–65.

23. Pillon B, Deweer B, Michon A, et al. Are explicit memory disorders of progressive supranuclear palsy related to damage to striatofrontal circuits? Comparison with

Alzheimer's, Parkinson's, and Huntington's diseases. Neurology 1994;44: 1264–70.

24. Navia BA, Cho ES, Petito CK, et al. The AIDS dementia complex: II. Neuropathology. Ann Neurol 1986;19:525–35.

25. Tisch S, Brew B. Parkinsonism in HIV-infected patients on highly active antiretroviral therapy. Neurology 2009;73:401–3.

26. Castellon SA, Hinkin CH, Myers HF. Neuropsychiatric disturbance is associated with executive dysfunction in HIV-1 infection. J Int Neuropsychol Soc 2000;6: 336–47.

27. Cole MA, Castellon SA, Perkins AC, et al. Relationship between psychiatric status and frontal-subcortical systems in HIV-infected individuals. J Int Neuropsychol Soc 2007;13:549–54.

28. Ayuso Mateos JL, Singh AN, Catalan J. Drug treatment of HIV associated neuropsychiatric syndromes. Neurologia 2000;15:164–71.

29. Bing EG, Burnam MA, Longshore D, et al. Psychiatric disorders and drug use among human immunodeficiency virus-infected adults in the United States. Arch Gen Psychiatry 2001;58:721–8.

30. Lyketsos CG, Schwartz J, Fishman M, et al. AIDS mania. J Neuropsychiatry Clin Neurosci 1997;9:277–9.

31. Nakimuli-Mpungu E, Musisi S, Mpungu SK, et al. Primary mania versus HIV-related secondary mania in Uganda. Am J Psychiatry 2006;163:1349–54 [quiz 1480].

32. Portegies P, Enting RH, de Gans J, et al. Presentation and course of AIDS dementia complex: 10 years of follow-up in Amsterdam, The Netherlands. AIDS 1993;7:669–75.

33. McArthur JC, Hoover DR, Bacellar H, et al. Dementia in AIDS patients: incidence and risk factors. Multicenter AIDS Cohort Study. Neurology 1993;43:2245–52.

34. Ellis RJ, Moore DJ, Childers ME, et al. Progression to neuropsychological impairment in human immunodeficiency virus infection predicted by elevated cerebrospinal fluid levels of human immunodeficiency virus RNA. Arch Neurol 2002;59: 923–8.

35. Stern Y, McDermott MP, Albert S, et al. Factors associated with incident human immunodeficiency virus—dementia. Arch Neurol 2001;58:473–9.

36. Navia BA, Jordan BD, Price RW. The AIDS dementia complex: I. Clinical features. Ann Neurol 1986;19:517–24.

37. Snider WD, Simpson DM, Nielsen S, et al. Neurological complications of acquired immune deficiency syndrome: analysis of 50 patients. Ann Neurol 1983;14:403–18.

38. McArthur JC. HIV dementia: an evolving disease. J Neuroimmunol 2004;157:3–10.

39. Brew BJ. Evidence for a change in AIDS dementia complex in the era of highly active antiretroviral therapy and the possibility of new forms of AIDS dementia complex. AIDS 2004;18(Suppl 1):S75–8.

40. Ernst T, Chang L. Effect of aging on brain metabolism in antiretroviral-naive HIV patients. AIDS 2004;18(Suppl 1):S61–7.

41. Dore GJ, Correll PK, Li Y, et al. Changes to AIDS dementia complex in the era of highly active antiretroviral therapy. AIDS 1999;13:1249–53.

42. Sevigny JJ, Albert SM, McDermott MP, et al. Evaluation of HIV RNA and markers of immune activation as predictors of HIV-associated dementia. Neurology 2004; 63:2084–90.

43. Cysique LA, Brew BJ, Halman M, et al. Undetectable cerebrospinal fluid HIV RNA and beta-2 microglobulin do not indicate inactive AIDS dementia complex

in highly active antiretroviral therapy-treated patients. J Acquir Immune Defic Syndr 2005;39:426–9.

44. Descamps M, Hyare H, Stebbing J, et al. Magnetic resonance imaging and spectroscopy of the brain in HIV disease. J HIV Ther 2008;13:55–8.

45. Paul RH, Ernst T, Brickman AM, et al. Relative sensitivity of magnetic resonance spectroscopy and quantitative magnetic resonance imaging to cognitive function among nondemented individuals infected with HIV. J Int Neuropsychol Soc 2008;14:725–33.

46. Paul RH, Brickman AM, Navia B, et al. Apathy is associated with volume of the nucleus accumbens in patients infected with HIV. J Neuropsychiatry Clin Neurosci 2005;17:167–71.

47. Chiang MC, Dutton RA, Hayashi KM, et al. 3D pattern of brain atrophy in HIV/AIDS visualized using tensor-based morphometry. Neuroimage 2007;34:44–60.

48. Lentz MR, Kim WK, Lee V, et al. Changes in MRS neuronal markers and T cell phenotypes observed during early HIV infection. Neurology 2009;72:1465–72.

49. Paul RH, Yiannoutsos CT, Miller EN, et al. Proton MRS and neuropsychological correlates in AIDS dementia complex: evidence of subcortical specificity. J Neuropsychiatry Clin Neurosci 2007;19:283–92.

50. Rottenberg DA, Sidtis JJ, Strother SC, et al. Abnormal cerebral glucose metabolism in HIV-1 seropositive subjects with and without dementia. J Nucl Med 1996;37:1133–41.

51. Rottenberg DA, Moeller JR, Strother SC, et al. The metabolic pathology of the AIDS dementia complex. Ann Neurol 1987;22:700–6.

52. Schmitt FA, Bigley JW, McKinnis R, et al. Neuropsychological outcome of zidovudine (AZT) treatment of patients with AIDS and AIDS-related complex. N Engl J Med 1988;319:1573–8.

53. Sidtis JJ, Gatsonis C, Price RW, et al. Zidovudine treatment of the AIDS dementia complex: results of a placebo-controlled trial. AIDS Clinical Trials Group. Ann Neurol 1993;33:343–9.

54. Portegies P, Solod L, Cinque P, et al. Guidelines for the diagnosis and management of neurological complications of HIV infection. Eur J Neurol 2004;11:297–304.

55. Sacktor NC, Lyles RH, Skolasky RL, et al. Combination antiretroviral therapy improves psychomotor speed performance in HIV-seropositive homosexual men. Multicenter AIDS Cohort Study (MACS). Neurology 1999;52:1640–7.

56. Brodt HR, Kamps BS, Gute P, et al. Changing incidence of AIDS-defining illnesses in the era of antiretroviral combination therapy. AIDS 1997;11:1731–8.

57. Marra CM, Zhao Y, Clifford DB, et al. Impact of combination antiretroviral therapy on cerebrospinal fluid HIV RNA and neurocognitive performance. AIDS 2009;23:1359–66.

58. Tozzi V, Balestra P, Salvatori MF, et al. Changes in cognition during antiretroviral therapy: comparison of 2 different ranking systems to measure antiretroviral drug efficacy on HIV-associated neurocognitive disorders. J Acquir Immune Defic Syndr 2009;52:56–63.

59. Uthman OA, Abdulmalik JO. Adjunctive therapies for AIDS dementia complex. Cochrane Database Syst Rev 2008;(3):CD006496.

60. Breitbart W, Rosenfeld B, Kaim M, et al. A randomized, double-blind, placebo-controlled trial of psychostimulants for the treatment of fatigue in ambulatory patients with human immunodeficiency virus disease. Arch Intern Med 2001;161:411–20.

61. Hinkin CH, Castellon SA, Hardy DJ, et al. Methylphenidate improves HIV-1-associated cognitive slowing. J Neuropsychiatry Clin Neurosci 2001;13:248–54.
62. Petito CK. Review of central nervous system pathology in human immunodeficiency virus infection. Ann Neurol 1988;23(Suppl):S54–7.
63. Dal Pan GJ, Glass JD, McArthur JC. Clinicopathologic correlations of HIV-1-associated vacuolar myelopathy: an autopsy-based case-control study. Neurology 1994;44:2159–64.
64. Berger JR, Sabet A. Infectious myelopathies. Semin Neurol 2002;22:133–42.
65. Di Rocco A, Simpson DM. AIDS-associated vacuolar myelopathy. AIDS Patient Care STDS 1998;12:457–61.
66. Sartoretti-Schefer S, Blattler T, Wichmann W. Spinal MRI in vacuolar myelopathy, and correlation with histopathological findings. Neuroradiology 1997;39:865–9.
67. Chong J, Di Rocco A, Tagliati M, et al. MR findings in AIDS-associated myelopathy. AJNR Am J Neuroradiol 1999;20:1412–6.
68. Tagliati M, Di Rocco A, Danisi F, et al. The role of somatosensory evoked potentials in the diagnosis of AIDS-associated myelopathy. Neurology 2000;54: 1477–82.
69. Petito CK, Navia BA, Cho ES, et al. Vacuolar myelopathy pathologically resembling subacute combined degeneration in patients with the acquired immunodeficiency syndrome. N Engl J Med 1985;312:874–9.
70. Petito CK, Vecchio D, Chen YT. HIV antigen and DNA in AIDS spinal cords correlate with macrophage infiltration but not with vacuolar myelopathy. J Neuropathol Exp Neurol 1994;53:86–94.
71. Rosenblum M, Scheck AC, Cronin K, et al. Dissociation of AIDS-related vacuolar myelopathy and productive HIV-1 infection of the spinal cord. Neurology 1989; 39:892–6.
72. Eilbott DJ, Peress N, Burger H, et al. Human immunodeficiency virus type 1 in spinal cords of acquired immunodeficiency syndrome patients with myelopathy: expression and replication in macrophages. Proc Natl Acad Sci U S A 1989;86: 3337–41.
73. Geraci A, Di Rocco A, Liu M, et al. AIDS myelopathy is not associated with elevated HIV viral load in cerebrospinal fluid. Neurology 2000;55:440–2.
74. Di Rocco A, Bottiglieri T, Werner P, et al. Abnormal cobalamin-dependent transmethylation in AIDS-associated myelopathy. Neurology 2002;58:730–5.
75. Tan SV, Guiloff RJ. Hypothesis on the pathogenesis of vacuolar myelopathy, dementia, and peripheral neuropathy in AIDS. J Neurol Neurosurg Psychiatry 1998;65:23–8.
76. Tan SV, Guiloff RJ, Henderson DC, et al. AIDS-associated vacuolar myelopathy and tumor necrosis factor-alpha (TNF alpha). J Neurol Sci 1996;138:134–44.
77. Di Rocco A, Werner P, Bottiglieri T, et al. Treatment of AIDS-associated myelopathy with L-methionine: a placebo-controlled study. Neurology 2004; 63:1270–5.
78. Bizaare M, Dawood H, Moodley A. Vacuolar myelopathy: a case report of functional, clinical, and radiological improvement after highly active antiretroviral therapy. Int J Infect Dis 2008;12:442–4.
79. Di Rocco A, Tagliati M. Remission of HIV myelopathy after highly active antiretroviral therapy. Neurology 2000;55:456.
80. Staudinger R, Henry K. Remission of HIV myelopathy after highly active antiretroviral therapy. Neurology 2000;54:267–8.
81. Rottnek M, Di Rocco A, Laudier D, et al. Axonal damage is a late component of vacuolar myelopathy. Neurology 2002;58:479–81.

82. Verma S, Estanislao L, Simpson D. HIV-associated neuropathic pain: epidemiology, pathophysiology and management. CNS Drugs 2005;19:325–34.
83. Letendre SL, Ellis RJ, Everall I, et al. Neurologic complications of HIV disease and their treatment. Top HIV Med 2009;17:46–56.
84. Lopez OL, Becker JT, Dew MA, et al. Risk modifiers for peripheral sensory neuropathy in HIV infection/AIDS. Eur J Neurol 2004;11:97–102.
85. Lichtenstein KA, Armon C, Baron A, et al. Modification of the incidence of drug-associated symmetrical peripheral neuropathy by host and disease factors in the HIV outpatient study cohort. Clin Infect Dis 2005;40:148–57.
86. Simpson DM. Selected peripheral neuropathies associated with human immunodeficiency virus infection and antiretroviral therapy. J Neurovirol 2002; 8(Suppl 2):33–41.
87. Cornblath DR, McArthur JC. Predominantly sensory neuropathy in patients with AIDS and AIDS-related complex. Neurology 1988;38:794–6.
88. Kennedy JM, Hoke A, Zhu Y, et al. Peripheral neuropathy in lentivirus infection: evidence of inflammation and axonal injury. AIDS 2004;18:1241–50.
89. Zhu Y, Antony J, Liu S, et al. CD8+ lymphocyte-mediated injury of dorsal root ganglion neurons during lentivirus infection: CD154-dependent cell contact neurotoxicity. J Neurosci 2006;26:3396–403.
90. Herzberg U, Sagen J. Peripheral nerve exposure to HIV viral envelope protein gp120 induces neuropathic pain and spinal gliosis. J Neuroimmunol 2001;116:29–39.
91. de la Monte SM, Gabuzda DH, Ho DD, et al. Peripheral neuropathy in the acquired immunodeficiency syndrome. Ann Neurol 1988;23:485–92.
92. Evans SR, Clifford DB, Kitch DW, et al. Simplification of the research diagnosis of HIV-associated sensory neuropathy. HIV Clin Trials 2008;9:434–9.
93. McArthur JC, Yiannoutsos C, Simpson DM, et al. A phase II trial of nerve growth factor for sensory neuropathy associated with HIV infection. AIDS Clinical Trials Group Team 291. Neurology 2000;54:1080–8.
94. Evans SR, Simpson DM, Kitch DW, et al. A randomized trial evaluating Prosaptide for HIV-associated sensory neuropathies: use of an electronic diary to record neuropathic pain. PLoS One 2007;2:e551.
95. Simpson DM, McArthur JC, Olney R, et al. Lamotrigine for HIV-associated painful sensory neuropathies: a placebo-controlled trial. Neurology 2003;60:1508–14.
96. Simpson DM, Brown S, Tobias J. Controlled trial of high-concentration capsaicin patch for treatment of painful HIV neuropathy. Neurology 2008;70:2305–13.
97. Abrams DI, Jay CA, Shade SB, et al. Cannabis in painful HIV-associated sensory neuropathy: a randomized placebo-controlled trial. Neurology 2007;68:515–21.
98. Ellis RJ, Toperoff W, Vaida F, et al. Smoked medicinal cannabis for neuropathic pain in HIV: a randomized, crossover clinical trial. Neuropsychopharmacology 2009;34:672–80.
99. Hahn K, Arendt G, Braun JS, et al. A placebo-controlled trial of gabapentin for painful HIV-associated sensory neuropathies. J Neurol 2004;251:1260–6.
100. Kieburtz K, Simpson D, Yiannoutsos C, et al. A randomized trial of amitriptyline and mexiletine for painful neuropathy in HIV infection. AIDS Clinical Trial Group 242 Protocol Team. Neurology 1998;51:1682–8.
101. Shlay JC, Chaloner K, Max MB, et al. Acupuncture and amitriptyline for pain due to HIV-related peripheral neuropathy: a randomized controlled trial. Terry Beirn Community Programs for Clinical Research on AIDS. JAMA 1998;280:1590–5.
102. Schifitto G, Yiannoutsos CT, Simpson DM, et al. A placebo-controlled study of memantine for the treatment of human immunodeficiency virus-associated sensory neuropathy. J Neurovirol 2006;12:328–31.

103. Simpson DM, Dorfman D, Olney RK, et al. Peptide T in the treatment of painful distal neuropathy associated with AIDS: results of a placebo-controlled trial. The Peptide T Neuropathy Study Group. Neurology 1996;47:1254–9.
104. Moore RD, Wong WM, Keruly JC, et al. Incidence of neuropathy in HIV-infected patients on monotherapy versus those on combination therapy with didanosine, stavudine and hydroxyurea. AIDS 2000;14:273–8.
105. Verma A. Epidemiology and clinical features of HIV-1 associated neuropathies. J Peripher Nerv Syst 2001;6:8–13.
106. Arenas-Pinto A, Bhaskaran K, Dunn D, et al. The risk of developing peripheral neuropathy induced by nucleoside reverse transcriptase inhibitors decreases over time: evidence from the Delta trial. Antivir Ther 2008;13:289–95.
107. Lee H, Hanes J, Johnson KA. Toxicity of nucleoside analogues used to treat AIDS and the selectivity of the mitochondrial DNA polymerase. Biochemistry 2003;42:14711–9.
108. Peltier AC, Russell JW. Recent advances in drug-induced neuropathies. Curr Opin Neurol 2002;15:633–8.
109. Zhu Y, Antony JM, Martinez JA, et al. Didanosine causes sensory neuropathy in an HIV/AIDS animal model: impaired mitochondrial and neurotrophic factor gene expression. Brain 2007;130:2011–23.
110. Canter JA, Haas DW, Kallianpur AR, et al. The mitochondrial pharmacogenomics of haplogroup T: MTND2*LHON4917G and antiretroviral therapy-associated peripheral neuropathy. Pharmacogenomics J 2008;8:71–7.
111. Berger AR, Arezzo JC, Schaumburg HH, et al. 2′,3′-dideoxycytidine (ddC) toxic neuropathy: a study of 52 patients. Neurology 1993;43:358–62.
112. Hagberg L, Malmvall BE, Svennerholm L, et al. Guillain-Barré syndrome as an early manifestation of HIV central nervous system infection. Scand J Infect Dis 1986;18:591–2.
113. de Castro G, Bastos PG, Martinez R, et al. Episodes of Guillain-Barré syndrome associated with the acute phase of HIV-1 infection and with recurrence of viremia. Arq Neuropsiquiatr 2006;64:606–8.
114. Teo EC, Azwra A, Jones RL, et al. Guillain-Barré syndrome following immune reconstitution after antiretroviral therapy for primary HIV infection. J HIV Ther 2007;12:62–3.
115. McLeod JG. Electrophysiological studies in the Guillain-Barré syndrome. Ann Neurol 1981;9(Suppl):20–7.
116. Cornblath DR. Treatment of the neuromuscular complications of human immunodeficiency virus infection. Ann Neurol 1988;23(Suppl):S88–91.
117. Bani-Sadr F, Neuville S, Crassard I, et al. Acute Guillain-Barré syndrome during the chronic phase of HIV infection and dramatic improvement under highly active antiretroviral therapy. AIDS 2002;16:1562.
118. Sloan DJ, Nicolson A, Miller AR, et al. Human immunodeficiency virus seroconversion presenting with acute inflammatory demyelinating polyneuropathy: a case report. J Med Case Reports 2008;2:370.
119. Gorshtein A, Levy Y. Intravenous immunoglobulin in therapy of peripheral neuropathy. Clin Rev Allergy Immunol 2005;29:271–9.
120. Wulff EA, Wang AK, Simpson DM. HIV-associated peripheral neuropathy: epidemiology, pathophysiology and treatment. Drugs 2000;59:1251–60.
121. Astrom KE, Mancall EL, Richardson EP Jr. Progressive multifocal leuko-encephalopathy; a hitherto unrecognized complication of chronic lymphatic leukaemia and Hodgkin's disease. Brain 1958;81:93–111.
122. Padgett BL, Walker DL. Prevalence of antibodies in human sera against JC virus, an isolate from a case of progressive multifocal leukoencephalopathy. J Infect Dis 1973;127:467–70.

123. Weber T, Trebst C, Frye S, et al. Analysis of the systemic and intrathecal humoral immune response in progressive multifocal leukoencephalopathy. J Infect Dis 1997;176:250–4.
124. Berger JR, Pall L, Lanska D, et al. Progressive multifocal leukoencephalopathy in patients with HIV infection. J Neurovirol 1998;4:59–68.
125. Engsig FN, Hansen AB, Omland LH, et al. Incidence, clinical presentation, and outcome of progressive multifocal leukoencephalopathy in HIV-infected patients during the highly active antiretroviral therapy era: a nationwide cohort study. J Infect Dis 2009;199:77–83.
126. Yousry TA, Major EO, Ryschkewitsch C, et al. Evaluation of patients treated with natalizumab for progressive multifocal leukoencephalopathy. N Engl J Med 2006;354:924–33.
127. Whiteman ML, Post MJ, Berger JR, et al. Progressive multifocal leukoencephalopathy in 47 HIV-seropositive patients: neuroimaging with clinical and pathologic correlation. Radiology 1993;187:233–40.
128. Du Pasquier RA, Koralnik IJ. Inflammatory reaction in progressive multifocal leukoencephalopathy: harmful or beneficial? J Neurovirol 2003;9(Suppl 1):25–31.
129. Hammarin AL, Bogdanovic G, Svedhem V, et al. Analysis of PCR as a tool for detection of JC virus DNA in cerebrospinal fluid for diagnosis of progressive multifocal leukoencephalopathy. J Clin Microbiol 1996;34:2929–32.
130. Wang Y, Kirby JE, Qian Q. Effective use of JC virus PCR for diagnosis of progressive multifocal leukoencephalopathy. J Med Microbiol 2009;58:253–5.
131. Royal W 3rd, Dupont B, McGuire D, et al. Topotecan in the treatment of acquired immunodeficiency syndrome-related progressive multifocal leukoencephalopathy. J Neurovirol 2003;9:411–9.
132. Enting RH, Portegies P. Cytarabine and highly active antiretroviral therapy in HIV-related progressive multifocal leukoencephalopathy. J Neurol 2000;247:134–8.
133. Hall CD, Dafni U, Simpson D, et al. Failure of cytarabine in progressive multifocal leukoencephalopathy associated with human immunodeficiency virus infection. AIDS Clinical Trials Group 243 Team. N Engl J Med 1998;338:1345–51.
134. Marra CM, Rajicic N, Barker DE, et al. A pilot study of cidofovir for progressive multifocal leukoencephalopathy in AIDS. AIDS 2002;16:1791–7.
135. Clifford DB, Yiannoutsos C, Glicksman M, et al. HAART improves prognosis in HIV-associated progressive multifocal leukoencephalopathy. Neurology 1999;52:623–5.
136. Giudici B, Vaz B, Bossolasco S, et al. Highly active antiretroviral therapy and progressive multifocal leukoencephalopathy: effects on cerebrospinal fluid markers of JC virus replication and immune response. Clin Infect Dis 2000;30:95–9.
137. Levine AJ, Hinkin CH, Ando K, et al. An exploratory study of long-term neurocognitive outcomes following recovery from opportunistic brain infections in HIV+ adults. J Clin Exp Neuropsychol 2008;30(7):836–43.
138. Griffiths P. Cytomegalovirus infection of the central nervous system. Herpes 2004;11(Suppl 2):95A–104A.
139. Staras SA, Dollard SC, Radford KW, et al. Seroprevalence of cytomegalovirus infection in the United States, 1988–1994. Clin Infect Dis 2006;43:1143–51.
140. Embil JA, Pereira LH, MacNeil JP, et al. Levels of cytomegalovirus seropositivity in homosexual and heterosexual men. Sex Transm Dis 1988;15:85–7.
141. Skolnik PR, Kosloff BR, Hirsch MS. Bidirectional interactions between human immunodeficiency virus type 1 and cytomegalovirus. J Infect Dis 1988;157:508–14.

142. McCutchan JA. Clinical impact of cytomegalovirus infections of the nervous system in patients with AIDS. Clin Infect Dis 1995;21(Suppl 2):S196–201.
143. Arribas JR, Storch GA, Clifford DB, et al. Cytomegalovirus encephalitis. Ann Intern Med 1996;125:577–87.
144. Fiala M, Singer EJ, Graves MC, et al. AIDS dementia complex complicated by cytomegalovirus encephalopathy. J Neurol 1993;240:223–31.
145. Miller RF, Fox JD, Thomas P, et al. Acute lumbosacral polyradiculopathy due to cytomegalovirus in advanced HIV disease: CSF findings in 17 patients. J Neurol Neurosurg Psychiatry 1996;61:456–60.
146. So YT, Olney RK. Acute lumbosacral polyradiculopathy in acquired immunodeficiency syndrome: experience in 23 patients. Ann Neurol 1994;35:53–8.
147. Cinque P, Bossolasco S, Bestetti A, et al. Molecular studies of cerebrospinal fluid in human immunodeficiency virus type 1-associated opportunistic central nervous system diseases—an update. J Neurovirol 2002;8(Suppl 2):122–8.
148. de Gans J, Tiessens G, Portegies P, et al. Predominance of polymorphonuclear leukocytes in cerebrospinal fluid of AIDS patients with cytomegalovirus polyradiculomyelitis. J Acquir Immune Defic Syndr 1990;3:1155–8.
149. van Den Pol AN, Mocarski E, Saederup N, et al. Cytomegalovirus cell tropism, replication, and gene transfer in brain. J Neurosci 1999;19:10948–65.
150. Wiley CA, Schrier RD, Denaro FJ, et al. Localization of cytomegalovirus proteins and genome during fulminant central nervous system infection in an AIDS patient. J Neuropathol Exp Neurol 1986;45:127–39.
151. Chiou SH, Liu JH, Chen SS, et al. Apoptosis of human retina and retinal pigment cells induced by human cytomegalovirus infection. Ophthalmic Res 2002;34:77–82.
152. Odeberg J, Wolmer N, Falci S, et al. Human cytomegalovirus inhibits neuronal differentiation and induces apoptosis in human neural precursor cells. J Virol 2006;80:8929–39.
153. Morgello S, Cho ES, Nielsen S, et al. Cytomegalovirus encephalitis in patients with acquired immunodeficiency syndrome: an autopsy study of 30 cases and a review of the literature. Hum Pathol 1987;18:289–97.
154. Jabs DA, Bolton SG, Dunn JP, et al. Discontinuing anticytomegalovirus therapy in patients with immune reconstitution after combination antiretroviral therapy. Am J Ophthalmol 1998;126:817–22.
155. Kaplan JE, Benson C, Holmes KH, et al. Guidelines for prevention and treatment of opportunistic infections in HIV-infected adults and adolescents: recommendations from CDC, the National Institutes of Health, and the HIV Medicine Association of the Infectious Diseases Society of America. MMWR Recomm Rep 2009;58:1–207 [quiz CE201–4].
156. Jarvis JN, Harrison TS. HIV-associated cryptococcal meningitis. AIDS 2007;21:2119–29.
157. Polacheck I, Platt Y, Aronovitch J. Catecholamines and virulence of *Cryptococcus neoformans*. Infect Immun 1990;58:2919–22.
158. Moosa MY, Coovadia YM. Cryptococcal meningitis in Durban, South Africa: a comparison of clinical features, laboratory findings, and outcome for human immunodeficiency virus (HIV)-positive and HIV-negative patients. Clin Infect Dis 1997;24:131–4.
159. Charlier C, Dromer F, Leveque C, et al. Cryptococcal neuroradiological lesions correlate with severity during cryptococcal meningoencephalitis in HIV-positive patients in the HAART era. PLoS One 2008;3:e1950.
160. Lortholary O, Poizat G, Zeller V, et al. Long-term outcome of AIDS-associated cryptococcosis in the era of combination antiretroviral therapy. AIDS 2006;20:2183–91.

161. Larsen RA, Leal MA, Chan LS. Fluconazole compared with amphotericin B plus flucytosine for cryptococcal meningitis in AIDS. A randomized trial. Ann Intern Med 1990;113:183–7.

162. Graybill JR, Sobel J, Saag M, et al. Diagnosis and management of increased intracranial pressure in patients with AIDS and cryptococcal meningitis. The NIAID Mycoses Study Group and AIDS Cooperative Treatment Groups. Clin Infect Dis 2000;30:47–54.

163. Nascimento LV, Stollar F, Tavares LB, et al. Risk factors for toxoplasmic encephalitis in HIV-infected patients: a case-control study in Brazil. Ann Trop Med Parasitol 2001;95:587–93.

164. Ho YC, Sun HY, Chen MY, et al. Clinical presentation and outcome of toxoplasmic encephalitis in patients with human immunodeficiency virus type 1 infection. J Microbiol Immunol Infect 2008;41:386–92.

165. Luft BJ, Remington JS. Toxoplasmic encephalitis in AIDS. Clin Infect Dis 1992; 15:211–22.

166. Bousson V, Brunereau L, Meyohas M, et al. [Brain imaging in AIDS]. J Radiol 1999;80:99–107 [in French].

167. Bhagavati S, Choi J. Frequent hemorrhagic lesions in cerebral toxoplasmosis in AIDS patients. J Neuroimaging 2009;19:169–73.

168. Ruiz A, Ganz WI, Post MJ, et al. Use of thallium-201 brain SPECT to differentiate cerebral lymphoma from toxoplasma encephalitis in AIDS patients. AJNR Am J Neuroradiol 1994;15:1885–94.

169. Pierce MA, Johnson MD, Maciunas RJ, et al. Evaluating contrast-enhancing brain lesions in patients with AIDS by using positron emission tomography. Ann Intern Med 1995;123:594–8.

170. Miro JM, Lopez JC, Podzamczer D, et al. Discontinuation of primary and secondary *Toxoplasma gondii* prophylaxis is safe in HIV-infected patients after immunological restoration with highly active antiretroviral therapy: results of an open, randomized, multicenter clinical trial. Clin Infect Dis 2006;43:79–89.

171. MacMahon EM, Glass JD, Hayward SD, et al. Epstein-Barr virus in AIDS-related primary central nervous system lymphoma. Lancet 1991;338:969–73.

172. Birx DL, Redfield RR, Tosato G. Defective regulation of Epstein-Barr virus infection in patients with acquired immunodeficiency syndrome (AIDS) or AIDS-related disorders. N Engl J Med 1986;314:874–9.

173. Petito CK, Cho ES, Lemann W, et al. Neuropathology of acquired immunodeficiency syndrome (AIDS): an autopsy review. J Neuropathol Exp Neurol 1986; 45:635–46.

174. Levy RM, Bredesen DE, Rosenblum ML. Neurological manifestations of the acquired immunodeficiency syndrome (AIDS): experience at UCSF and review of the literature. J Neurosurg 1985;62:475–95.

175. Wolf T, Brodt HR, Fichtlscherer S, et al. Changing incidence and prognostic factors of survival in AIDS-related non-Hodgkin's lymphoma in the era of highly active antiretroviral therapy (HAART). Leuk Lymphoma 2005;46:207–15.

176. Skiest DJ, Crosby C. Survival is prolonged by highly active antiretroviral therapy in AIDS patients with primary central nervous system lymphoma. AIDS 2003;17: 1787–93.

177. Bossolasco S, Cinque P, Ponzoni M, et al. Epstein-Barr virus DNA load in cerebrospinal fluid and plasma of patients with AIDS-related lymphoma. J Neurovirol 2002;8:432–8.

178. Fan H, Kim SC, Chima CO, et al. Epstein-Barr viral load as a marker of lymphoma in AIDS patients. J Med Virol 2005;75:59–69.

179. Gerstner E, Batchelor T. Primary CNS lymphoma. Expert Rev Anticancer Ther 2007;7:689–700.
180. Bossolasco S, Falk KI, Ponzoni M, et al. Ganciclovir is associated with low or undetectable Epstein-Barr virus DNA load in cerebrospinal fluid of patients with HIV-related primary central nervous system lymphoma. Clin Infect Dis 2006;42:e21–5.
181. Correa DD, DeAngelis LM, Shi W, et al. Cognitive functions in survivors of primary central nervous system lymphoma. Neurology 2004;62:548–55.
182. Harder H, Holtel H, Bromberg JE, et al. Cognitive status and quality of life after treatment for primary CNS lymphoma. Neurology 2004;62:544–7.
183. Riedel DJ, Pardo CA, McArthur J, et al. Therapy insight: CNS manifestations of HIV-associated immune reconstitution inflammatory syndrome. Nat Clin Pract Neurol 2006;2:557–65.
184. Vendrely A, Bienvenu B, Gasnault J, et al. Fulminant inflammatory leukoence-phalopathy associated with HAART-induced immune restoration in AIDS-related progressive multifocal leukoencephalopathy. Acta Neuropathol 2005;109:449–55.
185. York J, Bodi I, Reeves I, et al. Raised intracranial pressure complicating crypto-coccal meningitis: immune reconstitution inflammatory syndrome or recurrent cryptococcal disease? J Infect 2005;51:165–71.
186. Miller RF, Isaacson PG, Hall-Craggs M, et al. Cerebral CD8+ lymphocytosis in HIV-1 infected patients with immune restoration induced by HAART. Acta Neuropathol 2004;108:17–23.
187. Venkataramana A, Pardo CA, McArthur JC, et al. Immune reconstitution inflam-matory syndrome in the CNS of HIV-infected patients. Neurology 2006;67:383–8.
188. Langford TD, Letendre SL, Marcotte TD, et al. Severe, demyelinating leukoence-phalopathy in AIDS patients on antiretroviral therapy. AIDS 2002;16:1019–29.
189. Pfeffer G, Prout A, Hooge J, et al. Biopsy-proven immune reconstitution syndrome in a patient with AIDS and cerebral toxoplasmosis. Neurology 2009;73:321–2.
190. Shelburne SA, Visnegarwala F, Darcourt J, et al. Incidence and risk factors for immune reconstitution inflammatory syndrome during highly active antiretroviral therapy. AIDS 2005;19:399–406.
191. Robertson J, Meier M, Wall J, et al. Immune reconstitution syndrome in HIV: vali-dating a case definition and identifying clinical predictors in persons initiating antiretroviral therapy. Clin Infect Dis 2006;42:1639–46.

A Tale of Two Spirochetes: Lyme Disease and Syphilis

John J. Halperin, MD[a,b,*]

KEYWORDS

• Lyme disease • Neurosyphilis • Neuroborreliosis • Syphilis

Two spirochetal infections hold fascinating positions in the history of infectious diseases. Numerous historic and literary figures were believed to have neurosyphilis, which consequently has been blamed for otherwise inexplicable developments in Western European history. More recently, Lyme disease has served as a focal point for the divide between evidence-based medicine and traditional experiential approaches, highlighting issues of physician autonomy in an era of guideline development, and epitomizing the tension between patient advocacy and scientific medical care.

How is it that spirochetal infections can play such outsized roles? Several biologic and sociologic factors are probably relevant. Both can affect the nervous system, and for patients and most physicians, few things are more unnerving than disorders that may affect brain function. Both can be chronic. Although both *Treponema pallidum* and *Borrelia burgdorferi* are highly sensitive to antibiotics, without appropriate treatment, these slowly multiplying, not very immunogenic organisms can persist in relatively immune-protected sites for years, gradually resulting in end organ damage.

Most significant is the societal context in which these diseases first appeared. Syphilis invaded Europe when biologic understanding of disease was limited. In the absence of knowledge of other diseases, and with few tools to diagnose syphilis unequivocally, all manner of clinical phenomena were blamed on this infection. Lyme disease was described at a time of far greater scientific understanding. However, the inaccurate notion that this is a novel infection for which diagnostic tools are limited, and the availability of the Internet to enable widespread but uncritical proliferation of information have contributed to an unfortunate degree of misunderstanding. At a time when the population is inadequately scientifically literate but simultaneously suspicious of organized medicine and sympathetic to populist outpourings,

[a] Department of Neurology, Madison Avenue, Mount Sinai School of Medicine, NY, USA
[b] Department of Neurosciences, Overlook Hospital, 99 Beauvoir Avenue, Summit, NJ 07902, USA
* Department of Neurosciences, Overlook Hospital, 99 Beauvoir Avenue, Summit, NJ 07902.
E-mail address: john.halperin@atlantichealth.org

Neurol Clin 28 (2010) 277–291
doi:10.1016/j.ncl.2009.09.009
0733-8619/09/$ – see front matter
neurologic.theclinics.com

this has allowed the widespread acceptance of scientifically invalid information, culminating in state legislatures passing laws requiring insurance companies to pay for treatment that has been shown to be irrelevant, unhelpful, and, in fact, harmful.

LYME DISEASE

The terms *Lyme arthritis* and *Lyme disease* were coined in the mid-1970s when a large number of children near Lyme Connecticut were diagnosed with what seemed to be juvenile rheumatoid arthritis.[1] In response to vigorous advocacy by the children's parents, a series of epidemiologic studies rapidly identified the cause as a novel tick-borne spirochete, *B burgdorferi*. As more was learned about this infection, experts realized that it was remarkably similar to a group of disorders identified early in the twentieth century in Europe, and ultimately that all of these disorders were caused by infection with closely related organisms.

In Europe, four strains, all belonging to the *B burgdorferi sensu lato* group, have been identified: *B burgdorferi senso stricto, B garinii, B afzelii*, and *B spielmanii*.[2] In the United States, only the first has been found.[3–5] The general belief is that the disease was introduced into the United States when a herd of infected deer was imported from Europe early in the twentieth century. All four strains consist of motile corkscrew-shaped bacteria, typically approximately 0.2 to 0.3 µm in diameter, and 20 to 30 µm in length. Their entire genome has now been sequenced.

The clinical disorders described in Europe and those in the United States have some differences. Arthritis seems to be more common in patients in the United States, whereas painful radiculitis and encephalomyelitis are more frequent in Europe. However, rheumatism was described in one of the earliest European descriptions of this disorder.[6] Although these differences have several possible explanations, they are probably caused by a combination of bacterial strain differences and ascertainment bias. The systemic disease is largely treated by neurologists in Europe and by rheumatologists in the United States.

Regardless of the strain, transmission occurs virtually exclusively by bites of hard-shelled *Ixodes* ticks; *I scapularis* in North America, and *I persulcatus, I ricinus*, and others elsewhere in the world. The host–vector relationship depends on several unique features, including the feeding cycle of these ticks. Larval ticks hatch uninfected from eggs and then have their first blood meal, typically on small mammals such as field mice. If that host is infected, the tick can become infected, with spirochetes then residing in their gut. Months later, when as a nymph they have their second blood meal, they will have either a second opportunity to become infected or their first opportunity to infect a new host, which is more often a larger mammal, including potentially humans.

When ticks attach to feed, they inject saliva into the host, saliva that contains local anesthetics, anticoagulants, and other bioactive molecules to allow uninterrupted feeding for up to several days. When blood arrives in their gut, this triggers spirochete proliferation. Spirochetes then disseminate throughout the tick, particularly invading the tick salivary glands, a sequence of events that requires at least 24 hours. At that point, injection of additional saliva can result in injection of viable spirochetes. Consequently, infected ticks must remain attached for at least 24 hours before hosts are at significant risk for infection.[7]

After inoculation into the new host, spirochetes proliferate locally. Within days to, at most, weeks, this results in a local erythema, erythema migrans (EM), that has virtually unique characteristics. As spirochetes migrate outward, the area of erythema gradually expands, growing to many centimeters in diameter. Characteristically, EM grows demonstrably day-by-day, lasting many days to weeks. It is typically macular, circular to oval, and not particularly painful or pruritic. If it appears on a part of the body not normally visualized, such as the back, it may be missed entirely. In small children, whose bodies are fairly frequently scrutinized by parents, large series indicate the rash occurs in at least 90% of infected individuals.[8]

Spirochetes can also disseminate hematogenously from the site of inoculation, resulting in multifocal EM, with each focus representing a new, hematogenously disseminated nidus of infection that will blossom into a similar EM. This type of infection occurs in up to a quarter of patients in the United States, and a smaller fraction in European patients.

As with any bacterial infection, dissemination elicits a host inflammatory response, commonly marked by fever, headache, malaise, and muscle and joint aches. This response, often termed *flu-like*, does not include any respiratory or gastrointestinal symptoms. Although the spirochetes can spread to any part of the body, *B burgdorferi* seems to have several tropisms. Early involvement of the nervous system is probably the most common, with up to 15% of untreated individuals developing all or part of the triad of lymphocytic meningitis, cranial neuritis, and painful radiculitis.[9] Up to 5% will develop cardiac conduction abnormalities, up to and including third-degree heart block, occasionally requiring a temporary pacemaker. Joint involvement is similarly common, although it usually occurs later in disease, when it may present as a relapsing remitting large joint oligoarthritis.

Diagnosis

Although, unlike *T pallidum*, *B burgdorferi* can be cultured from infected patients, this approach is not practical. EM lesions contain innumerable spirochetes, but the rash is so characteristic that culture is rarely necessary. Unfortunately, in other circumstances the number of organisms present is so low that, even in research laboratories prepared to perform the studies, positive findings are very infrequent (approximately 10% in Lyme meningitis). Even polymerase chain reaction-based techniques add minimally to this test sensitivity.[10] Additionally, culture is technically challenging. A unique medium, BSK II, is required but not available in most laboratories. Cultures must be maintained at lower temperatures than usual and must be maintained for weeks because of the slow doubling time. Therefore, as in syphilis, diagnosis relies on demonstration of a measurable specific antibody response.

Although specific assay details vary, testing relies primarily on enzyme-linked immunosorbent assays (ELISAs), tests that measure total immunoreactivity to the antigens of the organism in question. Results are generally compared with a panel of uninfected controls and expressed as positive if the amount of antibody exceeds the mean by three standard deviations, or borderline if by two. ELISAs can be negative in as many as half of individuals tested very early in infection (first month or so), such as when EM occurs,[11] simply because it takes several weeks to develop a measurable antibody response. EM should be treated regardless of ELISA results, but if doubt exists the approach used with virtually all other serologic testing can be adopted: measuring acute and convalescent titers. By 6 weeks after infection, virtually all patients should be seropositive. Being on antimicrobial therapy does not directly affect the ELISA. If a patient is successfully treated and no further bacteria are stimulating an immune response, some patients will become seronegative. As with most other infections, others will continue to produce demonstrable antibody for years after the infection has been eradicated.

False-positives are a concern and fall into two groups. Some organisms, *T pallidum*, *T denticola* (an organism responsible for periodontal disease), and *Borrelia* responsible for relapsing fever, are so antigenically similar that differentiation can be difficult. Fortunately, little geographic overlap exists between relapsing fever and Lyme disease; syphilis can usually be differentiated using tests to measure reaginic antibodies, such as the venereal disease research laboratory (VDRL) or rapid plasma reagin (RPR) assays. These anticardiolipin antibodies are almost always produced in syphilis and are rarely if ever demonstrable in Lyme disease.

More common is cross-reactivity caused by more global B-cell stimulation. Patients who have lupus, subacute bacterial endocarditis,[12] parvovirus, and other disorders develop a significant polyclonal gammopathy that can result in cross-reactive false-positives on many serologic assays. This cross-reactivity can be most easily differentiated using a Western blot, a test performed by first separating the bacterial proteins by molecular weight and then identifying the specific proteins (bands) to which the patient's antibodies react. When interpreting these, one must remember that criteria (**Table 1**) derive from studies of large numbers of patients who have and do not have Lyme disease.[13] A statistical analysis of these results led to the conclusion that patients who have two of three specific IgM bands (acute disease) or 5 of 10 specific IgG bands (disease of >1–2 months duration) were virtually certain to have disease. However, the patients studied all had positive or borderline ELISA results; therefore, the criteria cannot be applied in patients who have negative ELISA results.

None of these bands represents an antigen unique to *B burgdorferi*; therefore, diagnosis is based on the observed combination of bands, not the presence of any single one. Furthermore, IgM criteria are only useful in early disease. IgM antibodies are notoriously cross-reactive; normally the IgM response is supplanted by an IgG response within 1 to 2 months. Therefore, if symptoms have been present for more than 1 or 2 months and only IgM bands are present, this laboratory finding is unlikely to be of any significance. Finally, the sensitivity of the Western blot criteria is incomplete, and therefore these criteria must be balanced against the clinical context. If a patient has facial palsy, is living in an endemic area, and has an ELISA five standard deviations greater than the positive cut-off, but has a negative Western blot, then the presumptive diagnosis is Lyme disease and treatment should be initiated.

Unfortunately, serologic testing generally is not a useful indicator of treatment adequacy. Because the normal role of the immune system is to continue to produce antibody to protect against reinfection, many patients will continue to be seropositive after successful treatment. In patients who have ongoing infection, Western blots tend to show an expanding array of antibody reactivities over time, but old and new serum samples must be assayed simultaneously to show this conclusively, requiring old samples to be maintained at −70°C indefinitely for future reference, which is not a generally practical approach.

One additional serologic technique is useful for diagnosing central nervous system (CNS) infection with *B burgdorferi*. As in many other infections, the CNS acts as a separate immunologic compartment; targeted B cells migrate across the blood–brain barrier, proliferate, and mature to locally produce antibodies against the inciting

Table 1
Western blot criteria for confirmation of positive ELISA in Lyme disease

	IgM (2/3 Required)	IgG (5/10 Required)
Bands	23, 39, 41	18, 23, 28, 30, 39, 41, 45, 58, 66, 93
Sensitivity	1/3 (acute disease)	9/10 (established disease)

organism. This phenomenon can be shown in several ways. Calculations of either IgG synthesis rate or an IgG index will show increased total concentration of IgG in the cerebrospinal fluid (CSF). When infection is present for a sufficient period, oligoclonal bands will be seen, reflecting the proliferation of clones of plasma cells targeting the inciting organism's antigens.

Most useful and specific is the demonstration of intrathecal production of antibody specific for the inciting organism[14] (grade B evidence). Comparing the amount of specific antibody targeted at *B burgdorferi* in CSF and serum, expressed as a proportion of total immunoglobulin in the two fluids, can provide specific evidence of infection. Because normally the amount of CSF antibody is small, false-positives are rare, limited primarily to neurosyphilis. The biggest drawback is that apparent intrathecal antibody synthesis can persist long after curative treatment, presumably as antibody concentrations in CSF and serum gradually decline in parallel.[15] Fortunately, treatment efficacy can often be assessed through improvement in CSF cell count and protein.

The biggest shortcoming of this method is that defining its sensitivity has been impossible, because no other unequivocal marker of CNS infection exists. Estimates range from nearly 100% in the European literature to approximately 50% in patients who have chronic disorders that may or may not have reflected active CNS infection.[16,17]

Clinical

Contrary to assertions of some internists and hapless candidates at the Neurology Board examination, Lyme disease does not cause every imaginable neurologic disorder. Although the specifics of neuroborreliosis can be approached several ways, these are most easily considered by dividing them into peripheral and CNS processes (**Table 2**).

The classic triad consisting of lymphocytic meningitis, cranial neuritis, and painful radiculitis, described by European authors almost 9 decades ago[18] and more recently in the United States by Reik and colleagues[9] and Pachner,[19] bridges this divide somewhat. The most common entity is probably lymphocytic meningitis, clinically very similar to viral meningitis. Several algorithms have been proposed to differentiate between viral and Lyme meningitis[20,21]; these are heavily influenced by the cooccurrence of other parts of the triad, primarily cranial neuritis. If a patient has two or more elements of the triad and had potential exposure to Lyme disease (particularly in the preceding 30–60 days), this diagnosis should be considered seriously. In addition,

Table 2 Neurologic disorders in Lyme disease and their pathophysiology grouped by pathophysiologic mechanism		
	Peripheral Nervous System	**Central Nervous System**
Diffuse inflammatory		Lymphocytic meningitis
Multifocal inflammatory	Mononeuropathy multiplex Cranial neuropathy Radiculopathy Plexopathy (Lumbosacral, brachial) Confluent mononeuropathy multiplex	Myelitis Encephalitis
Remote (not neuroinfection)		Encephalopathy

when compared with viral meningitis, which tends to have a more acute onset, Lyme meningitis symptoms tend to be present for a few more days before medical evaluation. CSF findings are indistinguishable, with a modest, lymphocyte-predominant pleocytosis, modest increase in protein, and normal to minimally decreased glucose.

Cranial neuritis occurs in approximately 8% to 10% of patients, often cooccurring with meningitis. The seventh (facial) cranial nerve is by far the most common site of involvement, with bilateral paralysis in as many as a quarter of patients who have facial nerve palsy (only sarcoid, Guillain-Barré syndrome, and HIV are similarly associated with bilateral involvement). Other cranial nerves can be involved but far less commonly, with most of the remaining 20% of Lyme-associated cranial neuropathies involving cranial nerve viii or the extraocular muscles.

The third element, which is probably significantly underdiagnosed, is painful radiculitis, known in Europe as Garin-Bujadoux-Bannwarth syndrome.[6,18] Clinical signs and symptoms are typically similar to those of a mechanical or diabetic radiculopathy, with severe dermatomal pain and corresponding sensory, motor, and reflex changes. This disorder may involve several adjacent dermatomes or just one, and frequently but not invariably cooccurs with meningitis. Truncal involvement occurs and can, like diabetic truncal radiculopathy, be confused with visceral pathology.

Other forms of peripheral nerve involvement have been described,[22] including brachial and lumbosacral plexopathies, typical mononeuropathy multiplex, and more diffuse neuropathies. More acute and focal disorders tend to occur earlier in disease, with more diffuse and insidiously progressive disorders occurring later. Whether this process reflects inoculum size, host immune response, a coinfection, or some other factor remains to be determined.

Detailed neurophysiologic testing indicates that the common thread of all these disorders is an underlying mononeuropathy multiplex, such as a cranial neuropathy, radiculopathy, or confluent mononeuropathy multiplex mimicking a more diffuse neuropathy.[23] Pathophysiologically, virtually all cases seem to have involved axon damage. A few isolated instances of demyelinating neuropathies have been reported[24]; whether these are causally related or coincidence is unclear.

Fortunately, parenchymal CNS involvement is rare. In the European literature, Bannwarth's syndrome occasionally includes spinal cord involvement at the level of root involvement. Rare cases of parenchymal encephalitis have been described in the European and United States' literature. These cases are more often subacute to chronic and manifest with focal abnormities on examination and MRI imaging; all have inflammatory CSF. In particular, patients who have been symptomatic for any interval, such as those who have other chronic CNS infections, have increased IgG synthesis and frequently have oligoclonal bands. In patients who have inflammatory CNS disorders who have this clear evidence of immune stimulation within the CNS, specific intrathecal production of anti–B burgdorferi antibody should invariably be present.

Patients who have active Lyme infection, particularly with evidence of active inflammation such as arthritis, often experience ongoing fatigue and malaise, and perceive cognitive and memory difficulties. These symptoms are identical to the toxic metabolic encephalopathies seen in innumerable other chronic infections or inflammatory states.[25] Unfortunately, some have asserted that these cognitive symptoms, in isolation, are strongly suggestive of Lyme disease, with or without laboratory support for the diagnosis. Because population studies indicate that these same symptoms occur for unexplained reasons in a significant number of individuals, even being sufficient to disrupt daily activities in a meaningful fashion in 2% of the otherwise healthy population,[26] this assumption is clearly inappropriate.

Neuro-imaging is infrequently helpful. In those rare patients with parenchymal involvement of the brain or spinal cord, MRI imaging demonstrates typical inflammatory lesions – bright on T2, contrast enhancing. SPECT imaging in these patients demonstrates hyperactivity in the inflammatory lesions.[27] Although a sophisticated quantitative analysis of brain SPECT images in a population of patients who had unequivocal Lyme disease and cognitive difficult detected some abnormalities,[28] qualitative brain SPECT scans in individual patients are not helpful.

Treatment

B burgdorferi is sensitive to common antibiotics; meaningful antimicrobial resistance has not been shown.[7] For most patients, oral regimens with doxycycline, amoxicillin or cefuroxime axetil given for between 2 and 4 weeks are highly effective (grade A evidence) (**Table 3**). Numerous studies in the European literature indicate that oral treatment with doxycycline is highly effective (grade A evidence, meta-analysis) in individuals who have Lyme meningitis, cranial neuritis, and radiculitis.[29] This treatment has not been tested in the United States but, in light of the known biology of the organism and its different strains, similar results seem likely.

In patients who have parenchymal CNS disease, other severe forms of involvement, or whose infection does not respond to oral regimens, 2- to 4-week parenteral regimens with ceftriaxone, cefotaxime, or penicillin are all highly effective (grade A evidence) (see **Table 3**). Longer courses of treatment have been shown to provide no lasting benefit, but rather pose considerable risk (grade A evidence).[30–32]

Table 3
Lyme disease treatment recommendations

Disorder	Adults	Children
Early Lyme disease	Doxycycline,[a] 100 mg PO bid; 21 d *OR*	≥8 y, 1–2 mg/kg bid
	Amoxicillin, 500 mg PO tid; 21 d *OR*	50 mg/kg/d in 3 divided doses
	Cefuroxime axetil, 500 mg PO bid; 21 d	30 mg/kg/d in 2 divided doses
Acute neuroborreliosis (meningitis, radiculitis, cranial neuritis)	Ceftriaxone,[b] 2 g/d, IV; 2–4 wk *OR*	75–100 mg/kg/d
	Cefotaxime, 2 g, q8h IV; 2–4 wk *OR*	150–200 mg/kg/d in 3–4 divided doses
	Penicillin, 20–24 million U/d, IV; 2–4 wk *OR*	300,000 U/kg/d
	Possibly doxycycline,[a] 100 mg, PO bid to qid for 3–4 wk	≥8 y 1–2 mg/kg bid
Encephalomyelitis	Ceftriaxone[b] *OR* cefotaxime *OR* penicillin IV, as above	
Chronic or recurrent neuroborreliosis (eg, treatment failure after 2 wk of treatment)	Ceftriaxone[b] *OR* cefotaxime IV, or pencillin as above	

Abbreviation: IV, intravenously.
[a] Doxycycline should not be used in pregnant women or children younger than 8 years.
[b] Ceftriaxone should not be used late in pregnancy.

SYPHILIS

Syphilis, much like tobacco years later, seems to have been an early and unfortunate export from the New World to the Old. First appearing in Europe at the time of Columbus' voyages to the New World, "the French Pox" was initially highly virulent, killing many of its immunologically naïve hosts. As the organism and its hosts evolved and selected each other, the disease developed into its current form.

T pallidum and *B burgdorferi* share several important biologic characteristics. Slowly dividing and fastidious, they are difficult (*B burgdorferi*) to impossible (*T pallidum*) to grow in vitro. Both expose few antigens on their surfaces and change the exposed epitopes over time so that even though hosts develop a targeted immune response, this response is not uniformly effective at eliminating the infection.

Like *B burgdorferi*, *T pallidum* has been well characterized. It is a motile corkscrew-shaped bacterium, approximately 0.25 μm in diameter and 6 to 20 μm in length. Although *T pallidum* elicits a prominent B-cell response, T-cell mediated immunity plays a key role in its elimination from infected hosts. In Lyme disease and syphilis, infection begins with a peculiarly asymptomatic cutaneous lesion, which then subsides spontaneously over time. Organisms then disseminate and show particular tropism for the CNS. Both bacteria remain highly sensitive to widely available antibiotics, and both illnesses have been blamed inappropriately for several unrelated disorders, generally because of widespread ignorance of relevant biologic information.

The incidence of syphilis (**Fig. 1**) has declined significantly over the years, attaining a fairly low level through the early 1980s, and increasing substantially in the early HIV era. As public health measures and education were implemented in the 1990s, the incidence again declined, with fewer than 12,000 cases of primary and secondary disease in 2006,[33] representing approximately half the number of reported cases of Lyme disease.[34] (In the same year there were approximately 18,000 cases of late syphilis, reflecting untreated infection from earlier years.)

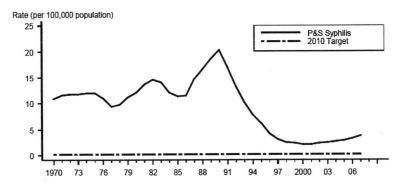

Note: The Healthy People 2010 (HP2010) target for primary and secondary syphilis is 0.2 case per 100,000 population.

Fig. 1. Trends in syphilis incidence. Reported rates of primary and secondary syphilis in the United States from 1970 to 2007. (*From* Centers for Disease Control and Prevention. Sexually transmitted disease surveillance 2007 supplement, syphilis surveillance report. U.S. Department of Health and Human Services, Centers for Disease Control and Prevention. Atlanta (GA): 2009.)

Clinical: General

Like Lyme disease, syphilis is transmitted virtually exclusively through intimate contact with a single vector species. With syphilis, infection is transmitted through sexual contact. The earliest evidence of infection, generally developing within up to 3 weeks of exposure and present in virtually all infected individuals, is an ulcerating indurated lesion at the site of inoculation, most often present on mucosal surfaces. Just like erythema migrans, the lesion persists for days to weeks. However, despite its ulcerated appearance and location, it is remarkably asymptomatic. If scrapings of the surface are examined by dark field microscopy, spirochetes are readily seen. This phase of acute, localized disease, generally referred to as *primary syphilis*, typically subsides over several weeks, even if untreated.

In many patients, acute disseminated infection, or *secondary syphilis*, occurs within approximately a month of the rash. During this phase, spirochetes disseminate throughout the body. In addition to the anticipated febrile illness and other symptoms typical of a bacteremia, most patients develop a disseminated maculopapular rash, analogous to disseminated EM. One of the unusual features of this rash is its tendency to involve the palms and soles, which are areas rarely involved in other exanthems. This phase also is commonly associated with significant lymphadenopathy, particularly the epitrochlear nodes, which are infrequently enlarged in other illnesses, and multiorgan involvement, including the liver and bones.

At this point, meningeal seeding is extremely common, resulting in syphilitic meningitis. Like Lyme meningitis, its onset or symptomatology is often less dramatic than bacterial or viral meningitis. Like neuroborreliosis, involvement of the cranial nerves is not uncommon.

The meningitis clears spontaneously, even without treatment. The disease can then progress into its latent phase. The first year is referred to as *early latent syphilis*, and beyond that as *late latent*. Although this timeframe may seem somewhat arbitrary, it is clinically useful in that patients are substantially more likely to transmit infection during the early latent period. Without antimicrobial therapy, approximately one third of patients will eventually develop symptomatic late syphilis, primarily with neurologic involvement or the other threatening late manifestation, syphilitic aortitis. The remaining two thirds seem to clear the infection.

Diagnosis

Much as in EM in early Lyme disease, diagnosis of the chancre is straightforward. Its appearance is virtually diagnostic. Scraping the surface and examining the resultant material under dark field microscopy, or with immunofluorescence, is simple and diagnostic. Similarly, the presence of a disseminated rash involving the palms and soles is highly suspicious of acute disseminated (secondary) syphilis. Beyond these clinical inferences, laboratory support for the diagnosis rests primarily on serologic testing. Although *B burgdorferi* can, with difficulty, be grown in vitro, *T pallidum* cannot. However, again similar to Lyme disease, serologic tests are extremely useful.

Although in recent years specific ELISAs have been developed,[35] screening usually relies on what are termed *reaginic* tests. Over the years, many of these procedures were developed, beginning with the Wasserman, and more recently including the VDRL and RPR. All measure anticardiolipin antibodies, which are antibodies that do not react directly with *T pallidum* but arise in most cases (for poorly understood reasons). These are reliable screening tests; they are very sensitive but not completely specific. False-negatives arise occasionally, particularly with a peculiar but rare phenomenon known as the *prozone reaction*, in which antibody is present in great excess, interfering with the reaction needed to produce a positive reaginic test.[36] Positives are confirmed with either the fluorescent treponemal antibody absorbed (FTA-abs; absorbed against nonpathogenic treponemata) or an ELISA, if available.

Treatment response is often measured by the decline in reaginic test titer; when treated early, many patients become seronegative after undergoing successful treatment. Patients who have disease of significant duration may be *serofast*, which means they may remain seropositive indefinitely.

Because neurosyphilis involves primarily the CNS (as opposed to the peripheral nervous system), examining the CSF can be informative. Unfortunately, because no definitive tool exists to establish the diagnosis of neurosyphilis with 100% accuracy, estimates of sensitivity and specificity of different measures are challenging.

Most individuals who have neurosyphilis have an active lymphocytic pleocytosis, typically consisting largely of plasma cells and B cells. Protein is typically moderately elevated, and glucose is generally essentially normal. Patients usually have increased immunoglobulin production in the CSF, with elevated IgG index and even oligoclonal bands.

The greatest specificity is derived from measuring reaginic antibodies in the CSF. The CSF VDRL is the most widely used. Although it is specific (presumably because it is such an insensitive test, false-positives caused by contamination from a traumatic tap rarely occur), its sensitivity is probably less than 50%.[37] The FTA enhances sensitivity, as may the *T pallidum* hemagglutination assay[38]; however, both sacrifice specificity because enough antibody may cross the blood–brain barrier to reflect false-positives. Efforts to derive antibody indices, such as in neuroborreliosis, have not yet improved diagnostic accuracy but may prove helpful in the future.

Clinical: Neurologic Disease

Nervous system infection is both common and varied in its manifestations, although distinct unifying themes are present (**Table 4**). CNS involvement occurs early; CSF shows significant abnormalities in more than 50% of patients who have early disease.[39] However, as in early Lyme disease, the clinical implications of this are unclear. Patients who have early disease seem to recover equally well after standard treatment, whether or not CSF is normal.[39]

Symptomatic syphilitic meningitis is typically the earliest evidence of nervous system involvement, usually occurring in the first year of infection. Its frequency ranges from 1% to 25% of patients who have neurosyphilis,[40] which is substantially less than that of a CSF pleocytosis. Symptoms are generally nonspecific, involving typical symptoms of aseptic meningitis, such as headache, nausea, and

Table 4
Symptoms of neurosyphilis during the different stages of the illness

Stage	Form	Onset	Symptoms
Secondary	Syphilitic meningitis	1st to 2nd y, post acute	Headache, cranial neuropathy
Tertiary	Meningovascular Parenchymatous	1st decade; peak at 7 y	Stroke-like
	Tabes	10–20 y	Dorsal root → post columns
	Genera paresis	10–20 y	Behavior, dementia, headache
	Gummatous	Late but variable	Focal mass, seizures

photosensitivity. Patients can have nuchal rigidity and even papilledema, and cranial neuropathies also occur. CSF findings are typical of aseptic meningitis, except that the CSF VDRL is usually positive.

Within the first 10 years of infection, some patients will develop meningovascular syphilis. These patients have chronic syphilitic meningitis with involvement of blood vessels that pass through the subarachnoid space. Inflammation of meningeal blood vessels is thought to be the primary event, causing the meningitis, rather than the other way around. Vessels develop endothelial edema, lymphocytic inflammatory infiltrates, fibroblast proliferation, and ultimately obliterative endarteritis[41] (Heubner's endarteritis). Stroke-like events result, although their onset may be less abrupt than in typical atherosclerotic large artery strokes,[42] which are typically embolic. The gradual development of arterial obstruction may allow time for development of collaterals, perhaps explaining why these patients seem to have a better prognosis than those whose strokes are due to atherosclerotic cerebrovascular disease.

Parenchymatous neurosyphilis tends to occur even later in infection, typically 10 to 20 years after onset. Parenchymatous neurosyphilis includes two different disorders: general paresis and tabes dorsalis. Although these disorders may cooccur, they differ in pathology and clinical manifestations. Before the penicillin era, both were common.

General paresis typically involves personality change; psychiatric manifestations such as delusions or mood changes; dementia and headaches; and more focal findings. The upper brainstem is commonly involved, causing irregularly shaped pupils that do not react to light but do to accommodation (Argyll Robertson pupils). Tremors, myoclonus, and even seizures can occur. Histopathologically, the involved cortex is rather bland, with atrophy, neuronal loss, and prominent astrocyte proliferation and gliosis. However, significant meningeal inflammation often overlies the affected cortex.

Although spirochetes have been described within the brain parenchyma, parenchymal inflammation is not prominent. Not surprisingly, CSF is typically inflammatory. Antimicrobial therapy can arrest the process but, given the underlying tissue changes, is unlikely to reverse the neurologic deficits.

Although tabes dorsalis is grouped with general paresis, it looks pathophysiologically different. The described pathology[41] consists primarily of atrophy in the dorsal roots and posterior columns; meningeal inflammation may occur early, but typically disappears. Approximately half of affected patients have bland CSF; CSF VDRL is positive in most. Pathologic studies do not typically show arachnoiditis affecting the symptomatic roots, suggesting that much of the pathology is more peripheral, perhaps closer to the dorsal root ganglion. Neurophysiologic studies suggest the pathology lies just proximal to the ganglion itself, in the distal part of the dorsal root.[43]

Clinically, patients have deficits that follow logically from the site of damage. The marked loss of proprioception leads to gait and lower-extremity ataxia. The loss of pain perception leads to repeated injuries, accentuated by the ataxic gait, leading to Charcot's joints, which are joints that are mechanically destroyed by repeated, unnoticed injuries. Patients also have prominent positive symptoms of a sensory neuropathy, involving lightning-like pains in the limbs or trunk. These episodes can be brief to more protracted. Most tabetic patients also have Argyll Robertson pupils.

Finally, rare patients will develop CNS gummas, which are syphilitic granulomata in the brain parenchyma. These present as mass lesions, with signs appropriate to location; seizures may occur. CSF can be normal if the gummas are not adjacent to the CSF space. Spirochetes have been visualized within gummas using various techniques.

Treatment

T pallidum has remained exquisitely sensitive to penicillin. Parenteral treatment is required at all stages. Dosing and form of penicillin depend on the stage of involvement (**Table 5**) (grade B evidence).

In primary and secondary syphilis,[44] a single dose of benzathine penicillin G intramuscularly, 2.4 mU, is effective in most individuals not infected with HIV. In children, a dose of 50,000 U/kg, up to the adult dose, is used. Because patients who have primary or secondary syphilis experience such a uniform response to this regimen, CSF must be examined only in individuals clinically suspected of having nervous system or ophthalmologic disease. Early latent syphilis (<1 year duration) is generally treated with a single dose (2.4 mU) of benzathine penicillin G intramuscularly. Late latent disease (or disease of unclear duration) is treated with 3 weekly injections.

Although most patients experience a response to these standard regimens, as in all infectious diseases, some do not. Response is best judged by clinical symptoms, either onset of new symptoms or failure to improve. and by reaginic antibody titers. If titers do not decline fourfold in 6 months, or if a sustained fourfold increase is seen, this is considered failed treatment. These patients should be evaluated for HIV infection (if they have not already) and probably should undergo CSF examination. If no evidence of CNS involvement is present, recommended retreatment consists of three weekly intramuscular injections of benzathine penicillin G, 2.4 MU.

The rare individuals who remain serofast despite this, and have neither progressive symptoms nor abnormal CSF, require no further treatment, although continued monitoring is advisable.

When the nervous system is involved[44,45] (or eye, which is functionally equivalent), higher-dose treatment is required, designed to sustain high CSF levels of penicillin.

Table 5
Syphilis treatment

	Recommended	Penicillin Allergic	Children
Primary, secondary	Benzathine penicillin G, 2.4 mU, IM × 1	Doxycycline, 100 mg orally bid × 10–14 d	Benzathine penicillin, 50,000 U/kg, to maximum of 2.4 mU
		Tetracycline 500 mg orally 4/d × 10–14 d	Doxycycline, tetracycline only if patient aged ≥8 y
Early latent	As above	As above	As above
Late latent	Benzathine penicillin G, 2.4 mU, IM weekly × 3 wk	As above, but for 4 wk	As above, but for 4 wk
Treatment failure, not CNS	As in late latent	As in late latent	As in late latent
Neurosyphilis	Aqueous penicillin G, 18–24 mU, daily × 10–14 d	Ceftriaxone, 2 g, daily × 10–14 d	(Rare because of required duration of infection)

Abbreviations: CNS, central nervous system; IM, intramuscularly.
Adapted from Centers for Disease Control and Prevention, Workowski K, Berman S. Sexually transmitted diseases treatment guidelines, 2006. MMWR Morb Mortal Wkly Rep 2006;55 (RR-11):1–94.

Recommended treatment consists of aqueous crystalline penicillin G, 18 to 24 million U/d (3–4 mU every 4 hours), intravenously for 10 to 14 days. An alternative treatment (although theoretically it may not achieve spirocheticidal levels in the CSF) is procaine penicillin, 2.4 mU, given daily intramuscularly, with oral probenecid, 500 mg, four times daily, both for 10 to 14 days.

Several regimens[44] are recommended for patients allergic to penicillin, although none has been shown to be as effective as penicillin. Ceftriaxone, 2 g, intravenously daily for 10 to 14 days can be used, although allergy cross-reactivity can occur and the evidence supporting this and other nonpenicillin regimens remains incomplete. Primary, secondary, and early latent syphilis can be treated orally with 2 weeks of doxycycline, 100 mg, twice daily or tetracycline, 500 mg, four times daily. For late latent disease, these courses are extended to 4 weeks.

Patients who have HIV pose a potential challenge. Several reports describe individuals infected with HIV whose neurosyphilis clearly relapsed despite obtaining full recommended therapy when they were not severely immunocompromised.[46] Recommendations call for the same treatment regimen as in individuals not infected with HIV, but much closer follow-up is required for possible treatment failure.

SUMMARY

Because neurosyphilis and neuroborreliosis share similar biologic characteristics, these two spirochetal infections have several of the same distinct clinical themes. Both can readily seed the nervous system and cause prolonged infections, despite the presence of an obvious humoral immune response. Both are readily diagnosed primarily using serologic tests, which are excellent but imperfect. In both, CNS infection is most readily confirmed through CSF examination. Both infections remain readily responsive to straightforward antimicrobial regimens. However, each has acquired a distinct mystique, leading to its being blamed for a broad range of unrelated disorders. Hopefully the final common thread will be that, just as increased scientific understanding resulted in clarification of the true biology of syphilis, continued development of understanding of Lyme disease, and the dissemination and acceptance of this information, will similarly result in its demystification.

REFERENCES

1. Steere AC, Malawista SE, Hardin JA, et al. Erythema chronicum migrans and Lyme arthritis. The enlarging clinical spectrum. Ann Intern Med 1977;86(6): 685–98.
2. Fingerle V, Schulte-Spechtel UC, Ruzic-Sabljic E, et al. Epidemiological aspects and molecular characterization of Borrelia burgdorferi s.l. from southern Germany with special respect to the new species Borrelia spielmanii sp. nov. Int J Med Microbiol 2008;298:279–90.
3. Benach JL, Bosler EM, Hanrahan JP, et al. Spirochetes isolated from the blood of two patients with Lyme disease. N Engl J Med 1983;308:740–2.
4. Steere AC, Grodzicki RL, Kornblatt AN, et al. The spirochetal etiology of Lyme disease. N Engl J Med 1983;308:733–40.
5. Asbrink E, Hederstedt B, Hovmark A. The spirochetal etiology of acrodermatitis chronica atrophicans Herxheimer. Acta Derm Venereol 1984;64:506–12.
6. Bannwarth A. Chronische lymphocytare meningitis, entzundliche polyneuritis und "rheumatismus". Arch Psychiatr Nervenkr 1941;113:284–376.
7. Wormser GP, Dattwyler RJ, Shapiro ED, et al. The clinical assessment, treatment, and prevention of Lyme disease, human granulocytic anaplasmosis, and

babesiosis: clinical practice guidelines by the Infectious Diseases Society of America. Clin Infect Dis 2006;43:1089–134.

8. Gerber MA, Shapiro ED, Burke GS, et al. Lyme disease in children in southeastern Connecticut. Pediatric Lyme Disease Study Group. N Engl J Med 1996;335(17):1270–4.

9. Reik L, Steere AC, Bartenhagen NH, et al. Neurologic abnormalities of Lyme disease. Medicine 1979;58(4):281–94.

10. Avery RA, Frank G, Eppes SC. Diagnostic utility of *Borrelia burgdorferi* cerebrospinal fluid polymerase chain reaction in children with Lyme meningitis. Pediatr Infect Dis J 2005;24(8):705–8.

11. Tugwell P, Dennis DT, Weinstein A, et al. Laboratory evaluation in the diagnosis of Lyme Disease. Ann Intern Med 1997;127:1109–23.

12. Kaell AT, Volkman DJ, Gorevic PD, et al. Positive Lyme serology in subacute bacterial endocarditis. A study of four patients. JAMA 1990;264(22):2916–8.

13. Centers for Disease Control and Prevention (CDC). Recommendations for test performance and interpretation from the Second National Conference on serologic diagnosis of Lyme Disease. MMWR Morb Mortal Wkly Rep 1995;44(31):590–1.

14. Halperin J, Logigian E, Finkel M, et al. Practice parameter for the diagnosis of patients with nervous system Lyme borreliosis (Lyme disease). Neurology 1996;46:619–27.

15. Hammers Berggren S, Hansen K, Lebech AM, et al. *Borrelia burgdorferi*-specific intrathecal antibody production in neuroborreliosis: a follow-up study. Neurology 1993;43(1):169–75.

16. Ljostad U, Skarpaas T, Mygland A. Clinical usefulness of intrathecal antibody testing in acute Lyme neuroborreliosis. Eur J Neurol 2007;14(8):873–6.

17. Blanc F, Jaulhac B, Fleury M, et al. Relevance of the antibody index to diagnose Lyme neuroborreliosis among seropositive patients. Neurology 2007;69(10):953–8.

18. Garin C, Bujadoux A. Paralysie par les tiques. [Paralysis by ticks]. J Med Lyon 1922;71:765–7 [in French].

19. Steere AC, Pachner AR, Malawista SE. Neurologic abnormalities of Lyme disease: successful treatment with high-dose intravenous penicillin. Ann Intern Med 1983;99:767–72.

20. Shah SS, Zaoutis TE, Turnquist J, et al. Early differentiation of Lyme from enteroviral meningitis. Pediatr Infect Dis J 2005;24(6):542–5.

21. Garro AC, Rutman M, Simonsen K, et al. Prospective validation of a clinical prediction model for Lyme meningitis in children. Pediatrics 2009;123(5):e829–34.

22. Halperin JJ. Diagnosis and treatment of the neuromuscular manifestations of Lyme disease. Curr Treat Options Neurol 2007;9(2):93–100.

23. Halperin JJ, Luft BJ, Volkman DJ, et al. Lyme neuroborreliosis—peripheral nervous system manifestations. Brain 1990;113:1207–21.

24. Muley SA, Parry GJ. Antibiotic responsive demyelinating neuropathy related to Lyme disease. Neurology 2009;72(20):1786–7.

25. Halperin JJ, Krupp LB, Golightly MG, et al. Lyme borreliosis-associated encephalopathy. Neurology 1990;40:1340–3.

26. Luo N, Johnson J, Shaw J, et al. Self-reported health status of the general adult U.S. population as assessed by the EQ-5D and Health Utilities Index. Med Care 2005;43(11):1078–86.

27. Kalina P, Decker A, Kornel E, et al. Lyme disease of the brainstem. Neuroradiology 2005;47(12):903–7.

28. Logigian EL, Johnson KA, Kijewski MF, et al. Reversible cerebral hypoperfusion in Lyme encephalopathy. Neurology 1997;49(6):1661–70.
29. Halperin JJ, Shapiro ED, Logigian EL, et al. Practice parameter: treatment of nervous system Lyme disease. Neurology 2007;69(1):91–102.
30. Klempner M, Hu L, Evans J, et al. Two controlled trials of antibiotic treatment in patients with persistent symptoms and a history of Lyme disease. N Engl J Med 2001;345:85–92.
31. Krupp LB, Hyman LG, Grimson R, et al. Study and treatment of post Lyme disease (STOP-LD): a randomized double masked clinical trial. Neurology 2003;60(12):1923–30.
32. Fallon B, Sackheim H, Keil J, et al. Double-blind placebo-controlled retreatment with IV ceftriaxone for Lyme encephalopathy: clinical outcome. Paper presented at the 10th International Conference on Lyme Borreliosis and other tick-borne diseases. Vienna, Austria, September 11–15, 2005.
33. Centers for Disease Control and Prevention. Sexually transmitted disease surveillance 2007 supplement, syphilis surveillance report. Atlanta (GA): U.S. Department of Health and Human Services, Centers for Disease Control and Prevention; 2009.
34. Bacon RM, Kugeler KJ, Mead PS. Surveillance for Lyme disease – United States, 1992–2006. MMWR Morb Mortal Wkly Rep 2008;57(SS10):1–9.
35. Martin IE, Lau A, Sawatzky P, et al. Serological diagnosis of syphilis: enzyme-linked immunosorbent assay to measure antibodies to individual recombinant *Treponema pallidum* antigens. J Immunoassay Immunochem 2008;29(2):143–51.
36. Lessig S, Tecoma E. Perils of the prozone reaction: neurosyphilis presenting as an RPR-negative subacute dementia. Neurology 2006;66:777.
37. Marra CM, Critchlow CW, Hook EW 3rd, et al. Cerebrospinal fluid treponemal antibodies in untreated early syphilis. Arch Neurol 1995;52(1):68–72.
38. Marra C, Tantalo L, Maxwell C, et al. Alternative cerebrospinal fluid tests to diagnose neurosyphilis in HIV-infected individuals. Neurology 2004;63:85–8.
39. Flood JM, Weinstock HS, Guroy ME, et al. Neurosyphilis during the AIDS epidemic, San Francisco, 1985–1992. J Infect Dis 1998;177(4):931–40.
40. Katz DA, Berger JR. Neurosyphilis in acquired immunodeficiency syndrome. Arch Neurol 1989;46(8):895–8.
41. Hook EW 3rd, Chansolme D. Neurosyphilis. In: Roos KL, editor. Principles of neurological infectious diseases. New York: McGraw Hill Medical Publishing Division; 2005. p. 215–31.
42. Flint A, Liberato B, Anziska Y, et al. Meningovascular syphilis as a cause of basilar artery stenosis. Neurology 2005;64:391–2.
43. Sonoo M, Katayama A, Miura T, et al. Tibial nerve SEPs localized the lesion site in a patient with early tabes dorsalis. Neurology 2005;64:1452–4.
44. Workowski K, Berman S. Sexually transmitted diseases treatment guidelines, 2006. MMWR Morb Mortal Wkly Rep 2006;55(RR-11):22–35.
45. Jay CA. Treatment of neurosyphilis. Curr Treat Options Neurol 2006;8(3):185–92.
46. Gordon S, Eaton M, George R, et al. The response of symptomatic neurosyphilis to high-dose intravenous penicillin G in patients with human immunodeficiency virus infection. N Engl J Med 1994;331:1469–73.

Neurologic Presentations of Fungal Infections

Amy C. Rauchway, DO*, Sameea Husain, DO,
John B. Selhorst, MD

KEYWORDS

• Neurologic • Fungal • Infection • Presentation

Fungal infections of the central nervous system (CNS) have a high rate of morbidity and mortality because of several factors. Most importantly, the last three decades have witnessed a rising prevalence of susceptible hosts from the growing numbers of organ transplants, chemotherapy patients, and intensive care unit hospitalizations. Additional developments include emerging fungal pathogens and resistance to antifungal agents.[1–3] Knowledge of CNS fungal infections including their symptoms and signs, required diagnostic studies, and treatment methods are imperative for all neurologists. This article provides an overview of the clinical features and laboratory findings of the major mycoses affecting the CNS and a focus on their neurologic presentations (**Table 1**).

OVERVIEW
Fungi and Mycoses

Fungi are ubiquitous.[4] They occur as yeasts, molds, and dimorphic organisms. Yeasts are small unicellular organisms that are often found in decaying material. Molds are comparatively larger and exist in the filamentous form of branching hyphae. Dimorphic fungi, which have specific geographic distributions, cause endemic mycoses. In nature, they are filamentous at 25°C and yeasts or spherules at 35°C in host tissue.[1] Exposure to fungi occurs commonly from inhalation, ingestion, and skin contact. A competent immune system usually defends mucosal surfaces and the skin against invasion and consequent disease.[5] Primary pathogens are capable of producing disease in immunocompetent individuals, whereas opportunistic fungi are pathogenic in immunocompromised hosts.[6] Fungal infections commonly begin in subcutaneous sites or within invaded organs and secondarily disseminate through the bloodstream into the CNS.[3–5] Mycoses also penetrate the CNS by direct extension from adjacent

Department of Neurology & Psychiatry, Saint Louis University School of Medicine, 1438 South Grand Boulevard, St Louis, MO 63104, USA
* Corresponding author.
E-mail address: rauchway@slu.edu (A.C. Rauchway).

Neurol Clin 28 (2010) 293–309
doi:10.1016/j.ncl.2009.09.013
0733-8619/09/$ – see front matter © 2010 Elsevier Inc. All rights reserved.

neurologic.theclinics.com

Table 1
Fundamental pathologic and clinical features of CNS fungal infections

Infection Organisms	Morphology of Organism	Major Sources of Infection	Neurologic Presentations	Diagnostic Studies[a]	Treatment Options
Candidiasis C albicans C glabrata	Yeast with pseudohyphae	Skin[b] Oropharynx[b] Gastrointestinal tract[b] Vagina[b]	Meningitis Cranial neuropathy Stroke Abscesses	Neuroimaging CSF[c] Blood culture[d] Serum assay[e] Biopsy	LFAmB with or without 5-FC followed by fluconazole Manage hydrocephalus
Cryptococcosis C neoformans C gattii	Encapsulated yeast	Lungs[b] Skin[b]	Meningitis Meningoencephalitis Cryptococcomas Abscesses Pseudocysts Hydrocephalus Stroke Dementia Cranial neuropathies	Neuroimaging CSF[c,f] Serum assay[f]	AmB with 5-FC followed by fluconazole Manage hydrocephalus
Zygomycosis Mucor Rhizopus Absidia	Broad nonseptate hyphae	Lungs[b] Sinus[b,g]	Orbital cellulitis Cranial neuropathies Strokes	Neuroimaging Biopsy	AmB with debridement
Aspergillosis A fumigatus A flavus A niger A terreus	Septate hyphae	Lungs[b] Sinus[b,g]	Meningitis Mycotic aneurysms Abscesses Aspergilloma Strokes Orbital cellulitis Spinal cord compression	Neuroimaging CSF[c] Serum assays[e,h] Biopsy	Voriconazole Consider surgical resection of lesions

Coccidioidomycosis C immitis	Dimorphic	Lungs[b]	Meningitis Seizures Abscesses Granuloma Strokes Myelopathy Cauda equina syndrome Cranial neuropathies Hydrocephalus	Neuroimaging CSF[c,i] Serum assay[i] Biopsy	Fluconazole Manage hydrocephalus
Histoplasmosis H capsulatum var. capsulatum	Dimorphic	Lungs[b]	Meningitis Stroke Encephalitis Hydrocephalus Cranial neuropathies	Neuroimaging CSF[c,j] Blood culture Serum assay[j] Urine assay[j]	LFAmB followed by itraconazole Manage hydrocephalus
Blastomycosis B dermatitidis	Dimorphic	Lungs[b]	Meningitis Abscesses	Neuroimaging CSF[c] Serum assays Biopsy	LFAmB followed by an oral triazole Manage hydrocephalus

Abbreviations: CSF, cerebrospinal fluid; 5-FC, flucytosine; LFAmB, lipid-based formulations of amphotericin B.

[a] Sensitivity and specificity for assays vary by disease and patient population.
[b] Hematogenous spread.
[c] Opening pressure, cell count with differential, total protein and glucose, Gram stain, microscopic examination of sediment, India ink preparation, fungal culture.
[d] Rapid detection by peptide nucleic acid fluorescence in situ hybridization assay.
[e] Beta-D-glucan assay.
[f] Cryptococcal antigen detection.
[g] Direct extension.
[h] Galactomannan enzyme immunoassay.
[i] Complement fixation and other serologic testing.
[j] Histoplasma antigen detection.

anatomic structures (eg, the sinuses or infected bone) or breach the blood-brain barrier because of trauma or neurosurgical procedures.[5,7] Fungal morphology and size, dose of inoculum,[8] virulence, antigenic composition, and the host's immune status determine disease severity and pathology, such as meningitis, meningoencephalitis, brain abscesses, cerebral infarction, or myelopathy.[9,10]

Epidemiology

Currently, the estimated annual incidences of invasive mycoses caused by opportunistic pathogens per million of the population are 72 to 228 infections for *Candida* species, 30 to 66 for *Cryptococcus neoformans*, and 12 to 34 for *Aspergillus* species.[2] Autopsy studies, however, suggest that the incidence of CNS mycoses is underestimated.[11] Because of underdiagnosis, especially in immunocompromised and critically ill patients, fungal meningitis and fungal abscesses are associated with high mortality.[2,7] Invasive yeast infections account for most of the serious mycoses both in immunocompromised and immunocompetent patients.[12] For example, *Candida* infections have mortality rates ranging between 10% and 49%. Moreover, extended hospital stays because of invasive *Candida* infections generate estimated annual costs of nearly $1 billion in the United States.[2,13]

Clinical Features

The most revealing aspect of a fungal infection is the clinical history, particularly the tempo of the illness and the context in which symptoms develop. An in-depth history necessarily includes the past medical and surgical history, geographic residence, travel exposure, occupation, leisure activities, and drug use. The potential for fungal invasions is highly associated with prolonged hospitalizations and interventions. These include solid organ or allogenic stem cell transplant; use of broad-spectrum antibiotics; immunosuppressants, such as chemotherapy, glucocorticoids, or parenteral nutrition; and placement of central venous catheters or intracranial pressure monitors.

Meningitis and Meningoencephalitis

Although all major fungal pathogens produce meningitis, yeast infections particularly cause meningitis or meningoencephalitis because of seeding of the microcirculation and spread from subpial infarction into the subarachnoid space.[9,10] Primary fungal pathogens are *C neoformans* and *Cryptococcus gattii*, *Coccidioides immitis*, *Blastomyces dermatitidis*, and *Histoplasma capsulatum*.[6,14,15] Opportunistic fungi that cause meningitis include *C neoformans*, *Candida* species, *Aspergillus* species, and the *Zygomycetes*.[6]

Fungal meningitis is sometimes acute or subacute, but often chronic. Solitary or multiple symptoms and signs include fever, headache, lethargy, confusion, photophobia, neck stiffness, or focal neurologic deficits. Increased intracranial pressure is an important complication, especially in patients with cryptococcal meningitis and manifests as nausea, vomiting, cranial nerve palsies, and papilledema.[14] Fungal meningitis also presents as a subacute dementia.[6] Symptoms vary in severity, but develop swiftly in some immunocompromised patients. If untreated, the initial meningeal infection is life-threatening within weeks. Meningoencephalitis develops with extension into the parenchyma from perivascular spaces and is heralded by diminished level of consciousness, confusion, seizures, and focal neurologic deficits.

Focal Cerebral Lesions

Yeasts and filamentous molds invade the brain parenchyma. Infection usually occurs by hematogenous spread or from implantation of surgical devices. *Candida*,

Aspergillus, Blastomyces dermatitidis, and cryptococcal species are commonly reported etiologic agents.[16] Invasion of an artery results in arteritis with subsequent embolization or occlusion, whereas direct extension from the paranasal sinuses, orbit, or middle ear leads to abscesses or granulomatous invasion in the frontal or temporal lobes.[4,9,17] Simultaneous infarction and meningitis provide clinical evidence of angioinvasive disease. Patients with space-occupying lesions have focal neurologic deficits and raised intracranial pressure. Mycoses commonly associated with abscess formation include *Zygomycetes, Aspergillus*, and *Candida* species.

Spinal Syndromes

Spinal cord disease caused by invasive mycoses is far less common than cerebral disease, and includes myelitis and epidural abscesses with cord compression and nerve root impingement. The authors have also encountered patients with cauda equina syndromes from *C neoformans* and *C immitis* caused by settling of fungal organisms in the lower spinal canal and matting of the spinal roots in a fungus ball or mycelium.

Laboratory Studies

The definitive diagnosis of an invasive fungal infection requires histopathologic identification in tissue or growth in culture. Biopsy is not always feasible, however, or is inconclusive. Additionally, cultures are time-taking and have a low yield. Radiologic studies define sites of tissue invasion, but do not identify the offending agent. Ancillary laboratory techniques are useful in providing a probable diagnosis and allow for earlier treatment.

Once a CNS fungal infection is suspected and radiologic studies have excluded risk of herniation, examination of cerebrospinal fluid (CSF) is imperative. Studies include cell count with differential, total protein and glucose, Gram stain, India ink preparation, fungal culture, fungal antigen tests, and antibody assays. Fungal meningitis classically presents with a lymphocytic or monocytic pleocytosis. Exceptions include infection caused by *Aspergillus* and *Blastomyces* in which a neutrophilic pleocytosis predominates. Eosinophilia in the CSF is characteristic of coccidiomycosis. Hypoglycorrachia and elevated CSF protein are common. Gram stain and India ink preparations are valuable, but often inconclusive. Concentrates of CSF specimens have proved useful in revealing *C neoformans* in patients with AIDS.[18] Fungal culture allows for a specific taxonomic identification that is useful in both tracking of outbreaks and epidemiologic trends[19] and selection of antifungal agents. A successful culture, however, often requires repeated samples and larger CSF volumes (10–45 mL) than usually obtained for bacterial cultures. Generally, antigen detection is more useful than antibody testing, especially in immunosuppressed patients who are unable to mount an antibody response. Importantly, antigen detection of *C neoformans* and *H capsulatum* in the CSF have high sensitivity and specificity.[15,20] Antibody testing of the CSF is helpful when the organism burden is too low to detect the pathogen by polymerase chain reaction. The presence of antibodies, however, does not differentiate between active and prior infection.[18]

Repeated blood cultures are rewarding for the diagnosis of candidiasis, cryptococcal, and sometimes other fungal infections. The peptide nucleic acid fluorescence in situ hybridization assay allows for the rapid identification of *Candida albicans* from blood cultures. Most molds fail to grow in blood culture.[18,19] Two serum immunoassays are useful for rapid detection of fungal cell wall components. The beta-D-glucan assay is nonspecific for *Candida* species and other opportunistic fungi, whereas the galactomannan immunoassay is specific for invasive *Aspergillus*.[20]

Treatment

Pharmacologic options for the treatment of invasive fungal infections have broadened over the past 5 years. Optimal antifungal drug regimens depend on efficacy, spectrum of activity, CNS penetration, safety profile, role in combination therapy, drug-drug interactions, route of administration, and drug resistance. There are three classes of antifungal drugs used for the primary treatment of CNS infection: (1) polyenes including amphotericin B deoxycholate (AmB) and three lipid-based formulations (LFAmB); (2) triazoles (fluconazole, itraconazole, voriconazole, posaconazole); and (3) flucytosine (5-FC), a pyrimidine analog that inhibits DNA replication and disrupts protein synthesis in the fungal cell. Caspofungin and micafungin are echinocandins, a newer class of antifungals, used for the alternative treatment of *Aspergillus*. Flucytosine is rarely used alone because of development of resistant strains, but remains the gold standard in combination with AmB for cryptococcal meningitis and is preferably added to AmB for *Candida* meningitis.[13,21,22] Drug resistance varies among antifungal drugs and is less problematic with polyenes and echinocandins compared with 5-FC and the triazoles.[21] Disease-specific recommendations for AmB, the triazoles, and other fungal agents are available in the Infectious Diseases Society of America guidelines (http://www.idsociety.org).

Amazingly, AmB, the mainstay of antifungal therapy, was introduced more than 50 years ago. Its longevity is attributed to the broad spectrum of coverage for fungal infections and rare reports of resistance. This polyene binds to ergosterol and creates pores in the fungal cell membrane, thereby resulting in cell death. AmB is administered intravenously and penetrates across the blood-brain barrier during active CNS infection.[22] Three LFAmBs have reduced the dose-limiting nephrotoxicity of AmB. Moreover, infusion-related side effects, such as fever, rigors, and chills, occur less frequently in LFAmBs than in AmB, but chest discomfort, respiratory distress, and flank pain are reported.[22]

Triazoles block fungal cell wall sterol biosynthesis by inhibiting the cytochrome P-450 dependent rate-limiting step in the ergosterol biosynthetic pathway. Depletion of ergosterol increases toxic metabolic intermediates, thereby inhibiting fungal growth. Clinicians should carefully review each patient's medications for drug-drug interactions because cytochrome P-450 inhibition is a serious complication.[21] The first United States approved triazole was fluconazole in 1990 for cryptococcal meningitis and candidiasis. Voriconazole, a second-generation triazole, is now the drug of choice for invasive aspergillosis. Adverse reactions remain a concern and include transient visual abnormalities, dose-limiting hepatotoxicity, and rash. Triazoles vary in their pharmacology and recommendations regarding use for life-threatening infections.[22] Itraconazole and posaconazole are oral formulations. Although caution is required in the use of combination antifungal therapy because of antagonistic effects found in animal and in vitro experiments, such therapy holds promise for invasive infections. Clinical evidence, although limited, suggests that combination antifungal therapy results in faster CSF sterilization than monotherapy, and underlies the current recommendations for the use of AmB with 5-FC in the treatment of cryptococcal meningitis.[23]

In addition to pharmacologic management, surgical resection also has a role in the management of invasive mycoses. For example, CNS aspergillosis has a mortality rate that approaches 100%. Neurosurgical intervention, in combination with voriconazole, improves survival in patients with CNS aspergillosis.[24] Surgical debridement of necrotic sinuses and sometimes orbital tissue is advocated for *Mucor* infections. Relief of elevated intracranial pressure by ventricular drainage or a ventriculoperitoneal

(VP) shunt is highly important in minimizing morbidity and mortality of patients with meningitis, especially in cryptococcal infection. Solitary brain abscesses with a mass effect on surrounding structures require excision. Lastly, diagnostic biopsy of potential fungal abscesses that remain unidentified after thorough serologic studies, cultures, and tissue samples of primary sites of infection is sometimes necessary.

PRESENTATIONS OF CNS FUNGAL INFECTIONS
Candidiasis

Candida meningitis was first recognized in 1933.[25] CNS infection was infrequently reported until the 1960s when the use of chemotherapeutic agents, glucocorticoids, and intravenous drugs increased the number of patients susceptible to opportunistic infections.[6] In the most recent three decades, *Candida* infections have burgeoned with the rise in the acuity of critical illnesses and use of intensive care units. Astonishingly, candidiasis is responsible for more than 90% of all clinical fungal infections.[26]

The skin, oral pharynx, gastrointestinal tract, and vagina are sources for hematogenous spread of *Candida* to the CNS. Meningitis is the most common form of CNS infection.[27] Typically, fever, headache, stiff neck, and altered consciousness develop over several days to several weeks.[28] Focal neurologic signs are uncommon. The less frequent acute-onset form resembles bacterial meningitis.[29] A more insidious form of meningitis occurs with the species *C glabrata*, in which obtundation worsens over weeks to months.[6] Basal meningitis results in cranial neuropathies or vascular infarction from an invasive arteritis.[30] Presentation is sometimes dictated by the patient's condition. For example, in prematures and newborns, acute meningitis is signaled by respiratory distress.[31] In patients with AIDS and an average CD4 count of 135/mm^3 or less, *Candida* meningitis is a concern for those with a subacute fever and headache.[28]

Space-occupying candidal abscesses are infrequent.[27] Multiple microabscesses, those less than 3 mm, are more common. These are manifested as a fluctuating encephalopathy.[28] Clinical attention is often focused on systemic invasive candidiasis, however, and CNS involvement is unrecognized before autopsy.[6,26] Candidiasis of the spinal cord and spinal roots is rare.

Diagnosis of neurocandidiasis is often achieved by establishing a diagnosis of an invasive infection with a biopsy of a systemic site. Neuroimaging is helpful to demonstrate hydrocephalus or microabcesses.[32] Meningeal enhancement is rare, but spinal fluid examination often reveals a moderate mononuclear or polynuclear pleocytosis with an elevated protein in patients with meningitis. *Candida* is identified by stains in a large minority and by culture in most of these patients.[28] Treatment is usually with LFAmB and oral 5-FC.[13,28] Hydrocephalus requires ventriculostomy or VP shunt.[6] Successful resolution of the infection is often dependent on early recognition of CNS involvement.

Cryptococcosis

Cryptococcus, aptly termed the "sugar-coated killer"[33] because of its thick polysaccharide capsule (**Fig. 1**A) and "once-sleeping giant"[34] because of its indolent nature, is a leading cause of fungal meningitis worldwide among those with HIV.[35] The organism is harbored in soil and bird excreta. Cryptococcosis primarily affects the immunosuppressed and infrequently invades immunocompetent patients. Infection remains difficult to diagnose and treat despite the enormous scientific advances made in understanding this encapsulated yeast. Only recently has the genome of *C neoformans* been sequenced, the cryptococcal taxonomy reorganized, and virulence factors

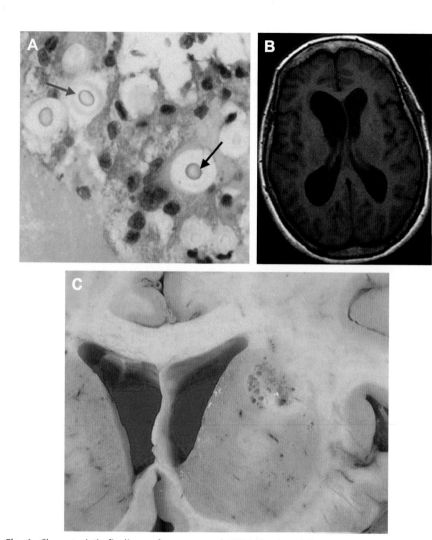

Fig. 1. Characteristic findings of cryptococcal CNS infection. (*A*) Brain biopsy (hematoxylin and eosin, ×400) shows multiple Cryptococci (*black arrow*) and inflammatory cells. The clear, mucoid appearance of the thick capsule (*red arrow*) results in a halo around the organism. (*Courtesy of* Dr Gretchen Johns, Mayo Clinic.) (*B*) MRI reveals dilated ventricles from communicating hydrocephalus in a patient with cryptococcal meningitis. (*C*) Multiple small gelatinous pseudocysts are evident in the basal ganglia. (*Courtesy of* Dr Beth Levy, Saint Louis University, St Louis, MO.)

genetically analyzed.[25,36,37] The current challenge is to develop pharmacologic interventions that target specific mediators of cryptococcal virulence and to systematize delivery of medical therapy to vulnerable populations.

Cryptococcus as a human pathogen was first clearly described by physicians Otto Busse and Abraham Buschke in 1894 and recognized as a cause of meningitis in the early 1900s.[38] The upward spike in prevalence that occurred in the 1980s with the HIV pandemic has been diminished by combination antiretroviral therapy in developed countries. Lately, cryptococcal infection has re-emerged because of the immune reconstitution inflammatory syndrome in the HIV population and an increase in solid organ transplant recipients.[21] In contrast, cryptococcosis remains an infection of elevated disproportion in developing countries.

Current taxonomic schemes are medically relevant because they differentiate two disease-causing species, four serotypes, and hybrid serotypes. These are C neoformans (serotypes A, D, and AD) and C gattii (serotypes B and C).[39] Hybrids AD and BC and BD are human pathogens. Serotypes A and D and AD are responsible for 98% of all cryptococcal infections.[8] C gattii, pathogenic in immunocompetent hosts, was found mostly in tropical and subtropical regions before an epidemic on Vancouver Island, Canada, in 1999. A hybrid of C neoformans and C gattii has been proposed as a candidate for a worldwide "superpathogen" with potential to infect immunocompetent individuals.[40]

Before 1981, the total number of cases of C neoformans in the United States was between 500 and 1000 cases annually.[38] Recent data show a staggering estimation of 957,900 yearly cases of cryptococcal meningitis in HIV-affected patients worldwide and an associated 624,725 deaths. In 2006, sub-Saharan Africa had the highest number of estimated cases at 720,000 yearly with associated deaths estimated at 500,000. The comparable annual figures for North America are 7800 cases with 700 deaths.[35]

The lungs serve as the primary site of infection, but most symptomatic infections are in the CNS, chiefly as meningitis. CNS disease usually occurs in isolation and infrequently presents with pneumonia or focal skin lesions.[41] Chronic granulomas or cryptococcomas occur in the parenchyma and occasionally in the choroid plexus and ventricles. Deep cerebral infarcts affecting the basal ganglia and thalamus are caused by an arteritis of small penetrating arteries.[16]

Headache, often mild, is the most common symptom and progresses slowly over days, weeks, or months.[42] Other symptoms of subacute meningoencephalitis, such as lethargy, confusion, and personality changes, arise. Fever is less common.[8] Occasionally, psychiatric symptoms or a subacute dementia is the only clinical finding. Hydrocephalus caused by elevated intracranial pressure occurs in two thirds of patients and is an important complication to recognize (**Fig. 1B**). Fungal infection and inflammation obstructs CSF outflow in the arachnoid villi and subarachnoid spaces, and requires urgent relief.[43] Nuchal rigidity and cranial neuropathies are more common in Africa among those with meningoencephalitis.[42] Immunocompetent patients tend to have localized, slowly progressive disease compared with those who are immunosuppressed.[8,16,42]

Radiologic findings include meningeal enhancement, abscesses, and cryptococcomas in intraparenchymal, intraventricular, or perivascular spaces. Clusters of pseudocysts in the basal ganglia and thalami strongly suggest cryptococcal infections (**Fig. 1C**). These cysts are composites of yeasts with little surrounding edema and are well-circumscribed, round-to-oval lesions of low density on CT and have CSF intensity on MRI.[16]

Lumbar puncture with manometry is necessary to diagnose cryptococcal meningitis after a large cerebral mass has been excluded by neuroimaging. Spinal fluid examination often reveals a mononuclear pleocytosis with a range of 20 to 200 cells/mm^3 in non-HIV patients and 0 to 50 cells/mm^3 in HIV cases. Typically, the protein is elevated and the glucose is decreased. India ink preparations are very worthwhile, especially in spun down, concentrated CSF specimens.[8] The thick capsule does not stain, but rather highlights the organism with a halo.[18] The organism is found in more than 50% of HIV-negative cases and 90% of patients with AIDS. Cryptococcal antigen assays in CSF specimens are positive in more than 90% of patients. Serum antigen has a high specificity in those with meningitis and HIV and is less sensitive in patients without HIV.[1,8] Lastly, the diagnosis is conclusively established by culture of organisms from the CSF, especially if large volumes of fluid are submitted.[8]

The goals of therapy are CSF sterilization; reduction of intracranial pressure; prevention of serious sequelae, such as blindness and cranial nerve abnormalities; and radiographic resolution of mass lesions. Current practice guidelines for treatment of cryptococcal CNS disease recommend combination therapy using an induction with AmB plus 5-FC followed by oral fluconazole.[21,41,44] Recommendations for reduction of elevated intracranial pressure include percutaneous lumbar or ventricular drainage or, if persistent, by VP shunt. Lipid formulations of AmB are given if renal impairment occurs.[44,45]

Zygomycosis

Several pathogens occur in this class of molds that have broad, nonseptate hyphae of uneven diameter and range from 6 to 50 μm in length.[46] Among a multitude of clinical conditions that compromise immune defense systems, poorly controlled diabetes mellitus is notoriously common in patients with mucormycosis.[47] Typically an airborne infection, primary disease begins as sinusitis or pneumonia. One feature of these organisms is their rapid growth and affinity to invade blood vessels. A serious complication is acute or subacute rhinocerebral zygomycosis (**Fig. 2**) and is linked to a tendency of these organisms for rapid growth and affinity to invade blood vessels.[48] As the infection spreads from an affected sinus, often the ethmoid, into the microvasculature of contiguous tissues, localized necrosis follows. Clinically, this necrotic slough is recognized as a black eschar (**Fig. 3**). Facial pain, headache, and feverishness are early symptoms. Extension of the infection into the apex of the orbit through the paper-thin wall of the ethmoid produces a dramatic orbital cellulitis with

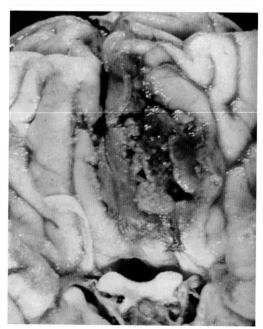

Fig. 2. Necrosis of the inferior frontal lobe was found in a patient with mucormycosis. (*Courtesy of* Dr Beth Levy, Saint Louis University, St Louis, MO.)

a characteristic diagnostic triad of acute proptosis, ophthalmoplegia, and blindness (**Fig. 4**). This dramatic syndrome is a medical emergency that requires prompt action to arrest further spread along orbital vessels and cranial nerves into the cavernous sinus and contiguous structures. Biopsy, usually by an otolaryngologist, and tissue demonstration of the invading mold confirms the diagnosis. Treatment requires aggressive surgical debridement of necrotic tissue and antifungal therapy with intravenous AmB.[49]

Aspergillosis

Aspergillus is a mold with septated hyphae that are 2 to 4 μm in diameter (**Fig. 5A**). *A fumigatus* is the most common pathogen, but *A flavus*, *A niger*, and *A terreus* also cause disease.[22] Invasive aspergillosis principally involves the sinopulmonary tract, reflecting inhalation as the most common route of entry of *Aspergillus* spores. Alternative entry sites are rarely the gastrointestinal tract and skin.[50] Chronic forms are necrotizing pulmonary or fibrocavitary aspergillosis that occur in immunocompetent patients, progress over months to years, and require prolonged antifungal therapy.[51,52] CNS involvement results from direct extension from a sinus, hematogenous dissemination from a primary pulmonary site, or embolization from an invaded artery.[53] Cerebral aspergillosis takes several pathologic forms, including meningitis, mycotic aneurysms, cerebral infarcts, multifocal cerebritis, or abscesses (**Fig. 5B**).

Suspicion of a fungal infection arises with the insidious evolution of persisting facial pain, headache, mental status changes, seizures, or focal neurologic deficits, especially in an immunocompromised or neutropenic patient.[54] Orbital infiltration is suggested by periorbital pain, proptosis, blurry vision, and diplopia. Stroke-like syndromes develop from spread into blood vessels, especially the internal carotid artery. Alternatively, focal deficits result from rapidly progressing parenchymal granulomas or brain abscesses. Pulmonary infections also extend through thoracic vertebrae into the epidural space and cause spinal cord compression.[53]

Several patterns of cerebral aspergillosis identifiable on CT and MRI include localized edema, hemorrhagic lesions, solid enhancing lesions referred to as

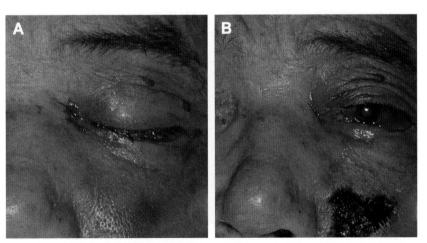

Fig. 3. In a patient with mucormycosis of the ethmoid and cancer of the lung, invasion of a thrombosed infraorbital artery is reflected in the development of an erythematous cheek (*A*) and necrotic eschar several days later (*B*).

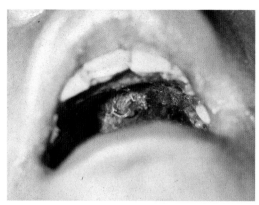

Fig. 4. A necrotic palate was observed in a diabetic woman with an acute cellulitis of the orbit from Rhizopus.

"aspergillomas" or "tumoral form," abscess-like ring enhancing masses, infarction, and mycotic aneurysms.[55] With neuroimaging, there is frequently a lack of contrast enhancement or perifocal edema caused by the immunosuppressed status of the patient.[56] Not infrequently, focal lesions are mistaken for pyogenic abscesses or brain tumors.[54] A definitive diagnosis requires brain tissue for histopathologic analysis.

Voriconazole is the recommended first-line agent for treatment of invasive aspergillosis.[22] AmB is also licensed in the United States for primary therapy of invasive aspergillosis. Because LFAmB, AmB colloidal dispersion, itraconazole, posaconazole, and caspofungin have demonstrated in vitro, in vivo, and clinical activity against *Aspergillus* species, they are used as alternative therapies for invasive aspergillosis.[22]

Coccidioidomycosis

In that portion of the Sonoran desert extending from northern Mexico into Arizona and California's Central Valley, *Coccidioides* species are endemic in the soil as a mold. The

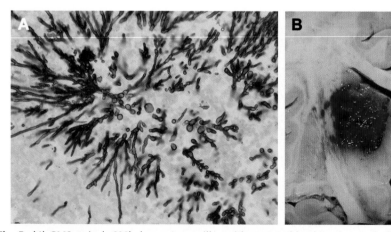

Fig. 5. (*A*) GMS stain (×600) shows Aspergillus with septated hyphae that typically branch no more than 45 degrees. (*Courtesy of* Department of Pathology, Saint Louis University, St Louis, MO.) (*B*) Hemorrhagic necrosis in the thalamus was caused by infection with Aspergillus. (*Courtesy of* Dr Beth Levy, Saint Louis University, St Louis, MO.)

airborne spores, conidia, are also found in some arid regions of Central and South America. Outdoor exposure accounts for men being four times more likely than women to become infected.

Infection is asymptomatic in over 60% of patients. Malaise, fever, diaphoresis, rashes, arthralgias, and a variably expressed pulmonary infection occur in the remainder of patients and persist for several weeks. Chorioretinal scars in 7.5% of patients supports a hematogenous dissemination, but an otherwise clinically evident extrapulmonary infection develops in only 1% of patients.[57,58] About one third of these patients acquire chronic meningitis with the initial fungemia.[59] Symptoms, however, are usually not expressed for several months. Hence, a history of recent travel to an endemic area is an important clue to recognizing this infection as a cause of an ill-defined pneumonitis or meningitis.[6,60] Furthermore, pregnant women, diabetics, steroid-treated, and immunosuppressed patients are more prone to develop meningitis.[61]

Headache, fever, altered mental status, nausea, vomiting, and weight loss as very common symptoms of chronic coccidioidomycosis. Frequent signs are nuchal rigidity, personality changes, seizures, papilledema, and focal neurologic deficits. Additional clues of coccidioidal infection are subcutaneous abscesses and persisting lung infections. As the meningitis progresses, hydrocephalus and cerebral granulomas and abscesses occur. Complications of the chronic meningitis include vasculitis, especially with involvement of veins, cranial neuropathies, myelopathies, and cauda equina syndromes. The differential diagnosis especially includes other causes of granulomatosis and more suppurative forms of meningitis. Chest radiographs are abnormal in over 90% of patients. Serum complement fixation antigen assays are nearly always positive, but persist long after an infection. Peripheral eosinophilia is found in one third of patients and is more indicative of an active process.

Neuroimaging often shows meningeal enhancement or hydrocephalus. The spinal fluid frequently has low glucose, elevated protein, and monocellular pleocytosis in which elevated eosinophils occur in 70% of specimens.[62] The fungus is cultured from nearly one half of sampled spinal fluids. It is important to recognize that complement fixation antigen assays are positive in over 85% of active meningeal infections. Diagnosis is definitively established by biopsy of infected tissue, usually skin nodules in which characteristic spherules are demonstrated.

Oral fluconazole or itraconazole is now the mainstay of treatment[63,64]; nephrotoxic AmB is reserved for more severe and acutely affected patients.

Histoplasmosis

Histoplasma capsulatum is a dimorphic fungus that grows as a mold in nature and bears both large and small spores.[46] It is carried by birds and bats commonly found in states bordering the Ohio and lower Mississippi River valleys. Primary infection occurs through inhalation into the pulmonary tree and is predominantly self-limiting. Disseminated histoplasmosis is rare and occurs mostly in immunocompromised patients and the aged. Involvement of the CNS occurs in 5% to 10% of patients who develop disseminated histoplasmosis.[65] Clinical syndromes include chronic meningitis, focal parenchymal lesions of the brain or spinal cord, stroke caused by septic emboli, and diffuse encephalitis. The most common neurologic symptoms are headache, altered sensorium, confusion, and cranial neuropathies. Focal neurologic deficits, seizures, or personality changes are found in 10% of patients.[66]

Imaging studies are normal or reveal low-signal, contrast-enhancing masses. Diagnosis is dependent on culture from the blood or detection of CSF or serum *Histoplasma* antigen.[65] Urine samples for *Histoplasma* antigen are useful because of a high sensitivity in patients with disseminated disease. Testing CSF for anti-*Histoplasma* antibodies has been shown to be helpful, particularly in immunocompetent persons. One of the important complications of this condition is hydrocephalus, which is often evident by CT scanning before chronic meningitis is diagnosed.

The treatment for histoplasmosis is with LFAmB over 4 to 6 weeks because of its reduced nephrotoxicity and higher concentrations in the brain than AmB. This is followed by itraconazole for at least 1 year and until clearance of CSF abnormalities, including detection of *Histoplasma* antigen.[67] Blood levels of itraconazole are used to ensure adequate drug exposure.

Blastomycosis

Blastomyces dermatitidis is a dimorphic fungus that has small spores borne on hyphae of the mold.[46] Geographic distribution of blastomycosis is restricted to southeastern and south central states that border the Mississippi and Ohio Rivers, the upper Midwestern states, and Canadian provinces near the Great Lakes and a small area of New York and Canada adjacent to the St Lawrence River.[67] Neurologic involvement occurs in 6% to 35% of individuals with disseminated blastomycosis. It is characterized by solitary or multiple CNS abscesses or chronic meningitis, which is often accompanied by a rapid clinical deterioration. Osteolytic infection of vertebrae is frequently painless as it spreads to the spinal canal and spinal cord.[53] Neuroimaging typically exhibits an intracranial dural-based granulomatous lesion.[68] Treatment of blastomycosis is LFAmB over 4 to 6 weeks. This is followed by an oral azole, such as fluconazole, itraconazole, or voriconazole, for at least 12 months and until resolution of CSF abnormalities.[69]

SUMMARY

Because of the increasing prevalence of fungal diseases affecting the CNS, neurologists should be fully acquainted with clues to their diagnosis and evolving methods of treatment. Fungal infections of the CNS primarily affect those who are immunosuppressed. Compromise of the body's defense system disposes patients to invasion by a fungus whether associated with requisite advanced medical therapies or an underlying illness, as in HIV infection. When the signs and symptoms of meningitis, strokes, focal neurologic deficits, and hydrocephalus in the setting of immunosuppression are evident, evaluation of a CNS fungal infection should be urgently pursued. Less frequently, CNS fungal infections occur in the immunocompetent. They are identified by careful diagnostic pursuit of patients with unexplained neurologic deficits. Timely recognition and medical treatment with antifungal agents are essential to reduce mortality and limit morbidity. Neurosurgical intervention is needed and often life-saving in some patients. Recommended treatment guidelines are readily available (http://www.idsociety.org).

REFERENCES

1. Black KE, Baden LR. Fungal infections of the CNS: treatment strategies for the immunocompromised patient. CNS Drugs 2007;21(4):293–318.
2. Pfaller MA, Pappas PG, Wingard JR. Invasive fungal pathogens: current epidemiological trends. Clin Infect Dis 2006;43(Suppl 1):S3–14.
3. Richardson M, Lass-Florl C. Changing epidemiology of systemic fungal infections. Clin Microbiol Infect 2008;14(Suppl 4):S5–24.

4. Shankar SK, Mahadevan A, Sundaram C, et al. Pathobiology of fungal infections of the central nervous system with special reference to the Indian scenario. Neurol India 2007;55(3):198–214.
5. Lucas S, Bell J, Chimelli L. Parasitic and fungal infections. In: Love S, Louis DN, Ellison DW, editors. Greenfield's neuropathology. 8th edition. London: Edward Arnold; 2008. p. 1488–511.
6. Perfect JR. Fungal meningitis. In: Scheld WM, Whitley RJ, Marra CM, editors. Infections of the central nervous system. 3rd edition. Philadelphia: Lippincott Williams & Wilkins; 2004. p. 691–713.
7. Chakrabarti A. Epidemiology of central nervous system mycoses. Neurol India 2007;55(3):191–7.
8. Satishchandra P, Mathew T, Gadre G, et al. Cryptococcal meningitis: clinical, diagnostic and therapeutic overviews. Neurol India 2007;55(3):226–32.
9. Murthy JMK. Fungal infections of the central nervous system: the clinical syndromes. Neurol India 2007;55(3):221–5.
10. Dotis J, Roilides E. Immunopathogenesis of central nervous system fungal infections. Neurol India 2007;55(3):216–20.
11. Bodey G, Bueltmann B, Duguid W, et al. Fungal infections in cancer patients: an international autopsy survey. Eur J Clin Microbiol Infect Dis 1992;11(2): 99–109.
12. Ostrosky-Zeichner L. Invasive yeast infections. In: Maertens JA, Marr KA, editors. Diagnosis of fungal infections. New York: Informa Healthcare; 2007. p. 221–38.
13. Pappas PG, Kauffman CA, Andes D, et al. Clinical practice guidelines for the management of candidiasis: 2009 update by the Infectious Diseases Society of America. Clin Infect Dis 2009;48(5):503–35.
14. Kauffman CA. Pearls in establishing a clinical diagnosis: signs and symptoms. In: Maertens JA, Marr KA, editors. Diagnosis of fungal infections. New York: Informa Healthcare; 2007. p. 1–17.
15. Scully EP, Baden LR, Katz JT. Fungal brain infections. Curr Opin Neurol 2008; 21(3):347–52.
16. Jain KK, Mittal SK, Kumar S, et al. Imaging features of central nervous system fungal infections. Neurol India 2007;55(3):241–50.
17. Cortez KJ, Walsh TJ. Space-occupying fungal lesions. In: Scheld WM, Whitley RJ, Marra CM, editors. Infections of the central nervous system. 3rd edition. Philadelphia: Lippincott Williams & Wilkins; 2004. p. 713–35.
18. Davis JA, Costello DJ, Venna N. Laboratory investigation of fungal infections of the central nervous system. Neurol India 2007;55(3):233–40.
19. Verweij PE, van der Lee HAL, Rijs AJMM. The role of conventional diagnostic tools. In: Maertens JA, Marr KA, editors. Diagnosis of fungal infections. New York: Informa Healthcare; 2007. p. 19–39.
20. Alexander BD, Pfaller MA. Contemporary tools for the diagnosis and management of invasive mycoses. Clin Infect Dis 2006;43(Suppl 1):S15–27.
21. Cannon RD, Lamping E, Holmes AR, et al. Efflux-mediated antifungal drug resistance. Clin Microbiol Rev 2009;22(2):291–321.
22. Walsh TJ, Anaissie EJ, Denning DW, et al. Treatment of aspergillosis: clinical practice guidelines of the Infectious Diseases Society of America. Clin Infect Dis 2008;46(3):327–60.
23. Ostrosky-Zeichner L. Combination antifungal therapy: a critical review of the evidence. Clin Microbiol Infect 2008;14(Suppl 4):S65–70.
24. Schwartz S, Ruhnke M, Ribaud P, et al. Improved outcome in central nervous system aspergillosis, using voriconazole treatment. Blood 2005;106(8):2641–5.

25. Espinel-Ingroff A. History of medical mycology in the United States. Clin Microbiol Rev 1996;9(2):235–72.
26. Berger JR. Fungal disease. In: Johnson RT, Griffin JW, McArthur JC, editors. Current therapy in neurologic disease. 6th edition. St Louis (Missouri): C.V. Mosby; 2002. p. 146–50.
27. Oyesiku NM, Schwarzmann SW, Alleyne CH Jr. Fungal infections of the brain. In: Osenbach RK, Zeidman SM, editors. Infection in neurological surgery: diagnosis and management. Philadelphia: Lippincott-Raven; 1999. p. 123–39.
28. Sanchez-Portocarrero J, Perez-Cecilia E, Corral O, et al. The central nervous system and infection by *Candida* species. Diagn Microbiol Infect Dis 2000;37: 169–79.
29. Vazquez JA, Sobel JD. Candidiasis. In: Dismukes WE, Pappas PG, Sobel JD, editors. Clinical mycology. New York: Oxford University Press; 2003. p. 143–87.
30. Burgert SJ, Classen DC, Burke JP, et al. Candidal brain abscess associated with vascular invasion: a devastating complication of vascular catheter-related candidemia. Clin Infect Dis 1995;21(1):202–5.
31. Fernandez M, Moylett EH, Noyola DE, et al. Candidal meningitis in neonates: a 10 year review. Clin Infect Dis 2000;31:458–63.
32. Lai PH, Lin SM, Pan HB, et al. Disseminated miliary cerebral candidiasis. AJNR Am J Neuroradiol 1997;18(7):1303–6.
33. Perfect JR. Cryptococcus neoformans: a sugar-coated killer with designer genes. FEMS Immunol Med Microbiol 2005;45(3):395–404.
34. Levitz SM, Boekhout T. *Cryptococcus*: the once-sleeping giant is fully awake. FEMS Yeast Res 2006;6(4):461–2.
35. Park BJ, Wannemuehler KA, Marston BJ, et al. Estimation of the current global burden of cryptococcal meningitis among persons living with HIV/AIDS. AIDS 2009;23(4):525–30.
36. Loftus BJ, Fung E, Roncaglia P, et al. The genome of the basidiomycetous yeast and human pathogen *Cryptococcus neoformans*. Science 2005;307(5713):1321–4.
37. Liu OW, Chun CD, Chow ED, et al. Systematic genetic analysis of virulence in the human fungal pathogen *Cryptococcus neoformans*. Cell 2008;135(1):174–88.
38. Casadevall A, Perfect JR. Cryptococcus neoformans. Washington, DC: American Society for Microbiology; 1998. p. 1–27.
39. Kwon-Chung KJ, Varma A. Do major species concepts support one, two or more species with *Cryptococcus neoformans*? FEMS Yeast Res 2006;6(4):574–87.
40. Bovers M, Hagen F, Kuramae E, et al. Unique hybrids between the fungal pathogens *Cryptococcus neoformans* and *Cryptococcus gatti*. FEMS Yeast Res 2006; 6(4):599–607.
41. Saag MS, Graybill RJ, Larsen RA, et al. Practice guidelines for the management of cryptococcal disease. Clin Infect Dis 2000;30(4):710–8.
42. Casadevall A, Perfect JR. Cryptococcus neoformans. Washington, DC: American Society for Microbiology; 1998. p. 407–56.
43. Denning DW, Armstrong RW, Lewis BH, et al. Elevated cerebrospinal fluid pressures in patients with cryptococcal meningitis and acquired immunodeficiency syndrome. Am J Med 1991;91(3):267–72.
44. Redmond A, Dancer C, Woods ML. Fungal infections of the central nervous system: a review of fungal pathogens and treatment. Neurol India 2007;55(3): 251–9.
45. Pukkila-Worley R, Mylonakis E. Epidemiology and management of cryptococcal meningitis: developments and challenges. Expert Opin Pharmacother 2008; 9(4):551–60.

46. Bennett JE. Fungal infections. In: Wilson J, Braunwald E, Isselbacher KJ, et al, editors. Harrison's principles of internal medicine. 12th edition. New York: McGraw-Hill Medical Publishing Division; 1991. p. 748–9.

47. Han SR, Choi CY, Joo M, et al. Isolated cerebral mucormycosis. J Korean Neurosurg Soc 2007;42(5):400–2.

48. Wu X, XU G, Wen W, et al. Clinical study on aggressive rhinocerebral mucormycosis. J Otolaryngol Head Neck Surg 2008;22(23):1060–2, 1067.

49. Sugar AM. Mucormycosis. Clin Infect Dis 1992;14(Suppl 1):S126–9.

50. Segal BH. Aspergillosis. N Engl J Med 2009;360(18):1870–84.

51. Denning DW, Riniotis K, Dobrashian R, et al. Chronic cavitary and fibrosing pulmonary and pleural aspergillosis: case series, proposed nomenclature change, and review. Clin Infect Dis 2003;37(Suppl 3):S265–80.

52. Sambatakou H, Dupont B, Lode H, et al. Voriconazole treatment for subacute invasive and chronic pulmonary aspergillosis. Am J Med 2006;119(6):527. e17–24.

53. Behari M, Tripathi M, Verma A. Fungal infections. In: Bradley W, Daroff RB, Fenichel GM, et al, editors. Neurology in clinical practice. 4th edition. London: Butterworth-Heinemann; 2004. p. 1548–9.

54. Azarpira N, Esfandiari M, Bagheri MH, et al. Cerebral aspergillosis presenting as a mass lesion. Braz J Infect Dis 2008;12(4):349–51.

55. Kastrup O, Wanke I, Maschke M. Neuroimaging of infections. NeuroRx 2005;2(2): 324–32.

56. Ruhnke M, Kofla G, Otto K, et al. CNS aspergillosis: recognition, diagnosis and management. CNS Drugs 2007;21(8):659–76.

57. Rodenbiker HT, Ganley JP, Galgiani JN, et al. Prevalence of chorioretinal scars associated with coccidioidomycosis. Arch Ophthalmol 1981;99:71–5.

58. Einstein HE, Johnson RH. Coccidiodomycosis: new aspects of epidemiology and therapy. Clin Infect Dis 1993;16:349–54.

59. Winn WA. The treatment of coccidioidal meningitis: the use of amphotericin B in a group of 25 patients. Calif Med 1964;101:78–89.

60. Panackal AA, Hajjeh RA, Cetron MS, et al. Fungal infections among returning travelers. Clin Infect Dis 2002;35:1088–95.

61. Van Bergen WS, Fleury FJ, Cheatle EL. Fatal maternal disseminated coccidioidomycosis in a nonendemic area. Am J Obstet Gynecol 1976;124:661–4.

62. Ragland AS, Arsura E, Ismail Y, et al. Eosinophilic pleocytosis in coccidioidal meningitis: frequency and significance. Am J Med 1993;195:254–7.

63. Galgiani JN. Coccidioidomycosis: changing perceptions and creating opportunities for its control. Ann N Y Acad Sci 2007;1111:1–18.

64. Parish JM, Blair JE. Coccidioidomycosis. Mayo Clin Proc 2008;83:343–9.

65. Wheat LJ, Freifeld AG, Kleiman MB, et al. Clinical practice guidelines for the management of patients with histoplasmosis: 2007 update by the Infectious Diseases Society of America. Clin Infect Dis 2007;45(7):807–25.

66. Cohen BA. Chronic meningitis. Curr Neurol Neurosci Rep 2005;5(6):429–39.

67. Sarosi GA. Blastomycosis. Am Rev Respir Dis 1979;120(4):911–38.

68. Kale HA, Narlawar RS, Maheswari S, et al. CNS blastomycosis, mimic of meningioma. Indian J Radiol Imaging 2002;12(4):483–4.

69. Chapman SW, Dismukes WE, Proia LA, et al. Clinical practice guidelines for the management of blastomycosis. Clin Infect Dis 2008;46(12):1801–12.

Neurologic Presentations of Infective Endocarditis

Mark D. Johnson, MD[a],*, Charles D. Johnson, MD, FACC[b]

KEYWORDS

• Stroke • Endocarditis • Mycotic aneurysm • Encephalopathy

As far back as the 1600s there are description of patients retrospectively suspected of having endocarditis.[1] Please verify. In the 1800s, Kirkes, followed by Virchow and Beckmann, showed evidence of embolization from the heart to other organs, including the cerebrum. These embolized particles at that time were associated with bacterial elements, which by 1877 prompted the use of the term, *infective endocarditis*.[2] Infectious aneurysms were first described by Church in 1869. He wrote about a 13-year-old boy who developed left hemiparesis and was found to have a mitral valve infection and a middle cerebral artery aneurysm rupture.[3] With the publication of the Gulstonian Lectures by Sir William Osler, the neurologic involvement (and the clinical triad of fever, heart murmur, and hemiplegia/stroke) became recognized as an important component of this protean disease.[4]

GENERAL EPIDEMIOLOGY AND ETIOLOGY

Neurologic complication data may be influenced by the changing epidemiology of infective endocarditis. In the postantibiotic era, a shift in causes of infective endocarditis has occurred. A common cause, rheumatic heart disease, has diminished in frequency, whereas conditions, such as cardiac valve replacement, mitral annulus calcification, calcific aortic valves, congenital cardiac defects, and mitral valve prolapse, have become more commonly recognized causes.[5] The mean age of development of infective endocarditis has shifted from approximately 30 years to the late 50s.[6] This shift has been caused by the highest incidence of infective endocarditis now in the 70- to 74-year age group.[7] The introduction of multiple new medical

[a] Division of Cerebrovascular Diseases, University of Texas Southwestern Medical Center, 5323 Harry Hines Avenue, Dallas, TX 75390-8897, USA
[b] Department of Medicine, Division of Cardiology, University of Puerto Rico School of Medicine, Medical Centre, P. O. Box 5067, Rio Piedras, PR 00936, USA
* Corresponding author.
E-mail address: mark.johnson@utsouthwestern.edu (M.D. Johnson).

Neurol Clin 28 (2010) 311–321
doi:10.1016/j.ncl.2009.09.001
0733-8619/09/$ – see front matter © 2010 Elsevier Inc. All rights reserved.

neurologic.theclinics.com

techniques and devices providing access to the bloodstream and location (hyperalimentation lines, intravenous catheters, prosthetic heart valves, intracardiac devices, hemodialysis, genitourinary, and gastroenterologic interventions) are permitting the potential introduction and harbor of bacterial sources of endocarditis.[8] Intravenous drug abuse is a well known source of infective endocarditis. Immunocompromised patients (those who have HIV-1 or are on chemotherapy) and nosocomial disease can be added as potential sources of infective endocarditis. The most common infectious agents in infective endocarditis continue to be *Staphylococcus* and *Streptococcus* species. Other causes of endocarditis include *Enterococci*, gram-negative, *Aspergillus*, and *Candida* species.

PRESENTATION

The diagnosis of infective endocarditis entails a combination of clinical, echocardiographic, and laboratory findings. It is useful to divide the presentation of endocarditis into patients with native cardiac valves, patients with prosthetic cardiac valves, patients with intravenous drug use, and patients with nosocomial infective endocarditis. In addition, prosthetic cardiac valve infections within 2 months of surgery are usually due to in-hospital acquired infections (early prosthetic-valve endocarditis). Infective endocarditis after 12 months is more commonly community acquired (late prosthetic-valve endocarditis). Endocarditis occurring within 2 to 12 months of surgery is usually secondary to a mixture of both types of infections.[9]

Fever, a new heart murmur, and skin/mucosal lesions may be detected in the evaluation of patients with suspected acute or subacute/chronic infective endocarditis. Examples of clinical markers are conjunctival/mucosal petechiae, Janeway's lesions (nontender erythematous hemorrhagic lesions in the palms and soles), Osler's nodes (tender subcutaneous nodules in digits or thenar eminence), petechiae, and splinter hemorrhages (initially red lines that change to brownish in 2 to 3 days).[9] In 1994, the Duke Endocarditis Service developed criteria for the diagnosis of infective endocarditis, which has since been validated.[10] More recently, in 2000, modified Duke criteria have been proposed that emphasize the use of transesophageal echocardiography.[11]

NEUROLOGIC PRESENTATIONS

Infective endocarditis is a major threat to the nervous system. Neurologic complications are the chief complaint or a major presenting symptom. Neurologic events can be a sudden catastrophic disaster. The mortality in patients with infective endocarditis without neurologic complications is 21% but rises to 58% in patients who have suffered neurologic damage.[8,9,12–18]

Neurologic complications of infective endocarditis have been estimated to occur in as many as 35% to 39% of cases.[19] Furthermore, a neurologic complication has been seen as the presenting symptom of infective endocarditis in close to half of cases. By the time patients receive their first dose of antibiotic, approximately 76% of them already have a neurologic clinical presentation.[20] Mortality is higher in patients with neurologic complications (50% vs 21%).[21] If the causative organism is *Staphylococcus aureus* and if the endocarditis extends to mitral and aortic valves, there is a significant association with a neurologic complication.[20]

Neurologic complications (**Table 1**) can be separated into embolic events (producing ischemic strokes or transient ischemic attacks [TIAs]), hemorrhagic strokes (secondary to multiple etiologies), central nervous system infectious processes, and other less specific presentations. Skinner emphasizes a staged sequence of pathophysiologic processes by which infectious endocarditis affects

Table 1	
Neurologic complications of infective endocarditis	
Stroke	**Cerebral Embolic Ischemic Infarction**
Intracranial hemorrhages	ICH SAH
Mycotic aneurysm	Septic
Infections	Brain abcess—macro, micro Cerebritis Meningoencephalitis Ventriculitis Ependymitis
Encephalopathy	Infectious Toxic-metabolic
Neuropsychiatric disorders Seizures Cranial nerve palsy Headache Peripheral neuropathy Myalgias	
Spine and spinal cord	Back pain Discitis Osteomyelitis Radiculitis Spinal cord infarction

From Refs.[8,9,12–18,22,34,35]

the central nervous system.[12] He describes a preclinical stage in which the release of inflammatory cytokines and other "humoral" responses affect the central nervous system and patients develop nonspecific symptoms of anorexia and fatigue. These early symptoms are followed by late preclinical diffuse vascular inflammatory processes that usually involve small vessels and cause generalized cognitive symptoms of inattention, somnolence, or irritability. At this stage, an immune complex vasculitis has been described that may affect the central nervous system and other organ-system, small-vessel trees. Skinner goes on to describe other stages, including the initial event, secondary event, and late-effects stages.[12] He warns that in the presence of infective endocarditis, when one neurologic event has occurred to be on the alert for a second more devastating event.

Central Nervous System Ischemic Embolic Events

After congestive heart failure, embolism is the most frequent systemic complication of infective endocarditis. Ischemic stroke is its most common embolic manifestation (65%).[13] Stroke is the presenting symptom in 14% to 19% of all cases of infective endocarditis.[15,22] Ischemic stroke or TIA results from cardiogenic valvular vegetation embolization and migration into the cerebral arteries. The emboli tend to lodge predominantly in the middle cerebral artery and its distal branches but any of the arteries of the cerebral vascular tree can be involved (**Fig. 1**). In terms of the endocarditis location, mitral valve endocarditis is more common in patients diagnosed with stroke. The vegetations found in these valves tend to be larger in size than the ones found in aortic valve endocarditis.[23,24] There are higher rates of cerebral embolization, neurologic complications, and mortality in infective endocarditis patients with *Staphylococcus aureus* organisms or with fungi and in patients with large vegetations

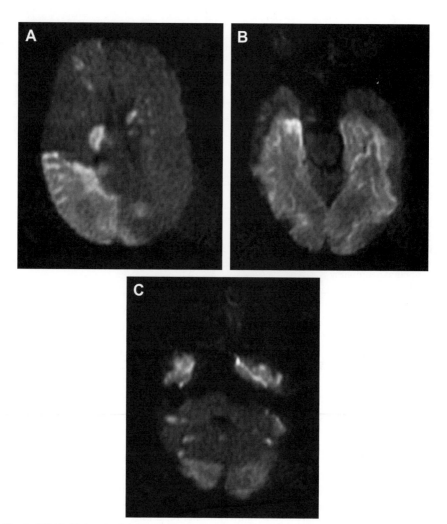

Fig. 1. (*A*) Multiple arterial distribution ischemic strokes in a patient with infective endocarditis. (*B*) Extensive bilateral occipitotemporal ischemic strokes in the same patient. (*C*) Bilateral embolic appearing cerebellar ischemic strokes in the same patient.

(10–15 mm).[22] Infection-related antiphospholipid antibodies in infective endocarditis may be a major risk factor for embolic events.[25]

In a recent publication, the incidence of stroke in patients with infective endocarditis is lower (9.6%) than in previous reports (21% to 39%).[24] The investigators attribute this lower rate of stroke to a rigorous coding system, and Duke criteria (diagnostic criteria for infective endocarditis) use with a careful chart review excluding other diagnoses as TIA or other infectious complications. Early antibiotic use is recommended because rapid reduction in embolic events has been noted in the days after initiating treatment. Events occurring at a rate of approximately 13 events per 1000 patient days in the first week decrease with antibiotic treatment to less than 1.2 events per 1000 patient days after 2 weeks of therapy.[26]

Recent studies have been looking prospectively at symptomatic and asymptomatic cerebrovascular complications (ischemic and hemorrhagic). These studies include

CT, MRI, and other biologic markers (spinal fluid) to assess for brain injury. The study using MRI and cerebrospinal fluid markers found that the overall frequency of symptomatic and asymptomatic cerebrovascular complications in, specifically, patients with left-sided infective endocarditis was markedly high, at 65%, with 30% "silent" in nature.[27] Another study was based on CT and clinical criteria for all patients diagnosed by Duke criteria found approximately 22% cerebrovascular complications. This and other studies have helped address the incidence of complications after cardiac repair surgery. The incidence is thought to be low in comparison to previous studies and not present in patients with asymptomatic cerebral embolism or TIAs.[28,29] The general management of patients with ischemic stroke continues mainly to be acute stroke care, reduction in complications, and antibiotic treatment.

Hemorrhagic Strokes

The overall incidence of hemorrhagic strokes in patients with infective endocarditis has remained between 3% and 7% throughout the past few decades.[28,30] These strokes can be divided into intracerebral hemorrhage (ICH) and subarachnoid hemorrhage (SAH) and they are associated with the highest mortality. Hemorrhagic infarctions (hemorrhagic transformation of an ischemic infarct due to septic emboli) are the most common cause of ICH.[12] In a recent prospective multicenter study, the incidence of primary ICH had been 2.4% and the incidence of hemorrhagic infarctions was 1.4% of all cases with infective endocarditis.[28] In this combined group of 19 patients with hemorrhagic strokes, 13 patients underwent catheter angiography, which revealed mycotic aneurysms (MAs) in seven patients. SAH secondary to MAs occurs in approximately 1% to 1.7% of cases of infective endocarditis with a high mortality rate.[12] Thus, MAs account for less than 3% of hemorrhages.[22] Aside from hemorrhagic transformation of ischemic strokes, other common causes of ICH include pyogenic arteritis, nonaneurysmal vascular wall necrosis, and concurrent antithrombotic medication use.[12,22]

Mycotic Aneurysms

It is estimated that MAs develop in approximately 2% to 5% of patients with infective endocarditis (**Fig. 2**).[3,31] Mechanisms of disease by which MAs can develop have been divided into (1) direct bacterial infection, (2) septic or bland embolic occlusion of the vasa vasorum, and (3) immune complex deposition injuring the arterial wall.[32] MAs tend to develop at arterial branch points, which are the common sites of embolic impaction, particularly in the distal middle cerebral artery branches at bifurcations. Bacterial pathogens associated with them have been *Streptococcus viridans* (approximately 50%) and *Staphylococcus aureus* (approximately 10%).[14,15] Occlusion of the vessel by septic emboli with secondary arteritis and vessel wall destruction is associated with *Staphylococcus aureus*. Vasa vasorum seeding and wall injury are associated with *Streptococcus viridans*.[15]

Clinical presentations vary widely from no symptoms, a slow leak that produces only a mild headache, meningeal irritation, altered sensorium, cranial neuropathies, seizures, sudden hemiparesis (usually face and arm > leg), and hemianopia. The overall mortality rate in infective endocarditis patients with MAs is 60%; in patients with MAs without rupture, the mortality rate is 30%; in patients with rupture, the mortality approaches 80%.[3,9,12–15,22,31]

The surgical management of MAs constitutes one of the challenges in patients with infective endocarditis. Currently no prospective randomized trial is available for guidance. For unruptured MAs, therapy comprises a prolonged course of antimicrobials/antibiotics. Approximately 80% of MAs resolve or decrease in size with antibiotics

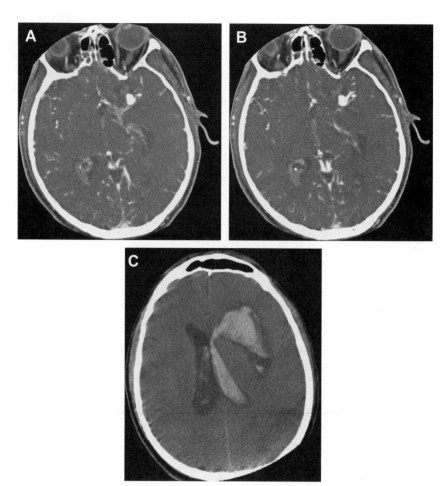

Fig. 2. (*A*) MA by CT angiography. (*B*) MA by CT angiography. (*C*) MA hemorrhage after CT angiography.

alone. A recommendation is of close angiographic imaging follow-up during the weeks of treatment (as often as every 1 to 2 weeks).[33] In patients without neurologic symptoms, if changes develop in the morphology of the aneurysm or there is an increase in size of the aneurysm, procedural intervention should be strongly considered whereas the medical therapy continues. An expert opinion approach to ruptured infectious intracranial aneurysm has been proposed.[22,33] If patients have a ruptured or morphologically evolving MA, a surgical or endovascular intervention is performed. If there is no mass effect, endovascular intervention may be attempted. If there is mass effect or if there is failure of the endovascular approach, surgical intervention is performed. Unfortunately, due to MAs having friable walls or fusiform configurations, either approach may include parent artery sacrifice with or without bypass.

Brain Abscess

Brain abscesses (macroabscesses) occur infrequently to rarely in infective endocarditis. They form as part of a continuum infectious inflammation called cerebritis, which may evolve into micro- or macroabscesses (**Fig. 3**). Most abscesses arise from sites where a preceding septic embolus had lodged. Microabscesses are more common and may also lead to headache, seizures, and encephalopathy. Management of brain abscesses is mainly with prolonged antibiotic treatment. Surgical excision may be practiced for solitary macroabscesses that do not respond to antibiotics. Occasionally, a large solitary abscess may require early surgical drainage.[8,12,15–17,22]

OTHER CENTRAL NERVOUS SYSTEM COMPLICATIONS OF INFECTIVE ENDOCARDITIS

Pruitt and colleagues,[16] Jones and Siekert,[8] Karchner,[15] and Prabhakaran[22] address other less well-recognized or less frequent neurologic manifestations of infective endocarditis. Acute or subacute encephalopathy occurs in up to 25% of patients. These patients have frequently been described to have psychiatric manifestations, which include personality changes, hallucinations, and paranoid ideation. A toxic/metabolic etiology is found in half of these patients. Seizures can be seen in up to 14% of patients with infective endocarditis and their causes include focal lesion and iatrogenic (medication effect on seizure threshold) and metabolic abnormalities. Other less

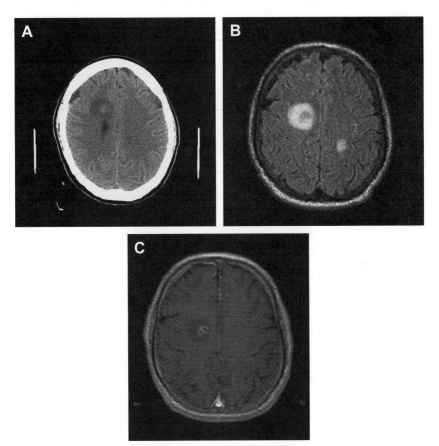

Fig. 3. (*A*) CT image of lesion suggestive of abscess. (*B*) MRI FLAIR image of same lesion: right, consistent with abscess, and left, consistent with an ischemic lesion. (*C*) MRI T1-weighted image with contrast consistent with evolving macroabscess.

common complications include septic meningitis (2%–20% of patients with infective endocarditis), cranial nerve neuropathy, cerebritis, meningoencephalitis, ventriculitis, and ependymitis. Spine and spinal cord involvement with back pain is reported in 9% to 10% of patients. The back pain has been related to vertebral osteomyelitis, discitis, and radiculitis. Other spinal cord involvement reported has been spinal cord embolic infarctions.[8,12,14–16,22,34,35]

ANTIPLATELET/ANTICOAGULATION AGENTS ISSUES

The use of antiplatelet and anticoagulant agents is in general not the therapeutic regimen to be used in the treatment of infective endocarditis. Most authorities believe that effective antibiotic treatment is the treatment of choice because the benefit of anticoagulation has not been shown, particularly in native-valve endocarditis. In the setting of an ischemic stroke and in ICHs, it is commonly agreed that anticoagulant agents should be stopped. A randomized, blinded, placebo-controlled trial was performed using aspirin (325 mg daily).[36] It did not reduce the risk of emboli and was likely associated with increased bleeding. In this trial, patients with "recent or actively evolving strokes" were excluded. In addition, the average onset of symptom onset to presentation was approximately 4 weeks. Alternatively, there is strong experimental data that the use of aspirin, particularly during the initial days of infection, supports the reduction of vegetation size and its likelihood of embolization.[37] In patients with infective endocarditis and without ischemic stroke, the current evidence-based recommendation is no routine use of antiplatelet agents (until further definitive evidence).[38] Doses lower than 325 mg of aspirin and the potential benefit of early introduction remain unproved considerations. In patients with infective endocarditis and ischemic stroke, there is no randomized trial to help guide treatment. Patients with prosthetic mechanical valves with infective endocarditis taking maintenance therapy are usually continued on this therapy in the absence of cerebral events. In these patients, if *Staphylococcus aureus* infection is confirmed, the discontinuation of anticoagulation is recommended with and without neurologic events. Starting anticoagulation in the latter case has been suggested after the septic phase has resolved. In general, if there is an ischemic stroke, restarting anticoagulation treatment after approximately 2 weeks is recommended. If it is a hemorrhagic stroke, 4 weeks is recommended.[14,15,22,36–39]

CARDIAC SURGERY IN PATIENTS WITH INFECTIVE ENDOCARDITIS AND NEUROLOGIC COMPLICATIONS

What is the optimal timing for heart valve surgery in these patients when needed—early or delayed? There seems to be considerable controversy surrounding this point. Timing for surgery depends on a patient's clinical status, the operative risk, and comorbidities. Timing of cardiac surgery after a cerebral embolic infarction recognizes a risk that depends on the size and location of the infarct and the risk of reperfusion injury after patients come off a bypass pump.[12]

In the past, investigators have recommended delaying cardiac surgery for at least 2 weeks after cerebral infarction and for at least 1 month after cerebral hemorrhage, holding that the risk for death or neurologic deterioration is high when surgery is done, during the initial 2 weeks after stroke.[31] More recently, the risk of surgery and the risk of early surgery in this setting are thought to be reduced. Ruttmann and associates state that early cardiac surgical treatment is favored in the absence of alternative treatment. They do recognize, however, the questionable safety of cardiopulmonary bypass in patients with acute neurologic injury, which has been suspected to worsen neurologic deficits and ischemia and could potentiate cerebral edema and secondary cerebral hemorrhage.[29] They note the conclusions of Piper and colleagues[40] that cardiac surgery ought to be performed within 72 hours and that stroke is not a contraindication for early valve replacement in acute infective endocarditis. Habib writes that recent guidelines recommend early surgery (<72 hours) in patients with focal deficits without hemorrhage, but that surgery must be delayed in cerebral hemorrhage or more severe neurologic symptoms, unless severe congestive heart failure dictates early intervention.[31,41]

In patients with infective endocarditis and ruptured MAs, the MA should be properly treated before valvular surgery is performed. In patients with unruptured MAs, treatment with a bioprosthetic valve that does not require anticoagulant therapy may be preferable to a mechanical valve in this situation.[14,22]

SUMMARY

Neurologic complications of bacterial endocarditis have been observed for centuries but its management has remained challenging at all times. The cerebrovascular complications of this disorder are the most feared and difficult to address. The management of MAs, recent ischemic/hemorrhagic strokes with and without brain abscesses, and mechanical valve patients continues as an ongoing challenge. Literature continues to appear, providing new alternatives in treatment and hope for improved therapy.

REFERENCES

1. Ronald A. Perspectives on the history of endocarditis. In: Chan KL, Embil JM, editors. Endocarditis: diagnosis and management. 1st edition. London: Springer-Verlag; 2006. p. 1–4.
2. Cavely W. Ulcerative or infecting endocarditis simulating typhoid fever. Med Times and Gaz 1877;2:509–11.
3. Phuong LK, Link M, Wijdicks E. Management of intracranial infectious aneurysms: a series of 16 cases. Neurosurgery 2002;51:1145–52.
4. Osler W. Gulstonian Lectures in malignant endocarditis. Lancet 1885;1:415–8, 459–64, 505–8.
5. Salgado AV. Central nervous system complications of infective endocarditis. Curr Conc Cerebrovasc Dis Stroke 1991;26:19–22.
6. Cabell CH, Abrutyn E. Progress toward a global understanding of infective endocarditis: lessons from the international collaboration on endocarditis. Cardiol Clin 2003;21:483.
7. Maor Y, Rubinstein E. Changing populations: the elderly, injection drug users, health-care-associated and immunocompromised patients. In: Chan KL, Embil JM, editors. Endocarditis: diagnosis and management. 1st edition. London: Springer-Verlag; 2006. p. 23–35.
8. Jones HR, Siekert RG. Neurological manifestations of infective endocarditis. Brain 1989;112:1295–315.
9. Mylonakis E, Calderwood SB. Infective endocarditis in adults. N Engl J Med 2001; 345(18):1318–30.
10. Durack DT, Lukes AS, Bright DK. New criteria for diagnosis of infective endocarditis: utilization of specific echocardiographic findings. Duke Endocarditis Service. Am J Med 1994;96(3):200–9.
11. Li JS, Sexton DJ, Mick N, et al. Proposed modifications to the Duke criteria for the diagnosis of infective endocarditis. Clin Infect Dis 2000;30:633–8.

12. Skinner CR. Neurological complications of endocarditis: pathophysiologic mechanisms and management issues. In: Chan KL, Embil JM, editors. Endocarditis: diagnosis and management. 1st edition. London: Springer-Verlag; 2006. p. 241–51.

13. Haldar SM, O'Gara PT. Infective rndocarditis. Chp.85. In: Fuster V, Walsh RA, O'Rourke RA, et al, editors. Hurst's the heart. 12th edition. New York: McGraw-Hill Medical; 2008. p. 1975–2004.

14. Bayer AS, Bolger AF, Taubert KA, et al. Diagnosis and management of infective endocarditis and its complications. Circulation 1998;98:2936–48.

15. Karchner AW. Infective endocarditis. In: Libby P, Bonow RO, Mann DL, editors. 8th edition, Braunwald's heart disease a textbook of cardiovascular medicine, vol. 2. Philadelphia: Saunders-Elsevier; 2008. p. 1720–1, 1730.

16. Pruitt AA, Rubin RH, Karchmer AW, et al. Neurologic complications of bacterial endocarditis. Medicine 1978;57:329–43.

17. Lerner P. Neurologic complications of infective endocarditis. Med Clin North Am 1985;69:385–98.

18. Kanter MC, Hart RS. Neurologic complications of infective endocarditis. Neurology 1991;41(7):1015–20.

19. Salgado AV, Furlan AJ, Keys TF, et al. Neurologic complications of endocarditis: a 12-year experience. Neurology 1989;39:173–8.

20. Heiro M, Nikoskelainen J, Engblom E, et al. Neurologic manifestations of infective endocarditis: a 17-year experience in a teaching hospital in Finland. Arch Intern Med. 2000;160:2781–7.

21. Chen C, Lo M, Hwang K, et al. Infective endocarditis with neurologic complications: 10-year experience. J Microbiol Immunol Infect 2001;34:119–24.

22. Prabhakaran S. Neurologic complications of endocarditis. Continuum Lifelong Learning in Neurology 2008;14:53–73.

23. Cabell CH, Pond KK, Peterson GE, et al. The risk of stroke and death in patients with aortic and mitral valve endocarditis. Am Heart J 2001;142:75–80.

24. Anderson DJ, Goldstein LB, Wilkinson WE, et al. Stroke location, characterization, severity, and outcome in mitral vs. aortic valve endocarditis. Neurology 2003;61:1341–6.

25. Kupferwasser LI, Hafner G, Mohr-Kahaly S, et al. The presence of infection-related antiphospholipid antibodies in infective endocarditis determines a major risk factor for embolic events. J Am Coll Cardiol 1999;33:1365–71.

26. Bashore TM, Cabeli C, Fowler V. Update on infective endocarditis. Current Problems in Cardiology 2006;31:274–352.

27. Snygg-Martin U, Gustafsson L, Rosengren L, et al. Cerebrovascular complications in patients with left-sided infective endocarditis are common: a prospective study using magnetic resonance imaging and neurochemical brain damage markers. Clin Infect Dis 2008;47:23–30.

28. Thuny F, Avierinos J, Tribolloy C, et al. Impact of cerebrovascular complications on mortality and neurologic outcome during infective endocarditis: a prospective multicentre study. Eur Heart J 2007;28:1155–61.

29. Ruttmann E, Willeit J, Ulmer H, et al. Neurologic outcome of septic cardioembolic stroke after infective endocarditis. Stroke 2006;37:2094–9.

30. Hart RG, Foster JW, Luther MF, et al. Stroke in infective endocarditis. Stroke 1990;21:695–700.

31. Habib G. Management of infective endocarditis. Heart 2006;92:124–30.

32. Fowler VG Jr, Scheld WM, Bayer Endocarditis AS, et al. In: Mandell GL, Bennett JE, Dolin R, editors. Principles and practice of infectious diseases. 6th edition. Philadelphia: Elsevier; 2005. p. 975–1022.

33. Peters PJ, Harrison T, Lennox JL. A dangerous dilemma: management of infectious intracranial aneurysms complicating endocarditis. Lancet Infect Dis 2006; 6:742–8.
34. Ziment I. Nervous system complications in bacterial endocarditis. Am J Med 1969;47:593–607.
35. Greenlee JE, Mandell GL. Neurologic manifestations of infective endocarditis: a review. Stroke 1973;4:958–63.
36. Chan KL, Dumesnil JG, Cujec B, et al. A randomized trial of aspirin on the risk of embolic events in patients with infective endocarditis. J Am Coll Cardiol 2003; 42(5):775–8.
37. Kupferwasser LI, Yeaman M, Shapiro S, et al. Acetylsalicylic acid reduces vegetation bacterial density, hematogenous bacterial dissemination, and frequency of embolic events in experimental staphylococcus aureus endocarditis through antiplatelet and antibacterial effects. Circulation 1999;99:2791–7.
38. Baddour LM, Wilson WR, Bayer AS, et al. Infective endocarditis: diagnosis, antimicrobial therapy, and management of complications. Circulation 2005;111:e421.
39. Tornos P, Almirante B, Mirabet S, et al. Infective endocarditis due to staphylococcus aureus. Arch Intern Med 1999;159:473–5.
40. Piper C, Wierner M, Schulte HD, et al. Stroke is not a contraindication for urgent valve replacement in acute infective endocarditis. J Heart Valve Dis 2001;10: 703–11.
41. Horskotte D, Fallth F, Gutschik E, et al. The Task force on infective endocarditis of the European Society of Cardiology. Guidelines on prevention, diagnosis and treatment of infective endocarditis. Eur Heart J 2004;25:267–76.

Index

Note: Page numbers of article titles are in **boldface** type.

A

Abscess(es), brain, infective endocarditis and, 316–317
Abuse
  alcohol
    epidemiology of, 199–203
    neuropharmacological treatment of, 209–210
  drug. See *Drug abuse.*
Achalasia
  defined, 75
  neurologic presentations of, 75–76
Acid-base disequilibrium, neurologic presentations of, **1–4**
  metabolic acidosis, 3
  metabolic alkalosis, 4
  respiratory acidosis, 1–2
  respiratory alkalosis, 2–3
Acidosis(es)
  metabolic, neurologic presentations of, 3
  neurologic symptoms and signs of, 2
  respiratory, neurologic presentations of, 1–2
ACR. See *American College of Rheumatology (ACR).*
Acute adrenal insufficiency, neurologic presentations of, 8–10
Acute cardioembolic stroke, management of, 29–31
Acute encephalopathy, radiation therapy and, 217
Acute hypoxia, neurologic presentations of, 37–39
Acute respiratory failure, neurologic presentations of, 37–38
Adrenal insufficiency, acute, neurologic presentations of, 8–10
AIDS, neurologic presentations of, **253–275.** See also *HIV.*
  CMV, 261–262
  cryptococcal meningitis, 262–263
  HIV-1–associated syndromes, 254–259
  HIV-associated neurocognitive disorder, 254–257
  HIV-associated peripheral neuropathies, 258–259
  HIV-associated vacuolar myelopathy, 257–258
  inflammatory demyelinating polyneuropathies, 259–260
  IRIS, 265
  PML, 260–261
  primary CNS lymphoma, 264–265
  toxoplasmosis encephalitis, 263–264
Alcohol, acute pharmacologic effects of, 206–207
Alcohol abuse

Neurol Clin 28 (2010) 323–337
doi:10.1016/S0733-8619(09)00100-5
0733-8619/09/$ – see front matter © 2010 Elsevier Inc. All rights reserved.
neurologic.theclinics.com

Moving?

Make sure your subscription moves with you!

To notify us of your new address, find your **Clinics Account Number** (located on your mailing label above your name), and contact customer service at:

Email: journalscustomerservice-usa@elsevier.com

800-654-2452 (subscribers in the U.S. & Canada)
314-447-8871 (subscribers outside of the U.S. & Canada)

Fax number: 314-447-8029

Elsevier Health Sciences Division
Subscription Customer Service
3251 Riverport Lane
Maryland Heights, MO 63043

*To ensure uninterrupted delivery of your subscription, please notify us at least 4 weeks in advance of move.

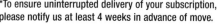
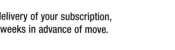